ADULT-GERONTOLOGY ACUTE CARE NURSE PRACTITIONER EXAM PREP 2024

Includes 450+ Practice Questions, Detailed Answer Explanations, and Prep Tips

Prestige Prep Publications

Table of Contents

INTRODUCTION

The Adult-Gerontology Acute Care Nurse Practitioner (AGACNP) exam is a rigorous certification examination designed to assess the knowledge and clinical skills of advanced practice registered nurses (APRNs) specializing in acute care for adult and geriatric patients.Successful completion of this exam leads to the credential of AGACNP-BC (Adult-Gerontology Acute Care Nurse Practitioner – Board Certified).

Who is it for?

This exam is targeted at registered nurses who have completed a graduate-level program focused on adult-gerontology acute care nurse practitioner education. Candidates must meet specific educational and clinical requirements as outlined by the certifying body.

Exam Format

The AGACNP exam is a computer-based test typically consisting of multiple-choice questions.It evaluates a candidate's understanding of advanced assessment, diagnosis, treatment, and management of acute and critically ill adult and geriatric patients.

Exam Topics

The exam covers a broad range of topics, including:
- Advanced pathophysiology
- Pharmacology
- Health assessment
- Diagnostic reasoning
- Critical care management
- Chronic illness management
- Gerontological care
- Healthcare policy and ethics

Minimum Requirements

To be eligible for the AGACNP exam, candidates must typically meet the following criteria:

- A Master's or Doctorate degree in Nursing
- Completion of an accredited AGACNP program
- A specified number of clinical hours in acute care settings
- Current, unencumbered RN licensure

Exam Cost

The cost of the AGACNP exam is determined by the certifying organization. Fees typically cover exam administration, score reporting, and certification maintenance.

Retake Policy

If a candidate fails the exam, they are usually allowed to retake it after a specified waiting period. The number of retakes permitted and any associated fees vary by certifying body.

Validation and Certificate Validity

Certification validates an individual's expertise in adult-gerontology acute care nursing. The AGACNP-BC credential is typically valid for a certain number of years, after which recertification is required to maintain the credential. Recertification often involves continuing education and professional development.

BENEFITS OF THE AGACNP CERTIFICATION

The AGACNP certification offers a multitude of advantages for advanced practice registered nurses specializing in acute care for adults and geriatrics.

Professional Advancement

- **Enhanced Career Opportunities:** Certification often leads to increased job opportunities and higher salaries in a competitive healthcare market.
- **Leadership Roles:** AGACNPs with certification are frequently sought after for leadership positions within acute care settings.
- **Specialization Recognition:** The certification validates expertise in adult-gerontology acute care, distinguishing certified nurses from their peers.

Patient Care

- **Improved Patient Outcomes:** AGACNPs with advanced knowledge and skills can provide high-quality, evidence-based care, leading to improved patient outcomes.
- **Critical Thinking and Decision-Making:** The rigorous exam preparation process enhances critical thinking and decision-making abilities, crucial in acute care settings.
- **Advocacy:** Certified AGACNPs can effectively advocate for their patients and contribute to shaping healthcare policies.

Personal Growth

- **Professional Recognition:** Achieving certification is a significant accomplishment that boosts professional confidence and credibility.
- **Lifelong Learning:** The certification process encourages continuous learning and staying updated with the latest advancements in the field.
- **Networking Opportunities:** Certification connects nurses with a network of colleagues, fostering professional growth and collaboration.

By investing time and effort in obtaining the AGACNP certification, nurses can significantly enhance their careers, improve patient care, and contribute to the advancement of the nursing profession.

TIPS FOR THE AGACNP EXAM PREPARATION

Creating a Solid Study Plan
- **Identify your learning style:** Are you a visual, auditory, or kinesthetic learner? Tailor your study methods accordingly.
- **Set realistic goals:** Break down the content into manageable chunks and create a study schedule.
- **Prioritize weak areas:** Focus on topics where you feel less confident.
- **Utilize resources:** Take advantage of textbooks, review courses, online resources, and practice questions.
- **Study groups:** Collaborate with peers to discuss complex concepts and fill in knowledge gaps.

Effective Study Techniques
- **Active recall:** Test yourself regularly through practice questions and flashcards.
- **Spaced repetition:** Review material at increasing intervals to enhance long-term memory.
- **Mind mapping:** Visually represent complex concepts to improve understanding.
- **Teach someone else:** Explaining concepts to others solidifies your knowledge.
- **Simulation:** Practice clinical scenarios to apply theoretical knowledge.

Mindfulness and Self-Care
- **Manage stress:** Incorporate relaxation techniques like meditation, deep breathing, or yoga.
- **Prioritize sleep:** Aim for 7-9 hours of quality sleep each night.
- **Exercise regularly:** Physical activity boosts mood and cognitive function.
- **Balanced diet:** Fuel your body with nutritious foods for optimal brain function.
- **Time management:** Create a study schedule that allows for breaks and leisure activities.
- **Support system:** Lean on friends, family, or mentors for emotional support.

Safety Tips

- **Ergonomics:** Set up a comfortable study space to prevent physical discomfort.
- **Eye care:** Take breaks to rest your eyes and prevent eyestrain.
- **Avoid distractions:** Find a quiet study environment and minimize interruptions.
- **Time management:** Set timers for study sessions to avoid burnout.

Crucial Steps Before the Exam

- **Review key concepts:** Revisit important topics and formulas.
- **Practice questions:** Familiarize yourself with the exam format and question types.
- **Get adequate sleep:** Ensure you are well-rested for optimal cognitive function.
- **Gather necessary materials:** Prepare your identification, exam admission ticket, and any required supplies.
- **Arrive early:** Allow ample time for check-in and finding your testing location.
- **Relaxation techniques:** Use deep breathing or meditation to manage anxiety.
- **Positive mindset:** Believe in your preparation and abilities.

PRACTICE QUESTIONS

1. A 78-year-old male presents to the emergency department with acute onset of chest pain, dyspnea, and hemoptysis. He has a history of deep vein thrombosis (DVT) and recent prolonged immobilization. Which of the following diagnostic tests would be most appropriate to confirm the suspected diagnosis?

    A. D-dimer
    B. Troponin I
    C. CT angiography of the chest
    D. Ventilation/perfusion (V/Q) scan

2. A 65-year-old woman with a history of hypertension and type 2 diabetes mellitus is admitted to the ICU with septic shock secondary to pneumonia. Which of the following interventions would be the most appropriate initial step in managing her fluid status?

    A. Administer a 500 mL bolus of 0.9% normal saline
    B. Initiate norepinephrine infusion
    C. Start hydrocortisone 50 mg IV every 6 hours
    D. Administer a 30 mL/kg bolus of crystalloid solution

3. A 50-year-old male with a history of alcoholism is admitted to the ICU with acute pancreatitis. Which of the following laboratory findings would be most consistent with this diagnosis?

    A. Elevated serum lipase and amylase
    B. Decreased serum calcium
    C. Elevated serum alanine aminotransferase (ALT) and aspartate aminotransferase (AST)
    D. All of the above

4. A 72-year-old female with a history of chronic obstructive pulmonary disease (COPD) is admitted to the ICU with acute respiratory failure. She is intubated and placed on mechanical ventilation. Which of the following ventilator settings would be most appropriate for this patient?

    A. Assist control mode, tidal volume of 8 mL/kg, PEEP of 5 cmH2O
    B. Pressure control mode, inspiratory pressure of 20 cmH2O, PEEP of 8 cmH2O
    C. Synchronized intermittent mandatory ventilation (SIMV) mode, tidal volume of 6 mL/kg, PEEP of 10 cmH2O
    D. Pressure support ventilation (PSV) mode, pressure support of 15 cmH2O, PEEP of 5 cmH2O

5. A 60-year-old male with a history of coronary artery disease is admitted to the ICU after undergoing coronary artery bypass graft (CABG) surgery. On postoperative day 2, he develops hypotension, tachycardia, and decreased urine output. Which of the following complications is most likely the cause of his symptoms?

    A. Cardiac tamponade
    B. Acute kidney injury
    C. Pulmonary embolism
    D. Myocardial infarction

6. A 45-year-old woman with a history of systemic lupus erythematosus (SLE) is admitted to the ICU with acute kidney injury (AKI). Which of the following would be the most appropriate initial diagnostic test to evaluate the cause of her AKI?

    A. Renal ultrasound
    B. Renal biopsy
    C. Urine protein-to-creatinine ratio
    D. Anti-nuclear antibody (ANA) titer

7. A 35-year-old male is admitted to the ICU with severe traumatic brain injury (TBI). Which of the following interventions would be most appropriate to prevent secondary brain injury?

    A. Maintain head of bed elevation at 30 degrees
    B. Hyperventilate to maintain PaCO2 between 25-30 mmHg
    C. Administer mannitol to reduce intracranial pressure (ICP)
    D. Initiate therapeutic hypothermia

8. A 55-year-old woman with a history of cirrhosis is admitted to the ICU with acute variceal bleeding. Which of the following medications would be most appropriate to reduce portal pressure and control bleeding?

    A. Octreotide
    B. Propranolol
    C. Lactulose
    D. Spironolactone

9. A 68-year-old male with a history of atrial fibrillation is admitted to the ICU with cardiogenic shock. Which of the following hemodynamic parameters would be most consistent with this diagnosis?

    A. Increased cardiac index, decreased systemic vascular resistance
    B. Decreased cardiac index, increased systemic vascular resistance
    C. Increased cardiac index, increased systemic vascular resistance
    D. Decreased cardiac index, decreased systemic vascular resistance

10. A 28-year-old male is admitted to the ICU with status epilepticus. Which of the following medications would be most appropriate to administer as a first-line treatment?

    A. Phenytoin
    B. Levetiracetam
    C. Lorazepam
    D. Valproic acid

11. A 25-year-old male presents to the emergency department with sudden onset of right-sided chest pain and shortness of breath. He is tall and thin, and a chest X-ray reveals a pneumothorax. Which of the following underlying conditions is most likely associated with this presentation?

    A. Cystic fibrosis
    B. Marfan syndrome
    C. Pulmonary embolism
    D. Sarcoidosis

12. A 68-year-old woman with a history of hypertension and coronary artery disease is admitted to the ICU with acute decompensated heart failure. Which of the following medications would be most appropriate to improve her cardiac output?

    A. Dobutamine
    B. Nitroglycerin
    C. Furosemide
    D. Metoprolol

13. A 48-year-old man with a history of intravenous drug use is admitted to the ICU with infective endocarditis. Which of the following physical exam findings would be most consistent with this diagnosis?

    A. Janeway lesions
    B. Osler nodes
    C. Roth spots
    D. All of the above

14. A 75-year-old man with a history of chronic kidney disease is admitted to the ICU with acute respiratory distress syndrome (ARDS). Which of the following interventions would be most appropriate to improve his oxygenation?

    A. Increase the FiO2 to 100%
    B. Initiate prone positioning
    C. Administer inhaled nitric oxide
    D. Increase the positive end-expiratory pressure (PEEP)

15. A 32-year-old woman with a history of asthma is admitted to the ICU with status asthmaticus. Which of the following arterial blood gas findings would be most consistent with this diagnosis?

    A. pH 7.35, PaCO2 45 mmHg, PaO2 70 mmHg, HCO3- 24 mEq/L
    B. pH 7.45, PaCO2 35 mmHg, PaO2 95 mmHg, HCO3- 22 mEq/L
    C. pH 7.25, PaCO2 60 mmHg, PaO2 55 mmHg, HCO3- 28 mEq/L
    D. pH 7.55, PaCO2 25 mmHg, PaO2 110 mmHg, HCO3- 18 mEq/L

16. A 50-year-old woman with a history of type 2 diabetes mellitus is admitted to the ICU with diabetic ketoacidosis (DKA). Which of the following laboratory findings would be most consistent with this diagnosis?

    A. Blood glucose of 200 mg/dL, serum bicarbonate of 20 mEq/L, anion gap of 12
    B. Blood glucose of 350 mg/dL, serum bicarbonate of 15 mEq/L, anion gap of 20
    C. Blood glucose of 150 mg/dL, serum bicarbonate of 25 mEq/L, anion gap of 8
    D. Blood glucose of 500 mg/dL, serum bicarbonate of 10 mEq/L, anion gap of 30

17. A 60-year-old man with a history of hypertension is admitted to the ICU with a subarachnoid hemorrhage (SAH). Which of the following complications is most likely to occur in this patient?

    A. Vasospasm
    B. Hydrocephalus
    C. Rebleeding
    D. All of the above

18. A 45-year-old woman with a history of alcohol abuse is admitted to the ICU with acute liver failure. Which of the following laboratory findings would be most consistent with this diagnosis?

    A. Elevated serum albumin
    B. Prolonged prothrombin time (PT)
    C. Decreased serum ammonia
    D. Normal serum bilirubin

19. A 55-year-old man with a history of smoking is admitted to the ICU with a diagnosis of small cell lung cancer. Which of the following paraneoplastic syndromes is most commonly associated with this type of cancer?

    A. Syndrome of inappropriate antidiuretic hormone secretion (SIADH)
    B. Cushing syndrome
    C. Lambert-Eaton myasthenic syndrome
    D. Hypercalcemia

20. A 70-year-old woman with a history of chronic obstructive pulmonary disease (COPD) is admitted to the ICU with an acute exacerbation. Which of the following interventions would be most appropriate to improve her respiratory status?

    A. Administer inhaled corticosteroids
    B. Administer inhaled bronchodilators
    C. Initiate noninvasive positive pressure ventilation (NIPPV)
    D. All of the above

21. A 40-year-old woman with a history of rheumatoid arthritis presents to the emergency department with complaints of fever, chills, and productive cough. She is found to have a right lower lobe consolidation on chest x-ray. Which of the following antibiotics would be most appropriate for empiric treatment of her suspected pneumonia?

    A. Azithromycin
    B. Ceftriaxone plus azithromycin
    C. Moxifloxacin
    D. Piperacillin/tazobactam

22. A 55-year-old man with a history of hypertension and hyperlipidemia presents to the emergency department with acute onset of severe chest painradiating to his back. He is diagnosed with an aortic dissection. Which of the following medications would be most appropriate for initial blood pressure management?

    A. Esmolol
    B. Nitroprusside
    C. Nicardipine
    D. Hydralazine

23. A 65-year-old woman with a history of heart failure with reduced ejection fraction (HFrEF) is admitted to the ICU with worsening dyspnea and peripheral edema. She is found to have elevated levels of B-type natriuretic peptide (BNP). Which of the following medications would be most appropriate to add to her regimen to improve her symptoms and reduce hospital readmission?

    A. Spironolactone
    B. Furosemide
    C. Sacubitril/valsartan
    D. Digoxin

24. A 30-year-old man with a history of ulcerative colitis is admitted to the ICU with severe abdominal pain, bloody diarrhea, and fever. He is diagnosed with toxic megacolon. Which of the following interventions would be most appropriate for initial management?

    A. Intravenous corticosteroids
    B. Bowel rest and nasogastric decompression
    C. Surgical colectomy
    D. Intravenous antibiotics and fluids

25. A 70-year-old woman with a history of atrial fibrillation is admitted to the ICU with ischemic stroke. She is found to have a large left middle cerebral artery (MCA) occlusion on CT angiography. Which of the following interventions would be most appropriate for revascularization?

    A. Intravenous tissue plasminogen activator (tPA)
    B. Mechanical thrombectomy
    C. Aspirin and clopidogrel
    D. Heparin drip

26. A 50-year-old man with a history of alcohol abuse is admitted to the ICU with acute pancreatitis. He develops acute respiratory distress syndrome (ARDS) and requires mechanical ventilation. Which of the following ventilator settings would be most appropriate for this patient?

    A. Low tidal volume ventilation (6 mL/kg)
    B. High positive end-expiratory pressure (PEEP)
    C. High respiratory rate
    D. Prone positioning

27. A 45-year-old woman with a history of systemic lupus erythematosus (SLE) is admitted to the ICU with lupus nephritis. She is found to have significant proteinuria and hematuria. Which of the following medications would be most appropriate to induce remission of her lupus nephritis?

    A. Mycophenolate mofetil
    B. Cyclophosphamide
    C. Rituximab
    D. Hydroxychloroquine

28. A 60-year-old man with a history of type 2 diabetes mellitus is admitted to the ICU with hyperosmolar hyperglycemic state (HHS). He is found to have a blood glucose of 1200 mg/dL and serum osmolality of 350 mOsm/kg. Which of the following interventions would be most appropriate for initial management?

    A. Intravenous insulin infusion
    B. Intravenous normal saline
    C. Subcutaneous insulin
    D. Oral hypoglycemic agents

29. A 25-year-old woman with a history of asthma is admitted to the ICU with status asthmaticus. She is treated with inhaled bronchodilators and systemic corticosteroids but fails to improve. Which of the following interventions would be most appropriate next?

    A. Intravenous magnesium sulfate
    B. Inhaled heliox
    C. Intravenous ketamine
    D. Endotracheal intubation and mechanical ventilation

30. A 75-year-old man with a history of hypertension and coronary artery disease is admitted to the ICU with cardiogenic shock. He is treated with inotropic and vasopressor support but remains hypotensive and oliguric. Which of the following interventions would be most appropriate next?

    A. Intra-aortic balloon pump (IABP)
    B. Impella device
    C. Extracorporeal membrane oxygenation (ECMO)
    D. Surgical revascularization

31. A 75-year-old man with a history of Parkinson's disease is admitted to the ICU with aspiration pneumonia. He is intubated and placed on mechanical ventilation. Which of the following medications would be most appropriate to manage his agitation and delirium?

    A. Haloperidol
    B. Quetiapine
    C. Dexmedetomidine
    D. Propofol

32. A 35-year-old woman with a history of Crohn's disease is admitted to the ICU with severe abdominal pain, fever, and leukocytosis. She is diagnosed with a perforated bowel. Which of the following surgical procedures would be most appropriate for her management?

    A. Laparoscopic appendectomy
    B. Exploratory laparotomy with bowel resection and anastomosis
    C. Hartmann's procedure (proctosigmoidectomy with end colostomy)
    D. Laparoscopic ileostomy

33. A 60-year-old man with a history of chronic lymphocytic leukemia (CLL) is admitted to the ICU with tumor lysis syndrome (TLS). Which of the following laboratory findings would be most consistent with this diagnosis?

    A. Hyperkalemia, hyperphosphatemia, hypocalcemia, hyperuricemia
    B. Hypokalemia, hypophosphatemia, hypercalcemia, hypouricemia
    C. Hyperkalemia, hypophosphatemia, hypocalcemia, hyperuricemia
    D. Hypokalemia, hyperphosphatemia, hypercalcemia, hypouricemia

34. A 45-year-old woman with a history of multiple sclerosis (MS) is admitted to the ICU with acute respiratory failure secondary to a myasthenic crisis. Which of the following medications would be most appropriate to improve her respiratory function?

    A. Pyridostigmine
    B. Edrophonium
    C. Neostigmine
    D. Plasmapheresis

35. A 50-year-old man with a history of alcoholism is admitted to the ICU with alcoholic hepatitis. He develops hepatic encephalopathy. Which of the following medications would be most appropriate to reduce ammonia levels and improve his mental status?

A. Lactulose
B. Rifaximin
C. Neomycin
D. All of the above

36. A 30-year-old woman with a history of systemic sclerosis (scleroderma) is admitted to the ICU with scleroderma renal crisis. Which of the following medications would be most appropriate to manage her hypertension and prevent kidney failure?

A. Captopril
B. Losartan
C. Amlodipine
D. Hydralazine

37. A 65-year-old man with a history of chronic kidney disease (CKD) is admitted to the ICU with acute hyperkalemia (serum potassium of 7.0 mEq/L). He is experiencing peaked T waves and widening of the QRS complex on his electrocardiogram (ECG). Which of the following interventions would be most appropriate to stabilize his cardiac membrane?

A. Intravenous calcium gluconate
B. Intravenous insulin and glucose
C. Inhaled beta-agonist
D. Hemodialysis

38. A 40-year-old woman with a history of Graves' disease is admitted to the ICU with thyroid storm. She is tachycardic, hypertensive, and febrile. Which of the following medications would be most appropriate to block the synthesis of thyroid hormones?

A. Propylthiouracil (PTU)
B. Methimazole
C. Propranolol
D. Iodine

39. A 55-year-old man with a history of hypertension and coronary artery disease is admitted to the ICU with acute ST-elevation myocardial infarction (STEMI). He is treated with percutaneous coronary intervention (PCI) but develops cardiogenic shock. Which of the following medications would be most appropriate to improve his cardiac contractility?

    A. Dobutamine
    B. Milrinone
    C. Dopamine
    D. Norepinephrine

40. A 25-year-old woman with no significant medical history is admitted to the ICU with septic shock secondary to a urinary tract infection (UTI). She is treated with broad-spectrum antibiotics and fluids but remains hypotensive and tachycardic. Which of the following interventions would be most appropriate to improve her blood pressure and perfusion?

    A. Norepinephrine
    B. Vasopressin
    C. Hydrocortisone
    D. All of the above

41. A 65-year-old woman with a history of hypertension and coronary artery disease is admitted to the ICU with acute decompensated heart failure (ADHF). Which of the following medications would be most appropriate to reduce cardiac preload in this patient?

    A. Milrinone
    B. Nitroglycerin
    C. Dobutamine
    D. Dopamine

42.   A 30-year-old man with a history of intravenous drug use presents to the emergency department with fever, chills, and a new heart murmur. He is diagnosed with infective endocarditis. Which of the following organisms is the most likely cause of his infection?

   A. Staphylococcus aureus
   B. Streptococcus pneumoniae
   C. Enterococcus faecalis
   D. Pseudomonas aeruginosa

43.   A 50-year-old man with a history of alcohol abuse is admitted to the ICU with acute pancreatitis. He develops acute kidney injury (AKI). Which of the following is the most likely cause of his AKI?

   A. Prerenal AKI due to hypovolemia
   B. Intrinsic AKI due to acute tubular necrosis
   C. Postrenal AKI due to ureteral obstruction
   D. All of the above

44.   A 45-year-old woman with a history of systemic lupus erythematosus (SLE) is admitted to the ICU with acute respiratory failure. She is found to have diffuse alveolar hemorrhage (DAH) on bronchoscopy. Which of the following medications would be most appropriate for her treatment?

   A. Cyclophosphamide
   B. Azathioprine
   C. Mycophenolate mofetil
   D. Rituximab

45.   A 70-year-old man with a history of chronic obstructive pulmonary disease (COPD) is admitted to the ICU with an acute exacerbation. He is intubated and placed on mechanical ventilation. Which of the following ventilator modes would be most appropriate for this patient?

   A. Assist control (AC)
   B. Pressure control (PC)
   C. Synchronized intermittent mandatory ventilation (SIMV)
   D. Pressure support ventilation (PSV)

46.   A 25-year-old woman with a history of asthma is admitted to the ICU with status asthmaticus. She is treated with inhaled bronchodilators, systemic corticosteroids, and intravenous magnesium sulfate but fails to improve. Which of the following interventions would be most appropriate next?

    A. Intravenous ketamine
    B. Inhaled heliox
    C. Noninvasive positive pressure ventilation (NIPPV)
    D. Endotracheal intubation and mechanical ventilation

47.   A 60-year-old man with a history of hypertension is admitted to the ICU with a subarachnoid hemorrhage (SAH). He develops cerebral vasospasm. Which of the following medications would be most appropriate to prevent and treat vasospasm?

    A. Nimodipine
    B. Nicardipine
    C. Verapamil
    D. Diltiazem

48.   A 45-year-old woman with a history of diabetes mellitus is admitted to the ICU with diabetic ketoacidosis (DKA). She is treated with intravenous insulin and fluids but develops hypokalemia (serum potassium of 2.5 mEq/L). Which of the following interventions would be most appropriate to correct her hypokalemia?

    A. Intravenous potassium chloride
    B. Oral potassium chloride
    C. Discontinue insulin infusion
    D. Administer kayexalate

49.   A 55-year-old man with a history of liver cirrhosis is admitted to the ICU with acute variceal bleeding. He is treated with endoscopic variceal ligation (EVL) and octreotide. Which of the following medications would be most appropriate to prevent rebleeding?

    A. Propranolol
    B. Nadolol
    C. Carvedilol
    D. All of the above

50. A 75-year-old woman with a history of atrial fibrillation is admitted to the ICU with ischemic stroke. She is not a candidate for reperfusion therapy. Which of the following medications would be most appropriate to prevent recurrent stroke?

    A. Aspirin
    B. Clopidogrel
    C. Warfarin
    D. Apixaban

51. A 35-year-old woman with a history of systemic lupus erythematosus (SLE) is admitted to the ICU with acute kidney injury (AKI). A renal biopsy reveals diffuse proliferative lupus nephritis (Class IV). Which of the following treatment options is most appropriate for induction therapy?

    A. Mycophenolate mofetil (MMF)
    B. Cyclophosphamide
    C. Rituximab
    D. Hydroxychloroquine

52. A 65-year-old man with a history of hypertension and coronary artery disease presents to the emergency department with sudden onset of severe tearing chest pain radiating to the back. His blood pressure is 200/110 mmHg, and his heart rate is 120 beats per minute. Which of the following diagnostic tests is most appropriate to confirm the suspected diagnosis?

    A. Chest X-ray
    B. Electrocardiogram (ECG)
    C. Computed tomography angiography (CTA) of the chest
    D. Transthoracic echocardiogram (TTE)

53.   A 40-year-old woman with a history of asthma presents to the ICU with acute respiratory failure requiring mechanical ventilation. She develops hypotension and tachycardia despite adequate fluid resuscitation. Which of the following medications would be most appropriate to improve her hemodynamic status?

    A. Norepinephrine
    B. Dobutamine
    C. Milrinone
    D. Vasopressin

54.   A 50-year-old man with a history of alcohol abuse is admitted to the ICU with acute pancreatitis. He develops acute respiratory distress syndrome (ARDS). Which of the following ventilation strategies is most likely to improve his oxygenation?

    A. High tidal volume ventilation
    B. Low positive end-expiratory pressure (PEEP)
    C. High respiratory rate
    D. Lung-protective ventilation with low tidal volumes and appropriate PEEP

55.   A 25-year-old woman with no significant medical history is admitted to the ICU with meningococcal meningitis. She develops disseminated intravascular coagulation (DIC). Which of the following laboratory findings would be most consistent with this diagnosis?

    A. Elevated platelet count
    B. Decreased fibrinogen level
    C. Normal prothrombin time (PT)
    D. Decreased D-dimer level

56. A 60-year-old man with a history of chronic kidney disease (CKD) is admitted to the ICU with acute hyperkalemia (serum potassium of 7.0 mEq/L). He is experiencing muscle weakness and peaked T waves on his electrocardiogram (ECG). Which of the following interventions would be most appropriate to shift potassium intracellularly?

    A. Intravenous calcium gluconate
    B. Intravenous insulin and glucose
    C. Oral sodium polystyrene sulfonate (Kayexalate)
    D. Hemodialysis

57. A 45-year-old woman with a history of rheumatoid arthritis is admitted to the ICU with septic shock secondary to pneumonia. She is intubated and mechanically ventilated. Which of the following hemodynamic goals is most appropriate for this patient during the initial resuscitation phase?

    A. Mean arterial pressure (MAP) > 65 mmHg
    B. Central venous pressure (CVP) 8-12 mmHg
    C. Urine output > 0.5 mL/kg/hour
    D. All of the above

58. A 70-year-old man with a history of atrial fibrillation is admitted to the ICU with acute ischemic stroke. He is not a candidate for reperfusion therapy. Which of the following medications would be most appropriate to prevent recurrent stroke in this patient?

    A. Aspirin
    B. Clopidogrel
    C. Warfarin
    D. Apixaban

59. A 35-year-old woman with a history of systemic lupus erythematosus (SLE) is admitted to the ICU with lupus nephritis. She is started on high-dose intravenous corticosteroids. Which of the following complications is most likely to occur due to her corticosteroid therapy?

    A. Hypoglycemia
    B. Hyperkalemia
    C. Hypernatremia
    D. Hypercalcemia

60. A 50-year-old man with a history of alcoholism is admitted to the ICU with acute variceal bleeding. He is treated with endoscopic variceal ligation (EVL) and octreotide. Which of the following prophylactic antibiotic regimens would be most appropriate to prevent spontaneous bacterial peritonitis (SBP) in this patient?

    A. Ciprofloxacin
    B. Ceftriaxone
    C. Trimethoprim-sulfamethoxazole (TMP-SMX)
    D. Amoxicillin-clavulanate

61. A 55-year-old woman presents to the emergency department with complaints of fever, chills, and right upper quadrant abdominal pain. She is diagnosed with acute cholangitis. Which of the following is the most appropriate initial intervention?

    A. Laparoscopic cholecystectomy
    B. Endoscopic retrograde cholangiopancreatography (ERCP)
    C. Percutaneous transhepatic cholangiography (PTC)
    D. Intravenous antibiotics and fluids

62. A 65-year-old man with a history of hypertension and diabetes mellitus presents to the ICU with ST-elevation myocardial infarction (STEMI). He is taken for emergent percutaneous coronary intervention (PCI). Which of the following adjunctive therapies is most likely to improve his outcomes?

    A. Therapeutic hypothermia
    B. Intra-aortic balloon pump (IABP)
    C. Glycoprotein IIb/IIIa inhibitors
    D. Thrombolytic therapy

63. A 40-year-old woman with a history of systemic sclerosis (scleroderma) is admitted to the ICU with worsening dyspnea and hypoxemia. A high-resolution computed tomography (HRCT) scan of the chest reveals ground-glass opacities and honeycombing. Which of the following is the most likely diagnosis?

    A. Interstitial lung disease (ILD)
    B. Pulmonary embolism (PE)
    C. Pulmonary hypertension (PH)
    D. Pneumonia

64. A 25-year-old man with a history of traumatic brain injury (TBI) is admitted to the ICU with increased intracranial pressure (ICP). Which of the following interventions is most likely to decrease his ICP?

   A. Mannitol infusion
   B. Hyperventilation
   C. Head-of-bed elevation to 30 degrees
   D. All of the above

65. A 70-year-old woman with a history of chronic kidney disease (CKD) is admitted to the ICU with metabolic acidosis. Her arterial blood gas (ABG) shows a pH of 7.25, PaCO2 of 30 mmHg, and HCO3- of 15 mEq/L. Which of the following is the most likely cause of her metabolic acidosis?

   A. Diabetic ketoacidosis (DKA)
   B. Uremic acidosis
   C. Lactic acidosis
   D. Salicylate toxicity

66. A 55-year-old man with a history of cirrhosis presents to the ICU with acute hepatic encephalopathy. Which of the following medications is most likely to improve his mental status?

   A. Lactulose
   B. Rifaximin
   C. Neomycin
   D. All of the above

67. A 30-year-old woman with a history of intravenous drug use presents to the ICU with fever, chills, and right upper quadrant abdominal pain. She is diagnosed with an amebic liver abscess. Which of the following medications is most appropriate for her treatment?

   A. Metronidazole
   B. Chloroquine
   C. Praziquantel
   D. Albendazole

68. A 65-year-old man with a history of hypertension and diabetes mellitus presents to the ICU with acute ST-elevation myocardial infarction (STEMI). He is not a candidate for reperfusion therapy. Which of the following medications would be most appropriate to reduce his risk of ventricular remodeling?

    A. Aspirin
    B. Clopidogrel
    C. Beta-blocker
    D. ACE inhibitor

69. A 40-year-old woman with a history of inflammatory bowel disease (IBD) presents to the ICU with toxic megacolon. Which of the following imaging modalities is most appropriate to confirm the diagnosis?

    A. Abdominal X-ray
    B. Computed tomography (CT) scan of the abdomen
    C. Magnetic resonance imaging (MRI) of the abdomen
    D. Ultrasound of the abdomen

70. A 25-year-oldman with a history of asthma presents to the ICU with status asthmaticus. He is treated with inhaled bronchodilators, systemic corticosteroids, and intravenous magnesium sulfate but fails to improve. Which of the following adjunctive therapies is most likely to improve his respiratory status?

    A. Heliox
    B. Ketamine
    C. Noninvasive positive pressure ventilation (NIPPV)
    D. Extracorporeal membrane oxygenation (ECMO)

71. A 48-year-old man with a history of end-stage renal disease (ESRD. on hemodialysis presents to the ICU with altered mental status and hypotension. His serum calcium level is 7.5 mg/dL. Which of the following is the most likely cause of his hypocalcemia?

    A. Decreased parathyroid hormone (PTH) production
    B. Vitamin D deficiency
    C. Hyperphosphatemia
    D. All of the above

72. A 35-year-old woman with a history of systemic lupus erythematosus (SLE) is admitted to the ICU with thrombotic thrombocytopenic purpura (TTP). Which of the following is the most appropriate treatment for this condition?

    A. Plasma exchange
    B. Corticosteroids
    C. Rituximab
    D. Splenectomy

73. A 60-year-old man with a history of hypertension and hyperlipidemia presents to the ICU with acute respiratory distress syndrome (ARDS) following a motor vehicle accident. Which of the following ventilator settings is most appropriate for this patient?

    A. High tidal volume ventilation
    B. Low positive end-expiratory pressure (PEEP)
    C. High respiratory rate
    D. Lung-protective ventilation with low tidal volumes and appropriate PEEP

74. A 50-year-old woman with a history of breast cancer presents to the ICU with altered mental status, polyuria, and polydipsia. Her serum calcium level is 15 mg/dL. Which of the following is the most likely cause of her hypercalcemia?

    A. Primary hyperparathyroidism
    B. Humoral hypercalcemia of malignancy
    C. Vitamin D intoxication
    D. Milk-alkali syndrome

75. A 25-year-old man with no significant medical history presents to the ICU with severe community-acquired pneumonia (CAP). He is intubated and mechanically ventilated. Which of the following antibiotic regimens is most appropriate for empiric treatment?

    A. Ceftriaxone and azithromycin
    B. Piperacillin/tazobactam and vancomycin
    C. Meropenem and vancomycin
    D. Levofloxacin and azithromycin

76. A 70-year-old woman with a history of heart failure with preserved ejection fraction (HFpEF) is admitted to the ICU with acute decompensated heart failure. Which of the following medications is most likely to improve her symptoms?

    A. Furosemide
    B. Spironolactone
    C. Sacubitril/valsartan
    D. Digoxin

77. A 45-year-old man with a history of alcoholism is admitted to the ICU with alcoholic hepatitis. He develops hepatorenal syndrome (HRS). Which of the following is the most appropriate treatment for HRS?

    A. Terlipressin
    B. Midodrine and octreotide
    C. Albumin
    D. All of the above

78. A 30-year-old woman with a history of systemic lupus erythematosus (SLE) is admitted to the ICU with diffuse alveolar hemorrhage (DAH). Which of the following medications is most likely to improve her respiratory status?

    A. Cyclophosphamide
    B. Azathioprine
    C. Mycophenolate mofetil
    D. Rituximab

79. A 60-year-old man with a history of chronic kidney disease (CKD) on hemodialysis is admitted to the ICU with septic shock. Which of the following antibiotics is most appropriate for empiric treatment?

    A. Vancomycin and piperacillin/tazobactam
    B. Cefepime and metronidazole
    C. Meropenem and vancomycin
    D. Levofloxacin and azithromycin

80. A 50-year-old woman with a history of rheumatoid arthritis is admitted to the ICU with acute respiratory distress syndrome (ARDS) secondary to pneumonia. She is intubated and mechanically ventilated. Which of the following ventilation strategies is most likely to improve her oxygenation?

    A. High tidal volume ventilation
    B. Low positive end-expiratory pressure (PEEP)
    C. High respiratory rate
    D. Lung-protective ventilation with low tidal volumes and appropriate PEEP

81. A 72-year-old man with a history of hypertension and coronary artery disease is admitted to the ICU with new-onset atrial fibrillation with rapid ventricular response (RVR). His heart rate is 150 beats per minute, and his blood pressure is 90/60 mmHg. Which of the following medications is most appropriate for rate control in this patient?

    A. Diltiazem
    B. Amiodarone
    C. Metoprolol
    D. Digoxin

82. A 35-year-old woman with a history of systemic lupus erythematosus (SLE) is admitted to the ICU with acute lupus myocarditis. Which of the following diagnostic findings is most consistent with this diagnosis?

    A. Elevated troponin levels
    B. ST-segment elevations on ECG
    C. Pericardial effusion on echocardiogram
    D. All of the above

83. A 60-year-old man with a history of cirrhosis presents to the ICU with hepatic encephalopathy. He is found to have elevated ammonia levels. Which of the following dietary modifications is most appropriate for this patient?

    A. High-protein diet
    B. Low-protein diet
    C. High-carbohydrate diet
    D. Low-carbohydrate diet

84. A 50-year-old woman with a history of chronic kidney disease (CKD) is admitted to the ICU with uremic pericarditis. Which of the following is the most appropriate treatment for this condition?

    A. Pericardiocentesis
    B. Corticosteroids
    C. Nonsteroidal anti-inflammatory drugs (NSAIDs)
    D. Dialysis

85. A 25-year-old man with no significant medical history presents to the ICU with acute respiratory distress syndrome (ARDS) following a near-drowning incident. Which of the following ventilator settings is most likely to improve his oxygenation?

    A. High tidal volume ventilation
    B. Low positive end-expiratory pressure (PEEP)
    C. High respiratory rate
    D. Lung-protective ventilation with low tidal volumes and high PEEP

86. A 70-year-old woman with a history of heart failure with reduced ejection fraction (HFrEF) is admitted to the ICU with cardiogenic shock. Which of the following mechanical circulatory support devices is most appropriate for this patient?

    A. Intra-aortic balloon pump (IABP)
    B. Impella
    C. TandemHeart
    D. Extracorporeal membrane oxygenation (ECMO)

87. A 45-year-old man with a history of alcoholism is admitted to the ICU with acute pancreatitis. He develops acute kidney injury (AKI) and requires renal replacement therapy (RRT). Which of the following modalities of RRT is most appropriate for this patient?

    A. Continuous venovenous hemofiltration (CVVH)
    B. Intermittent hemodialysis (IHD)
    C. Peritoneal dialysis (PD)
    D. Sustained low-efficiency dialysis (SLED)

88. A 30-year-old woman with a history of systemic lupus erythematosus (SLE) is admitted to the ICU with lupus nephritis. She is started on high-dose intravenous corticosteroids and cyclophosphamide. Which of the following laboratory tests is most important to monitor for potential complications of her therapy?

A. Complete blood count (CBC)
B. Liver function tests (LFTs)
C. Electrolytes
D. All of the above

89. A 60-year-old man with a history of hypertension and hyperlipidemia presents to the ICU with acute ischemic stroke. He is not a candidate for reperfusion therapy. Which of the following medications is most appropriate to prevent secondary stroke in this patient?

A. Aspirin
B. Clopidogrel
C. Warfarin
D. Apixaban

90. A 50-year-old woman with a history of diabetes mellitus presents to the ICU with diabetic ketoacidosis (DKA). She is treated with intravenous insulin and fluids. Which of the following electrolyte abnormalities is most likely to occur during the treatment of DKA?

A. Hypokalemia
B. Hyperkalemia
C. Hyponatremia
D. Hypernatremia

91. A 45-year-old woman with a history of rheumatoid arthritis presents to the ICU with new-onset shortness of breath, tachycardia, and hypotension. A chest x-ray reveals bilateral pleural effusions. Which of the following is the most likely diagnosis?

A. Acute respiratory distress syndrome (ARDS)
B. Pulmonary embolism (PE)
C. Congestive heart failure (CHF)
D. Pleural effusion secondary to rheumatoid arthritis

92. A 75-year-old man with a history of chronic obstructive pulmonary disease (COPD) presents to the ICU with acute respiratory failure. He is intubated and placed on mechanical ventilation. After 24 hours, his oxygenation deteriorates despite increasing ventilator support. Which of the following interventions should be considered next?

    A. Inhaled nitric oxide
    B. Prone positioning
    C. Extracorporeal membrane oxygenation (ECMO)
    D. High-frequency oscillatory ventilation (HFOV)

93. A 30-year-old woman with a history of intravenous drug use presents to the ICU with infective endocarditis. Blood cultures grow methicillin-resistant Staphylococcus aureus (MRSA). Which of the following antibiotic regimens is most appropriate for this patient?

    A. Vancomycin and gentamicin
    B. Daptomycin
    C. Linezolid
    D. Ceftaroline

94. A 65-year-old man with a history of hypertension and diabetes mellitus presents to the ICU with acute ischemic stroke. He is not a candidate for reperfusion therapy. Which of the following medications should be initiated within 48 hours of symptom onset to reduce the risk of recurrent stroke?

    A. Aspirin
    B. Clopidogrel
    C. Warfarin
    D. Statin

95. A 50-year-old woman with a history of cirrhosis presents to the ICU with acute variceal bleeding. She is treated with endoscopic variceal ligation (EVL) and octreotide. Which of the following is the most appropriate long-term management strategy for this patient?

    A. Nonselective beta-blocker (e.g., propranolol)
    B. Endoscopic variceal band ligation (EVL) every 2-4 weeks
    C. Transjugular intrahepatic portosystemic shunt (TIPS)
    D. Liver transplantation

96. A 40-year-old man with no significant medical history presents to the ICU with acute pancreatitis. He develops acute kidney injury (AKI) and requires renal replacement therapy (RRT). Which of the following modalities of RRT is most appropriate for this patient?

    A. Continuous venovenous hemofiltration (CVVH)
    B. Intermittent hemodialysis (IHD)
    C. Peritoneal dialysis (PD)
    D. Sustained low-efficiency dialysis (SLED)

97. A 75-year-old man with a history of Parkinson's disease is admitted to the ICU with aspiration pneumonia. He is intubated and placed on mechanical ventilation. Which of the following strategies is most likely to reduce his risk of ventilator-associated pneumonia (VAP)?

    A. Oral chlorhexidine gluconate rinse
    B. Elevation of the head of the bed to 30 degrees
    C. Daily "sedation vacations" and assessment of readiness to extubate
    D. All of the above

98. A 35-year-old woman with a history of systemic lupus erythematosus (SLE) is admitted to the ICU with diffuse alveolar hemorrhage (DAH). Which of the following interventions is most likely to improve her oxygenation?

    A. Intravenous corticosteroids
    B. Plasma exchange
    C. Intravenous cyclophosphamide
    D. All of the above

99. A 60-year-old man with a history of hypertension and diabetes mellitus presents to the ICU with acute decompensated heart failure (ADHF). He is treated with intravenous diuretics and vasodilators but remains hypotensive and oliguric. Which of the following inotropic agents is most appropriate for this patient?

    A. Dobutamine
    B. Milrinone
    C. Dopamine
    D. Norepinephrine

100. A 50-year-old woman with a history of rheumatoid arthritis presents to the ICU with septic shock secondary to pneumonia. She is intubated and mechanically ventilated. Which of the following bundles of care is most likely to improve her outcomes?

    A. Early goal-directed therapy (EGDT)
    B. Surviving Sepsis Campaign bundle
    C. ARDSNet protocol
    D. All of the above

101. A 68-year-old man with a history of hypertension and coronary artery disease presents to the ICU with new-onset chest pain and ST-segment elevations in leads II, III, and aVF on his electrocardiogram (ECG). He is diagnosed with an inferior ST-elevation myocardial infarction (STEMI). Which coronary artery is most likely occluded in this patient?

    A. Left anterior descending (LAD) artery
    B. Left circumflex (LCx) artery
    C. Right coronary artery (RCA)
    D. Left main coronary artery (LMCA)

102. A 55-year-old woman with a history of type 2 diabetes mellitus and obesity is admitted to the ICU with acute pancreatitis. Which of the following laboratory tests is most sensitive and specific for the diagnosis of acute pancreatitis?

    A. Serum amylase
    B. Serum lipase
    C. Serum alanine aminotransferase (ALT)
    D. Serum aspartate aminotransferase (AST)

103. A 45-year-old man with a history of intravenous drug use is admitted to the ICU with infective endocarditis. He develops septic embolic stroke. Which of the following diagnostic tests is most appropriate to evaluate for the presence of vegetations on his heart valves?

    A. Transthoracic echocardiogram (TTE)
    B. Transesophageal echocardiogram (TEE)
    C. Cardiac magnetic resonance imaging (MRI)
    D. Cardiac computed tomography (CT) scan

104. A 70-year-old woman with a history of chronic obstructive pulmonary disease (COPD) is admitted to the ICU with acute respiratory failure. She is intubated and placed on mechanical ventilation. After 48 hours, she develops ventilator-associated pneumonia (VAP). Which of the following organisms is the most likely cause of her VAP?

    A. Pseudomonas aeruginosa
    B. Staphylococcus aureus
    C. Klebsiella pneumoniae
    D. Escherichia coli

105. A 35-year-old man with no significant medical history presents to the ICU with severe community-acquired pneumonia (CAP). He is intubated and mechanically ventilated. Which of the following ventilator modes is most appropriate for this patient?

    A. Assist control (AC)
    B. Pressure control (PC)
    C. Synchronized intermittent mandatory ventilation (SIMV)
    D. Pressure support ventilation (PSV)

106. A 65-year-old woman with a history of heart failure with reduced ejection fraction (HFrEF) is admitted to the ICU with acute decompensated heart failure. She is treated with intravenous diuretics and vasodilators, but her symptoms do not improve. Which of the following inotropic agents is most appropriate for this patient?

    A. Dobutamine
    B. Milrinone
    C. Dopamine
    D. Norepinephrine

107. A 40-year-old man with a history of alcoholism is admitted to the ICU with acute alcoholic hepatitis. He develops hepatorenal syndrome (HRS). Which of the following is the most important prognostic factor for survival in HRS?

    A. Serum creatinine level
    B. Serum bilirubin level
    C. Model for End-Stage Liver Disease (MELD) score
    D. Response to treatment with terlipressin

108. A 25-year-old woman with a history of asthma is admitted to the ICU with status asthmaticus. She is treated with inhaled bronchodilators, systemic corticosteroids, and intravenous magnesium sulfate, but her condition continues to deteriorate. Which of the following interventions should be considered next?

    A. Intravenous ketamine
    B. Inhaled heliox
    C. Noninvasive positive pressure ventilation (NIPPV)
    D. Endotracheal intubation and mechanical ventilation

109. A 55-year-old man with a history of hypertension and hyperlipidemia presents to the ICU with an acute aortic dissection. He is hemodynamically stable. Which of the following is the most appropriate initial management strategy for this patient?

    A. Surgical repair
    B. Endovascular repair
    C. Medical therapy with beta-blockers and blood pressure control
    D. Percutaneous transluminal angioplasty (PTA)

110. A 70-year-old woman with a history of chronic kidney disease (CKD) is admitted to the ICU with uremic pericarditis. She develops cardiac tamponade. Which of the following is the most appropriate treatment for this condition?

    A. Pericardiocentesis
    B. Corticosteroids
    C. Nonsteroidal anti-inflammatory drugs (NSAIDs)
    D. Dialysis

111. A 58-year-old man with a history of hypertension and coronary artery disease presents to the ICU with acute decompensated heart failure (ADHF). Which of the following medications would be most appropriate to reduce afterload in this patient?

    A. Nitroglycerin
    B. Furosemide
    C. Dobutamine
    D. Nesiritide

112. A 42-year-old woman with a history of systemic lupus erythematosus (SLE) is admitted to the ICU with lupus nephritis. Which of the following laboratory findings would be most consistent with this diagnosis?

    A. Decreased serum creatinine
    B. Proteinuria and hematuria
    C. Normal complement levels
    D. Negative antinuclear antibody (ANA) titer

113. A 75-year-old man with a history of chronic obstructive pulmonary disease (COPD) is admitted to the ICU with an acute exacerbation. He is intubated and placed on mechanical ventilation. Which of the following ventilator settings is most likely to improve his ventilation-perfusion (V/Q) mismatch?

    A. High tidal volume ventilation
    B. Low positive end-expiratory pressure (PEEP)
    C. High respiratory rate
    D. Lung-protective ventilation with low tidal volumes and high PEEP

114. A 30-year-old woman with no significant medical history presents to the ICU with severe community-acquired pneumonia (CAP). She is intubated and mechanically ventilated. Which of the following interventions is most likely to reduce her risk of ventilator-associated pneumonia (VAP)?

    A. Oral chlorhexidine gluconate rinse
    B. Elevation of the head of the bed to 30 degrees
    C. Daily "sedation vacations" and assessment of readiness to extubate
    D. All of the above

115. A 65-year-old man with a history of heart failure with reduced ejection fraction (HFrEF) is admitted to the ICU with cardiogenic shock. He is treated with inotropic and vasopressor support but remains hypotensive and oliguric. Which of the following mechanical circulatory support devices is most appropriate for this patient?

    A. Intra-aortic balloon pump (IABP)
    B. Impella
    C. TandemHeart
    D. Extracorporeal membrane oxygenation (ECMO)

116. A 40-year-old man with a history of alcoholism is admitted to the ICU with acute variceal bleeding. He is treated with endoscopic variceal ligation (EVL) and octreotide. Which of the following is the most appropriate long-term management strategy for this patient?

    A. Nonselective beta-blocker (e.g., propranolol)
    B. Endoscopic variceal band ligation (EVL) every 2-4 weeks
    C. Transjugular intrahepatic portosystemic shunt (TIPS)
    D. Liver transplantation

117. A 25-year-old woman with a history of asthma is admitted to the ICU with status asthmaticus. She is treated with inhaled bronchodilators, systemic corticosteroids, and intravenous magnesium sulfate but fails to improve. Which of the following adjunctive therapies is most likely to improve her respiratory status?

    A. Heliox
    B. Ketamine
    C. Noninvasive positive pressure ventilation (NIPPV)
    D. Extracorporeal membrane oxygenation (ECMO)

118. A 55-year-old man with a history of hypertension and hyperlipidemia presents to the ICU with an acute aortic dissection. He is hemodynamically stable. Which of the following is the most appropriate diagnostic test to evaluate the extent of the dissection?

    A. Chest X-ray
    B. Computed tomography angiography (CTA) of the chest
    C. Transesophageal echocardiogram (TEE)
    D. Magnetic resonance imaging (MRI) of the chest

119. A 70-year-old woman with a history of chronic kidney disease (CKD) is admitted to the ICU with uremic pericarditis. She develops cardiac tamponade. Which of the following hemodynamic findings is most consistent with cardiac tamponade?

    A. Increased cardiac output
    B. Decreased central venous pressure (CVP)
    C. Pulsus paradoxus
    D. Widened pulse pressure

120. A 50-year-old woman with a history of rheumatoid arthritis presents to the ICU with septic shock secondary to pneumonia. She is intubated and mechanically ventilated. Which of the following interventions is most likely to improve her mortality?

    A. Early goal-directed therapy (EGDT)
    B. Low-dose corticosteroids
    C. Tight glycemic control
    D. All of the above

121. A 62-year-old male with a history of hypertension and coronary artery disease is admitted to the ICU with ST-elevation myocardial infarction (STEMI). During his hospital course, he develops new-onset holosystolic murmur at the apex radiating to the axilla. Which of the following complications is most likely responsible for this new murmur?

    A. Ventricular septal rupture
    B. Papillary muscle rupture
    C. Free wall rupture
    D. Acute pericarditis

122. A 38-year-old female with a history of systemic lupus erythematosus (SLE) presents to the ICU with altered mental status, seizures, and hypertension. Which of the following diagnostic tests would be most helpful in confirming the suspected diagnosis of posterior reversible encephalopathy syndrome (PRES)?

    A. Electroencephalogram (EEG)
    B. Lumbar puncture
    C. Magnetic resonance imaging (MRI) of the brain
    D. Computed tomography (CT) scan of the head

123. A 70-year-old male with a history of chronic kidney disease (CKD) and type 2 diabetes mellitus presents to the ICU with diabetic ketoacidosis (DKA). Which of the following electrolyte abnormalities is most commonly associated with DKA?

    A. Hyperkalemia
    B. Hypokalemia
    C. Hypernatremia
    D. Hyponatremia

124. A 55-year-old woman with a history of liver cirrhosis presents to the ICU with acute variceal bleeding. Which of the following endoscopic therapies is most effective in controlling acute variceal bleeding?

    A. Endoscopic variceal sclerotherapy (EVS)
    B. Endoscopic variceal band ligation (EVL)
    C. Balloon tamponade
    D. Transjugular intrahepatic portosystemic shunt (TIPS)

125. A 45-year-old man with no significant medical history presents to the ICU with acute respiratory distress syndrome (ARDS) following a near-drowning incident. Which of the following ventilator strategies is most likely to improve his oxygenation while minimizing lung injury?

    A. High tidal volume ventilation with high PEEP
    B. Low tidal volume ventilation with high PEEP
    C. High tidal volume ventilation with low PEEP
    D. Low tidal volume ventilation with low PEEP

126. A 30-year-old woman with a history of asthma presents to the ICU with status asthmaticus. She is intubated and mechanically ventilated. Which of the following ventilator settings is most appropriate to manage her airflow obstruction and air trapping?

    A. Low respiratory rate and short inspiratory time
    B. High respiratory rate and short inspiratory time
    C. Low respiratory rate and long inspiratory time
    D. High respiratory rate and long inspiratory time

127. A 60-year-old man with a history of hypertension and hyperlipidemia presents to the ICU with an acute aortic dissection. He undergoes successful endovascular repair of the dissection. Which of the following medications is most appropriate for long-term blood pressure control in this patient?

    A. Beta-blockers
    B. Calcium channel blockers
    C. Angiotensin-converting enzyme (ACE) inhibitors
    D. Angiotensin II receptor blockers (ARBs)

128. A 50-year-old woman with a history of rheumatoid arthritis presents to the ICU with septic shock secondary to pneumonia. She is initiated on norepinephrine for vasopressor support. Which of the following is a potential adverse effect of norepinephrine?

A. Tachycardia
B. Hypotension
C. Bradycardia
D. Hyperglycemia

129. A 75-year-old man with a history of chronic kidney disease (CKD) is admitted to the ICU with metabolic acidosis. His arterial blood gas (ABG) shows a pH of 7.20, PaCO2 of 30 mmHg, and HCO3- of 12 mEq/L. Which of the following is the most appropriate initial intervention for this patient?

A. Sodium bicarbonate infusion
B. Intravenous insulin and glucose
C. Hemodialysis
D. Thiamine supplementation

130. A 45-year-old man with a history of alcoholism is admitted to the ICU with acute alcoholic hepatitis. He develops severe coagulopathy and bleeding. Which of the following blood products is most appropriate to correct his coagulopathy?

A. Fresh frozen plasma (FFP)
B. Cryoprecipitate
C. Platelets
D. Prothrombin complex concentrate (PCC)

131. A 78-year-old woman with a history of hypertension and coronary artery disease is admitted to the ICU with acute decompensated heart failure. She is currently on lisinopril, metoprolol, and furosemide. Which of the following medications would be most appropriate to add to her regimen to improve her symptoms and reduce hospital readmission?

A. Spironolactone
B. Sacubitril/valsartan
C. Ivabradine
D. Digoxin

132. A 45-year-old man with no significant medical history is admitted to the ICU with severe acute pancreatitis. He develops acute respiratory distress syndrome (ARDS). Which of the following interventions is most likely to improve his oxygenation and reduce mortality?

    A. High tidal volume ventilation
    B. Low positive end-expiratory pressure (PEEP)
    C. Prone positioning
    D. Inhaled nitric oxide

133. A 32-year-old woman with a history of systemic lupus erythematosus (SLE) is admitted to the ICU with acute kidney injury (AKI). A renal biopsy reveals diffuse proliferative lupus nephritis (Class IV). Which of the following immunosuppressive agents is considered the standard of care for induction therapy in this patient?

    A. Mycophenolate mofetil (MMF)
    B. Cyclophosphamide
    C. Rituximab
    D. Belimumab

134. A 68-year-old man with a history of atrial fibrillation is admitted to the ICU with an acute ischemic stroke. He is not a candidate for intravenous thrombolysis or mechanical thrombectomy. Which of the following medications should be initiated within 24 hours of symptom onset to reduce the risk of early recurrent stroke?

    A. Aspirin
    B. Clopidogrel
    C. Warfarin
    D. Apixaban

135. A 55-year-old woman with a history of cirrhosis presents to the ICU with acute variceal bleeding. She undergoes successful endoscopic variceal ligation (EVL). Which of the following medications should be initiated to prevent rebleeding?

    A. Propranolol
    B. Nadolol
    C. Carvedilol
    D. Any of the above

136. A 40-year-old man with a history of alcohol abuse is admitted to the ICU with severe alcoholic hepatitis. He develops hepatic encephalopathy. Which of the following medications is most effective in reducing ammonia levels and improving mental status in this patient?

    A. Lactulose
    B. Rifaximin
    C. Neomycin
    D. L-ornithine L-aspartate (LOLA)

137. A 28-year-old woman with a history of asthma presents to the ICU with status asthmaticus. She is intubated and mechanically ventilated. Which of the following ventilator settings is most likely to reduce her risk of barotrauma and dynamic hyperinflation?

    A. High tidal volume ventilation
    B. Low respiratory rate
    C. High inspiratory flow rate
    D. Low inspiratory:expiratory (I:E) ratio

138. A 62-year-old man with a history of hypertension and coronary artery disease is admitted to the ICU with an acute inferior ST-elevation myocardial infarction (STEMI). He undergoes successful percutaneous coronary intervention (PCI) with placement of a drug-eluting stent in the right coronary artery (RCA). Which of the following medications should be added to his regimen to reduce the risk of stent thrombosis?

    A. Aspirin
    B. Clopidogrel
    C. Ticagrelor
    D. Prasugrel

139. A 50-year-old woman with a history of type 2 diabetes mellitus presents to the ICU with hyperosmolar hyperglycemic state (HHS). She is started on an intravenous insulin infusion. Which of the following electrolyte abnormalities should be monitored closely during the treatment of HHS?

    A. Hypokalemia
    B. Hyperkalemia
    C. Hypophosphatemia
    D. All of the above

140. A 75-year-old man with a history of chronic kidney disease (CKD) is admitted to the ICU with acute pulmonary edema. He is intubated and placed on mechanical ventilation. Which of the following diuretics is most appropriate for this patient given his CKD?

    A. Furosemide
    B. Bumetanide
    C. Torsemide
    D. Ethacrynic acid

141. A 68-year-old woman with a history of hypertension and coronary artery disease presents to the ICU with new-onset chest pain and ST-segment depressions in leads V1-V4 on her electrocardiogram (ECG). She is diagnosed with non-ST-elevation myocardial infarction (NSTEMI). Which of the following medications is NOT routinely recommended for the initial management of NSTEMI?

    A. Aspirin
    B. Ticagrelor
    C. Enoxaparin
    D. Fibrinolytic therapy

142. A 45-year-old man with a history of intravenous drug use is admitted to the ICU with infective endocarditis complicated by a large vegetation on the mitral valve. Which of the following is an absolute indication for surgical intervention in this patient?

    A. New-onset heart failure
    B. Persistent bacteremia despite appropriate antibiotic therapy
    C. Embolic events despite appropriate antibiotic therapy
    D. All of the above

143. A 75-year-old man with a history of chronic obstructive pulmonary disease (COPD) is admitted to the ICU with an acute exacerbation. He is intubated and placed on mechanical ventilation. After 72 hours, he develops ventilator-associated pneumonia (VAP). Which of the following is the most appropriate empiric antibiotic regimen for this patient?

    A. Piperacillin/tazobactam and vancomycin
    B. Cefepime and metronidazole
    C. Meropenem and vancomycin
    D. Levofloxacin and azithromycin

144. A 30-year-old woman with no significant medical history presents to the ICU with severe community-acquired pneumonia (CAP) and septic shock. Which of the following interventions has been shown to improve mortality in patients with septic shock?

    A. Early goal-directed therapy (EGDT)
    B. Low-dose corticosteroids
    C. Tight glycemic control
    D. All of the above

145. A 65-year-old woman with a history of heart failure with preserved ejection fraction (HFpEF) is admitted to the ICU with acute decompensated heart failure. She is treated with intravenous diuretics and vasodilators, but her symptoms do not improve. Which of the following interventions may be considered for this patient if she remains refractory to medical therapy?

    A. Impella
    B. Intra-aortic balloon pump (IABP)
    C. Ultrafiltration
    D. Inhaled nitric oxide

146. A 40-year-old man with a history of alcoholism is admitted to the ICU with alcoholic hepatitis. He develops acute kidney injury (AKI). Which of the following is the most likely type of AKI in this patient?

    A. Prerenal AKI
    B. Intrinsic AKI
    C. Postrenal AKI
    D. Hepatorenal syndrome

147. A 25-year-old woman with a history of asthma is admitted to the ICU with status asthmaticus. She is intubated and mechanically ventilated. Which of the following arterial blood gas (ABG) findings is most concerning for impending respiratory arrest?

    A. pH 7.35, PaCO2 45 mmHg
    B. pH 7.45, PaCO2 35 mmHg
    C. pH 7.25, PaCO2 60 mmHg
    D. pH 7.55, PaCO2 25 mmHg

148. A 55-year-old man with a history of hypertension and hyperlipidemia presents to the ICU with an acute Stanford type A aortic dissection. Which of the following is the most appropriate initial management strategy for this patient?

    A. Medical therapy with beta-blockers and blood pressure control
    B. Endovascular repair
    C. Surgical repair
    D. Percutaneous transluminal angioplasty (PTA)

149. A 70-year-old woman with a history of chronic kidney disease (CKD) is admitted to the ICU with uremic pericarditis. She develops cardiac tamponade. Which of the following echocardiographic findings is most consistent with cardiac tamponade?

    A. Right atrial collapse
    B. Left ventricular hypertrophy
    C. Mitral valve prolapse
    D. Aortic stenosis

150. A 50-year-old woman with a history of rheumatoid arthritis presents to the ICU with septic shock secondary to pneumonia. She is initiated on norepinephrine and vasopressin for vasopressor support. Which of the following is a potential adverse effect of vasopressin?

    A. Hypernatremia
    B. Hyponatremia
    C. Hyperglycemia
    D. Hypoglycemia

151. A 55-year-old male with a history of alcohol abuse presents to the ICU with hematemesis and melena. Endoscopy reveals esophageal varices. Which of the following medications is most effective in reducing portal hypertension and preventing variceal rebleeding?

    A. Octreotide
    B. Propranolol
    C. Nadolol
    D. Spironolactone

152. A 38-year-old female with a history of systemic lupus erythematosus (SLE) is admitted to the ICU with acute kidney injury (AKI) and nephrotic syndrome. Which of the following is the most likely histological finding on renal biopsy?

    A. Minimal change disease
    B. Focal segmental glomerulosclerosis (FSGS)
    C. Membranous nephropathy
    D. Diffuse proliferative lupus nephritis

153. A 75-year-old man with a history of chronic obstructive pulmonary disease (COPD) presents to the ICU with an acute exacerbation and hypercapnic respiratory failure. Which of the following noninvasive ventilation (NIV) modes is most appropriate for this patient?

    A. Continuous positive airway pressure (CPAP)
    B. Bilevel positive airway pressure (BiPAP)
    C. Adaptive servo-ventilation (ASV)
    D. High-flow nasal cannula (HFNC)

154. A 30-year-old woman with no significant medical history presents to the ICU with septic shock secondary to a pelvic abscess. Which of the following is the most appropriate initial fluid resuscitation strategy for this patient?

    A. 30 mL/kg crystalloid bolus over 30 minutes
    B. 500 mL crystalloid bolus over 15 minutes
    C. 1000 mL colloid bolus over 30 minutes
    D. 250 mL albumin bolus over 15 minutes

155. A 65-year-old man with a history of heart failure with reduced ejection fraction (HFrEF) is admitted to the ICU with cardiogenic shock. He is treated with inotropic and vasopressor support but remains hypotensive and oliguric. Which of the following mechanical circulatory support devices is most appropriate for this patient if he has severe aortic insufficiency?

    A. Intra-aortic balloon pump (IABP)
    B. Impella
    C. TandemHeart
    D. Extracorporeal membrane oxygenation (ECMO)

156. A 40-year-old man with a history of alcoholism is admitted to the ICU with severe alcoholic hepatitis and acute liver failure. Which of the following laboratory findings is most indicative of poor prognosis and increased mortality in this patient?

  A. Elevated serum bilirubin
  B. Prolonged prothrombin time (PT)
  C. Elevated serum ammonia
  D. Decreased serum albumin

157. A 25-year-old woman with a history of asthma is admitted to the ICU with status asthmaticus. She is intubated and mechanically ventilated. Which of the following bronchodilators is most appropriate for this patient?

  A. Albuterol
  B. Ipratropium bromide₁
  C. Magnesium sulfate
  D. All of the above

158. A 55-year-old man with a history of hypertension and hyperlipidemia presents to the ICU with an acute Stanford type B aortic dissection. He is hemodynamically stable. Which of the following is the most appropriate initial management strategy for this patient?

  A. Surgical repair
  B. Endovascular repair
  C. Medical therapy with beta-blockers and blood pressure control
  D. Percutaneous transluminal angioplasty (PTA)

159. A 70-year-old woman with a history of chronic kidney disease (CKD) is admitted to the ICU with uremic pericarditis. She develops cardiac tamponade. Which of the following physical exam findings is most characteristic of cardiac tamponade?

  A. Hypertension
  B. Pulsus paradoxus
  C. Widened pulse pressure
  D. Kussmaul's sign

160. A 50-year-old woman with a history of rheumatoid arthritis presents to the ICU with septic shock secondary to pneumonia. She is initiated on norepinephrine for vasopressor support. Which of the following laboratory tests is most important to monitor for potential complications of norepinephrine therapy?

    A. Serum lactate
    B. Troponin
    C. Creatinine kinase (CK)
    D. All of the above

161. A 72-year-old woman with a history of hypertension and type 2 diabetes mellitus is admitted to the ICU with septic shock secondary to a urinary tract infection. She is initiated on norepinephrine for vasopressor support. Which of the following laboratory parameters should be monitored closely to assess the adequacy of tissue perfusion in this patient?

    A. Central venous pressure (CVP)
    B. Pulmonary capillary wedge pressure (PCWP)
    C. Serum lactate
    D. Mixed venous oxygen saturation (SvO2)

162. A 48-year-old man with a history of alcohol abuse is admitted to the ICU with acute pancreatitis. He develops severe hypocalcemia (serum calcium of 6.5 mg/dL). Which of the following electrocardiogram (ECG) findings is most likely to be seen in this patient?

    A. Prolonged QT interval
    B. Shortened QT interval
    C. Peaked T waves
    D. U waves

163. A 35-year-old woman with no significant medical history is admitted to the ICU with Guillain-Barré syndrome (GBS). Which of the following is the most appropriate treatment for GBS?

    A. Intravenous immunoglobulin (IVIG)
    B. Plasma exchange (PLEX)
    C. Corticosteroids
    D. Either A or B

164. A 65-year-old man with a history of coronary artery disease is admitted to the ICU with cardiogenic shock following an acute myocardial infarction. He is intubated and mechanically ventilated. Which of the following ventilator settings is most appropriate to reduce cardiac workload in this patient?

    A. High tidal volume ventilation
    B. Low respiratory rate
    C. High inspiratory flow rate
    D. Low inspiratory:expiratory (I:E) ratio

165. A 50-year-old woman with a history of systemic lupus erythematosus (SLE) is admitted to the ICU with acute respiratory failure secondary to diffuse alveolar hemorrhage (DAH). Which of the following medications is most likely to control her bleeding and improve respiratory function?

    A. High-dose corticosteroids
    B. Cyclophosphamide
    C. Rituximab
    D. Plasma exchange

166. A 40-year-old man with a history of human immunodeficiency virus (HIV) infection is admitted to the ICU with Pneumocystis pneumonia (PCP). Which of the following is the most appropriate treatment for this patient?

    A. Trimethoprim-sulfamethoxazole (TMP-SMX)
    B. Pentamidine
    C. Clindamycin and primaquine
    D. Atovaquone

167. A 75-year-old man with a history of hypertension and diabetes mellitus is admitted to the ICU with septic shock secondary to a urinary tract infection. He is initiated on norepinephrine and vasopressin for vasopressor support. Which of the following laboratory tests is most important to monitor for potential complications of vasopressin therapy?

    A. Serum sodium
    B. Serum potassium
    C. Serum glucose
    D. Serum creatinine

168. A 30-year-old woman with a history of systemic sclerosis (scleroderma) is admitted to the ICU with scleroderma renal crisis (SRC.. Which of the following medications is most appropriate for the management of hypertension in this patient?

A. Angiotensin-converting enzyme (ACE) inhibitor
B. Angiotensin II receptor blocker (ARB)
C. Calcium channel blocker
D. Beta-blocker

169. A 60-year-old man with a history of cirrhosis presents to the ICU with acute variceal bleeding. He is treated with endoscopic variceal ligation (EVL) and octreotide. Which of the following is the most appropriate prophylactic antibiotic regimen for this patient to prevent spontaneous bacterial peritonitis (SBP)?

A. Ciprofloxacin
B. Norfloxacin
C. Trimethoprim-sulfamethoxazole (TMP-SMX)
D. Cefotaxime

170. A 55-year-old woman with a history of rheumatoid arthritis presents to the ICU with septic arthritis of the knee. Which of the following is the most appropriate initial management for this patient?

A. Joint aspiration and antibiotics
B. Surgical drainage and debridement
C. Intra-articular corticosteroid injection
D. Immobilization and physical therapy

171. A 65-year-old woman with a history of rheumatoid arthritis is admitted to the ICU with new-onset fever, confusion, and nuchal rigidity. Lumbar puncture reveals elevated white blood cell count with a predominance of neutrophils, low glucose, and elevated protein in the cerebrospinal fluid. Which of the following is the most likely diagnosis?

A. Bacterial meningitis
B. Viral meningitis
C. Fungal meningitis
D. Tuberculous meningitis

172. A 45-year-old man with a history of IV drug use presents to the ICU with fever, chills, and a new murmur. Echocardiography reveals a large vegetation on the tricuspid valve. Which of the following is the most likely organism causing this patient's infective endocarditis?

    A. Staphylococcus aureus
    B. Streptococcus viridans
    C. Enterococcus faecalis
    D. Pseudomonas aeruginosa

173. A 70-year-old man with a history of chronic obstructive pulmonary disease (COPD) presents to the ICU with an acute exacerbation and hypercapnic respiratory failure. Despite optimal medical management, his respiratory status continues to deteriorate. Which of the following interventions should be considered next?

    A. Noninvasive ventilation (NIV)
    B. Invasive mechanical ventilation
    C. High-flow nasal cannula (HFNC)
    D. Tracheostomy

174. A 30-year-old woman with no significant medical history presents to the ICU with severe community-acquired pneumonia (CAP). She is intubated and mechanically ventilated. Which of the following is the most important parameter to monitor to assess the effectiveness of mechanical ventilation in this patient?

    A. Tidal volume
    B. Respiratory rate
    C. Peak inspiratory pressure
    D. Arterial blood gas (ABG)

175. A 65-year-old woman with a history of heart failure with preserved ejection fraction (HFpEF) is admitted to the ICU with acute decompensated heart failure. She is treated with intravenous diuretics, but her urine output remains low. Which of the following medications would be most appropriate to add to her regimen to increase urine output?

    A. Spironolactone
    B. Sacubitril/valsartan
    C. Dopamine
    D. Nesiritide

176. A 40-year-old man with a history of alcoholism is admitted to the ICU with alcoholic hepatitis and acute liver failure. He develops hepatorenal syndrome (HRS). Which of the following interventions is most likely to improve his renal function?

    A. Albumin infusion
    B. Terlipressin
    C. Midodrine and octreotide
    D. Hemodialysis

177. A 25-year-old woman with a history of asthma is admitted to the ICU with status asthmaticus. She is treated with inhaled bronchodilators, systemic corticosteroids, and intravenous magnesium sulfate. However, her peak expiratory flow rate (PEFR) remains low. Which of the following interventions should be considered next?

    A. Inhaled heliox
    B. Intravenous ketamine
    C. Subcutaneous terbutaline
    D. Endotracheal intubation and mechanical ventilation

178. A 55-year-old man with a history of hypertension and hyperlipidemia presents to the ICU with an acute Stanford type A aortic dissection. Which of the following is the most appropriate definitive treatment for this patient?

    A. Medical therapy with beta-blockers and blood pressure control
    B. Endovascular repair
    C. Surgical repair
    D. Percutaneous transluminal angioplasty (PTA)

179. A 70-year-old woman with a history of chronic kidney disease (CKD) is admitted to the ICU with uremic pericarditis. Which of the following is the most common presenting symptom of uremic pericarditis?

A. Chest pain
B. Dyspnea
C. Pericardial friction rub
D. Fever

180. A 50-year-old woman with a history of rheumatoid arthritis presents to the ICU with septic shock secondary to pneumonia. She is initiated on norepinephrine for vasopressor support. Which of the following is a potential adverse effect of norepinephrine that should be monitored closely?

A. Hypotension
B. Bradycardia
C. Peripheral ischemia
D. Hypoglycemia

181. A 68-year-old woman with a history of hypertension, type 2 diabetes mellitus, and chronic kidney disease is admitted to the ICU with septic shock. She is initiated on norepinephrine but remains hypotensive despite adequate fluid resuscitation. Which of the following vasopressors would be the most appropriate second-line agent for this patient?

A. Epinephrine
B. Vasopressin
C. Phenylephrine
D. Dobutamine

182. A 35-year-old man with a history of ulcerative colitis is admitted to the ICU with toxic megacolon. He is febrile, tachycardic, and hypotensive. Which of the following is the most appropriate initial management for this patient?

A. Emergency colectomy
B. Intravenous corticosteroids
C. Intravenous antibiotics and fluids
D. Nasogastric decompression and bowel rest

183. A 50-year-old woman with a history of systemic lupus erythematosus (SLE) is admitted to the ICU with acute respiratory distress syndrome (ARDS). Which of the following is the most likely pathophysiologic mechanism underlying ARDS in this patient?

    A. Increased alveolar-capillary permeability
    B. Decreased surfactant production
    C. Pulmonary embolism
    D. Aspiration pneumonitis

184. A 75-year-old man with a history of coronary artery disease is admitted to the ICU with cardiogenic shock after an acute myocardial infarction. He is intubated and mechanically ventilated. Which of the following hemodynamic goals should be targeted during the initial resuscitation phase?

    A. Mean arterial pressure (MAP) > 65 mmHg
    B. Cardiac index (CI) > 2.2 L/min/m2
    C. Central venous pressure (CVP) 8-12 mmHg
    D. All of the above

185. A 45-year-old woman with a history of cirrhosis presents to the ICU with acute variceal bleeding. She is treated with endoscopic variceal ligation (EVL) and octreotide. Which of the following is the most common complication of EVL?

    A. Bleeding
    B. Infection
    C. Stricture formation
    D. Esophageal perforation

186. A 28-year-old man with no significant medical history is admitted to the ICU with traumatic brain injury (TBI) after a motor vehicle accident. He has a Glasgow Coma Scale (GCS) score of 6. Which of the following interventions is most likely to improve his neurological outcome?

    A. Hyperventilation
    B. Mannitol infusion
    C. Hypothermia
    D. Decompressive craniectomy

187. A 62-year-old woman with a history of hypertension and diabetes mellitus presents to the ICU with septic shock secondary to a urinary tract infection. She is initiated on norepinephrine and fluids, but her lactate level remains elevated.Which of the following interventions should be considered next?

    A. Transfusion of packed red blood cells (PRBCs)
    B. Initiation of hydrocortisone
    C. Addition of dobutamine
    D. Increase in norepinephrine dose

188. A 35-year-old man with a history of asthma presents to the ICU with status asthmaticus. He is intubated and mechanically ventilated. Despite aggressive bronchodilator therapy, his peak airway pressures remain high. Which of the following interventions may be considered to reduce his airway resistance and improve ventilation?

    A. Inhaled helium-oxygen mixture (heliox)
    B. Intravenous magnesium sulfate
    C. Inhaled corticosteroids
    D. All of the above

189. A 50-year-old woman with a history of systemic lupus erythematosus (SLE) is admitted to the ICU with acute lupus myocarditis. Which of the following medications is most appropriate for the treatment of lupus myocarditis?

    A. High-dose corticosteroids
    B. Cyclophosphamide
    C. Mycophenolate mofetil
    D. Rituximab

190. A 75-year-old man with a history of chronic kidney disease (CKD) is admitted to the ICU with acute pulmonary edema. He is intubated and mechanically ventilated. Which of the following modalities of renal replacement therapy (RRT) is most appropriate for this patient?

    A. Continuous venovenous hemofiltration (CVVH)
    B. Intermittent hemodialysis (IHD)
    C. Peritoneal dialysis (PD)
    D. Sustained low-efficiency dialysis (SLED)

191. A 58-year-old male presents to the ICU with new-onset atrial fibrillation with rapid ventricular response (RVR). His heart rate is 165 beats per minute, and his blood pressure is 80/40 mmHg. He has a history of COPD and heart failure with reduced ejection fraction (HFrEF). Which of the following medications is most appropriate for initial rate control in this patient?

    A. Amiodarone
    B. Diltiazem
    C. Digoxin
    D. Esmolol

192. A 42-year-old woman with a history of systemic lupus erythematosus (SLE) presents to the ICU with altered mental status, seizures, and hypertension. A brain MRI reveals diffuse white matter lesions consistent with posterior reversible encephalopathy syndrome (PRES). Which of the following is the most appropriate initial management strategy for this patient?

    A. Aggressive blood pressure control
    B. Intravenous immunoglobulin (IVIG)
    C. Plasma exchange
    D. Corticosteroid therapy

193. A 75-year-old man with a history of chronic obstructive pulmonary disease (COPD) is admitted to the ICU with an acute exacerbation and hypercapnic respiratory failure. He is intubated and placed on mechanical ventilation. Which of the following ventilator settings is most likely to reduce his work of breathing and improve gas exchange?

    A. Pressure-controlled ventilation (PCV)
    B. Volume-controlled ventilation (VCV)
    C. Pressure support ventilation (PSV)
    D. Airway pressure release ventilation (APRV)

194. A 30-year-old woman with no significant medical history presents to the ICU with severe community-acquired pneumonia (CAP). She is intubated and mechanically ventilated. Despite appropriate antibiotic therapy and supportive care, her condition deteriorates, and she develops septic shock. Which of the following adjunctive therapies may be considered to improve her hemodynamic status?

    A. Low-dose hydrocortisone
    B. Vitamin C
    C. Thiamine
    D. All of the above

195. A 65-year-old man with a history of heart failure with reduced ejection fraction (HFrEF) is admitted to the ICU with cardiogenic shock. He is treated with inotropic and vasopressor support but remains hypotensive and oliguric. Which of the following interventions would be most appropriate to consider if he remains refractory to medical therapy?

    A. Impella
    B. Intra-aortic balloon pump (IABP)
    C. Extracorporeal membrane oxygenation (ECMO)
    D. Ventricular assist device (VAD)

196. A 40-year-old man with a history of alcoholism is admitted to the ICU with acute pancreatitis. He develops acute kidney injury (AKI). Which of the following biomarkers is most specific for the diagnosis of acute tubular necrosis (ATN), a common cause of AKI in this setting?

    A. Blood urea nitrogen (BUN)
    B. Serum creatinine
    C. Fractional excretion of sodium (FeNa)
    D. Urine neutrophil gelatinase-associated lipocalin (NGAL)

197. A 25-year-old woman with a history of asthma is admitted to the ICU with status asthmaticus. She is intubated and mechanically ventilated. Which of the following is the most important predictor of successful extubation in this patient?

    A. Peak expiratory flow rate (PEFR)
    B. Forced expiratory volume in 1 second (FEV1)
    C. Rapid shallow breathing index (RSBI)
    D. Negative inspiratory force (NIF)

198. A 55-year-old man with a history of hypertension and hyperlipidemia presents to the ICU with an acute Stanford type B aortic dissection. He is hemodynamically stable and is treated with medical therapy. Which of the following imaging modalities is most appropriate for long-term surveillance of his aortic dissection?

    A. Chest X-ray
    B. Computed tomography angiography (CTA) of the chest
    C. Transesophageal echocardiogram (TEE)
    D. Magnetic resonance imaging (MRI) of the chest

199. A 70-year-old woman with a history of chronic kidney disease (CKD) is admitted to the ICU with uremic pericarditis. Which of the following is the most effective treatment for uremic pericarditis?

    A. Hemodialysis
    B. Pericardiocentesis
    C. Corticosteroids
    D. Nonsteroidal anti-inflammatory drugs (NSAIDs)

200. A 50-year-old woman with a history of rheumatoid arthritis presents to the ICU with septic shock secondary to pneumonia. She is initiated on norepinephrine for vasopressor support. Which of the following hemodynamic parameters should be monitored closely to assess the effectiveness of her therapy?

    A. Mean arterial pressure (MAP)
    B. Central venous pressure (CVP)
    C. Cardiac index (CI)
    D. All of the above

201. A 68-year-old woman with a history of hypertension and coronary artery disease is admitted to the ICU with new-onset chest pain and ST-segment depressions in leads V1-V4 on her electrocardiogram (ECG). She is diagnosed with non-ST-elevation myocardial infarction (NSTEMI). During her hospital course, she develops acute limb ischemia. Which of the following is the most likely cause of this complication?

    A. Cholesterol embolism
    B. Deep vein thrombosis (DVT)
    C. Peripheral arterial disease (PAD)
    D. Acute compartment syndrome

202. A 45-year-old man with a history of intravenous drug use is admitted to the ICU with infective endocarditis complicated by a perivalvular abscess. Which of the following is the most appropriate antibiotic regimen for this patient?

    A. Vancomycin and gentamicin for 4-6 weeks
    B. Daptomycin for 4-6 weeks
    C. Ceftaroline for 4-6 weeks
    D. Penicillin G for 4 weeks

203. A 75-year-old man with a history of chronic obstructive pulmonary disease (COPD) is admitted to the ICU with an acute exacerbation. He is intubated and placed on mechanical ventilation. Which of the following weaning strategies is most likely to reduce his duration of mechanical ventilation and risk of complications?

    A. Daily spontaneous awakening trial (SAT) and spontaneous breathing trial (SBT)
    B. Once-daily SBT only
    C. Intermittent mandatory ventilation (IMV)
    D. Pressure support ventilation (PSV) only

204. A 30-year-old woman with no significant medical history presents to the ICU with severe community-acquired pneumonia (CAP) and septic shock. She is initiated on norepinephrine for vasopressor support. Which of the following is the most appropriate target for mean arterial pressure (MAP) in this patient?

    A. MAP > 60 mmHg
    B. MAP > 65 mmHg
    C. MAP > 70 mmHg
    D. MAP > 75 mmHg

205. A 65-year-old woman with a history of heart failure with preserved ejection fraction (HFpEF) is admitted to the ICU with acute decompensated heart failure. She is treated with intravenous diuretics, but her urine output remains low. Which of the following interventions should be considered next to improve her diuresis?

    A. Continuous renal replacement therapy (CRRT)
    B. Ultrafiltration
    C. High-dose loop diuretics
    D. Vasodilator therapy

206. A 40-year-old man with a history of alcoholism is admitted to the ICU with alcoholic hepatitis. He develops acute kidney injury (AKI) due to hepatorenal syndrome (HRS). Which of the following is the most accurate definition of HRS?

    A. AKI caused by direct nephrotoxicity of alcohol
    B. AKI caused by hypovolemia due to gastrointestinal bleeding
    C. AKI characterized by renal vasoconstriction in the setting of advanced liver disease
    D. AKI caused by obstruction of the urinary tract

207. A 25-year-old woman with a history of asthma is admitted to the ICU with status asthmaticus. Despite aggressive bronchodilator therapy, her respiratory status continues to deteriorate. Which of the following adjunctive therapies has been shown to improve outcomes in patients with severe asthma exacerbations?

    A. Magnesium sulfate
    B. Ketamine
    C. Heliox
    D. All of the above

208. A 55-year-old man with a history of hypertension and hyperlipidemia presents to the ICU with an acute Stanford type B aortic dissection. He is hemodynamically stable and is treated with medical therapy. Which of the following blood pressure goals is most appropriate for this patient?

  A. Systolic blood pressure (SBP) < 120 mmHg
  B. SBP < 130 mmHg
  C. SBP < 140 mmHg
  D. SBP < 150 mmHg

209. A 70-year-old woman with a history of chronic kidney disease (CKD) is admitted to the ICU with uremic pericarditis. She develops cardiac tamponade. Which of the following is the most definitive treatment for cardiac tamponade?

  A. Pericardiocentesis
  B. Pericardial window
  C. Pericardiectomy
  D. Corticosteroids

210. A 50-year-old woman with a history of rheumatoid arthritis presents to the ICU with septic shock secondary to pneumonia. She is initiated on norepinephrine for vasopressor support and broad-spectrum antibiotics. After 48 hours, her blood cultures remain negative. Which of the following should be considered in the management of this patient?

  A. Change empiric antibiotic therapy
  B. Add antifungal therapy
  C. Search for an alternative source of infection
  D. All of the above

211. A 78-year-old man with a history of hypertension and coronary artery disease is admitted to the ICU with new-onset atrial fibrillation with rapid ventricular response (RVR). His heart rate is 150 beats per minute, and his blood pressure is 90/60 mmHg. He has a history of COPD and heart failure with reduced ejection fraction (HFrEF). Which of the following medications is the most appropriate for initial rate control in this patient?

    A. Amiodarone
    B. Diltiazem
    C. Digoxin
    D. Esmolol

212. A 42-year-old woman with a history of systemic lupus erythematosus (SLE) presents to the ICU with altered mental status, seizures, and hypertension. A brain MRI reveals diffuse white matter lesions consistent with posterior reversible encephalopathy syndrome (PRES). Which of the following is the most likely cause of PRES in this patient?

    A. Hypertension
    B. Immunosuppressive therapy
    C. Active lupus flare
    D. All of the above

213. A 75-year-old man with a history of chronic obstructive pulmonary disease (COPD) is admitted to the ICU with an acute exacerbation and hypercapnic respiratory failure. He is intubated and placed on mechanical ventilation. Which of the following ventilator settings is most likely to reduce his risk of ventilator-induced lung injury (VILI)?

    A. High tidal volume ventilation
    B. High plateau pressure
    C. Low positive end-expiratory pressure (PEEP)
    D. Lung-protective ventilation with low tidal volumes and appropriate PEEP

214. A 30-year-old woman with no significant medical history presents to the ICU with severe community-acquired pneumonia (CAP). She is intubated and mechanically ventilated. Despite appropriate antibiotic therapy and supportive care, her condition deteriorates, and she develops septic shock. Which of the following interventions may be considered to improve her oxygen delivery?

A. Transfusion of packed red blood cells (PRBCs)
B. Inotropic support with dobutamine
C. Increase in the fraction of inspired oxygen (FiO2)
D. All of the above

215. A 65-year-old man with a history of heart failure with reduced ejection fraction (HFrEF) is admitted to the ICU with cardiogenic shock. He is treated with inotropic and vasopressor support but remains hypotensive and oliguric. Which of the following interventions would be most appropriate to consider if he remains refractory to medical therapy and has a contraindication to Impella or ECMO?

A. Intra-aortic balloon pump (IABP)
B. TandemHeart
C. Ventricular assist device (VAD)
D. Percutaneous left ventricular assist device (pLVAD)

216. A 40-year-old man with a history of alcoholism is admitted to the ICU with acute pancreatitis. He develops acute kidney injury (AKI) due to acute tubular necrosis (ATN). Which of the following electrolyte abnormalities is most commonly associated with ATN?

A. Hyperkalemia
B. Hypokalemia
C. Hypernatremia
D. Hyponatremia

217. A 25-year-old woman with a history of asthma is admitted to the ICU with status asthmaticus. She is intubated and mechanically ventilated. Which of the following strategies is most likely to reduce her peak airway pressures and improve ventilation?

    A. Administration of neuromuscular blocking agents
    B. Use of inhaled anesthetics
    C. Increasing the respiratory rate
    D. Increasing the tidal volume

218. A 55-year-old man with a history of hypertension and hyperlipidemia presents to the ICU with an acute Stanford type B aortic dissection. He is hemodynamically stable and is treated with medical therapy. Which of the following medications is most appropriate for pain control in this patient?

    A. Morphine
    B. Fentanyl
    C. Hydromorphone
    D. All of the above

219. A 70-year-old woman with a history of chronic kidney disease (CKD) is admitted to the ICU with uremic pericarditis. Which of the following echocardiographic findings is most specific for the diagnosis of pericardial effusion?

    A. Diastolic collapse of the right ventricle
    B. Left ventricular hypertrophy
    C. Mitral valve prolapse
    D. Aortic stenosis

220. A 50-year-old woman with a history of rheumatoid arthritis presents to the ICU with septic shock secondary to pneumonia. She is initiated on norepinephrine for vasopressor support. Which of the following is the most common site of infection in patients with rheumatoid arthritis who develop septic shock?

    A. Lung
    B. Urinary tract
    C. Skin and soft tissue
    D. Gastrointestinal tract

221. A 68-year-old woman with a history of hypertension, diabetes mellitus, and atrial fibrillation is admitted to the ICU with new-onset left-sided weakness and facial droop. A head CT scan reveals a right middle cerebral artery (MCA) infarction. Which of the following is the most appropriate treatment for this patient if she presents within the thrombolysis window?

    A. Aspirin
    B. Clopidogrel
    C. Intravenous tissue plasminogen activator (tPA)
    D. Warfarin

222. A 45-year-old man with a history of intravenous drug use is admitted to the ICU with infective endocarditis complicated by a perivalvular abscess. He undergoes successful surgical valve replacement and debridement of the abscess. Which of the following complications should be monitored closely in the postoperative period?

    A. Arrhythmias
    B. Heart failure
    C. Stroke
    D. All of the above

223. A 75-year-old man with a history of chronic obstructive pulmonary disease (COPD) is admitted to the ICU with an acute exacerbation. He is intubated and placed on mechanical ventilation. After 72 hours, his sputum culture grows Pseudomonas aeruginosa. Which of the following antibiotics is most appropriate for the treatment of Pseudomonas aeruginosa pneumonia?

    A. Piperacillin/tazobactam
    B. Cefepime
    C. Meropenem
    D. Levofloxacin

224. A 30-year-old woman with no significant medical history presents to the ICU with septic shock secondary to a pelvic abscess. She is initiated on norepinephrine for vasopressor support. Which of the following is the most appropriate goal for central venous pressure (CVP) in this patient?

    A. CVP 0-5 mmHg
    B. CVP 5-10 mmHg
    C. CVP 8-12 mmHg
    D. CVP > 12 mmHg

225. A 65-year-old woman with a history of heart failure with preserved ejection fraction (HFpEF) is admitted to the ICU with acute decompensated heart failure. She is treated with intravenous diuretics, but her urine output remains low. Which of the following interventions should be considered next to improve her diuresis if she has a contraindication to ultrafiltration?

    A. Continuous renal replacement therapy (CRRT)
    B. High-dose loop diuretics
    C. Vasodilator therapy
    D. Inotropic therapy

226. A 40-year-old man with a history of alcoholism is admitted to the ICU with alcoholic hepatitis and acute liver failure. He develops hepatorenal syndrome (HRS). Which of the following laboratory findings is most characteristic of HRS?

    A. Increased serum creatinine
    B. Decreased urine sodium
    C. Dilute urine
    D. All of the above

227. A 25-year-old woman with a history of asthma is admitted to the ICU with status asthmaticus. She is intubated and mechanically ventilated. Which of the following ventilator settings is most appropriate to manage her airflow obstruction and air trapping?

    A. Low respiratory rate and short inspiratory time
    B. High respiratory rate and short inspiratory time
    C. Low respiratory rate and long inspiratory time
    D. High respiratory rate and long inspiratory time

228. A 55-year-old man with a history of hypertension and hyperlipidemia presents to the ICU with an acute Stanford type B aortic dissection. He is hemodynamically stable and is treated with medical therapy. Which of the following classes of medications is most appropriate for long-term blood pressure control in this patient?

    A. Beta-blockers
    B. Calcium channel blockers
    C. Angiotensin-converting enzyme (ACE) inhibitors
    D. Angiotensin II receptor blockers (ARBs)

229. A 70-year-old woman with a history of chronic kidney disease (CKD) is admitted to the ICU with uremic pericarditis. Which of the following diagnostic tests is most sensitive for detecting pericardial effusion?

    A. Chest X-ray
    B. Electrocardiogram (ECG)
    C. Echocardiogram
    D. Computed tomography (CT) scan of the chest

230. A 50-year-old woman with a history of rheumatoid arthritis presents to the ICU with septic shock secondary to pneumonia. She is initiated on norepinephrine for vasopressor support and broad-spectrum antibiotics. After 72 hours, her blood cultures remain negative. Which of the following should be considered in the management of this patient?

    A. Discontinue antibiotics and observe
    B. Change empiric antibiotic therapy
    C. Add antifungal therapy
    D. Continue current therapy and re-evaluate in 48 hours

231. A 55-year-old woman with a history of obesity and obstructive sleep apnea (OSA) is admitted to the ICU following bariatric surgery. On postoperative day 2, she develops acute respiratory failure requiring reintubation. Which of the following is the most likely cause of her respiratory failure?

    A. Pulmonary embolism
    B. Pneumonia
    C. Atelectasis
    D. Obesity hypoventilation syndrome

232. A 48-year-old man with a history of alcohol abuse is admitted to the ICU with acute alcoholic hepatitis. Which of the following scoring systems is used to assess the severity of alcoholic hepatitis and predict mortality?

    A. MELD score
    B. Child-Pugh score
    C. Glasgow Alcoholic Hepatitis Score (GAHS)
    D. Maddrey Discriminant Function (DF)

233. A 75-year-old man with a history of hypertension and coronary artery disease is admitted to the ICU with cardiogenic shock. He is initiated on dobutamine for inotropic support. Which of the following is a potential adverse effect of dobutamine?

    A. Bradycardia
    B. Hypotension
    C. Tachyarrhythmias
    D. Hyperkalemia

234. A 30-year-old woman with no significant medical history is admitted to the ICU with septic shock secondary to pyelonephritis. Despite adequate fluid resuscitation and norepinephrine, her mean arterial pressure (MAP) remains below 65 mmHg. Which of the following interventions should be considered next?

    A. Add vasopressin
    B. Initiate hydrocortisone
    C. Start an epinephrine infusion
    D. Increase the dose of norepinephrine

235. A 65-year-old woman with a history of heart failure with preserved ejection fraction (HFpEF) is admitted to the ICU with acute decompensated heart failure. She is treated with intravenous diuretics, but her urine output remains low. Which of the following medications should be avoided in this patient due to the risk of worsening renal function?

    A. Nesiritide
    B. Spironolactone
    C. Sacubitril/valsartan
    D. Acetazolamide

236. A 40-year-old man with a history of alcoholism is admitted to the ICU with acute pancreatitis complicated by acute respiratory distress syndrome (ARDS). Which of the following is the most important initial intervention to improve his oxygenation?

    A. High-flow nasal cannula (HFNC)
    B. Noninvasive positive pressure ventilation (NIPPV)
    C. Intubation and mechanical ventilation with lung-protective strategy
    D. Inhaled nitric oxide

237. A 25-year-old woman with a history of asthma is admitted to the ICU with status asthmaticus. She is intubated and mechanically ventilated. Which of the following is a potential complication of mechanical ventilation in this patient?

    A. Pneumothorax
    B. Pneumomediastinum
    C. Hypotension
    D. All of the above

238. A 55-year-old man with a history of hypertension and hyperlipidemia presents to the ICU with an acute Stanford type B aortic dissection. He is hemodynamically stable and is treated with medical therapy. Which of the following medications should be used with caution in this patient due to the risk of reflex tachycardia?

    A. Hydralazine
    B. Labetalol
    C. Esmolol
    D. Metoprolol

239. A 70-year-old woman with a history of chronic kidney disease (CKD) is admitted to the ICU with uremic pericarditis. She undergoes pericardiocentesis, and 500 mL of bloody fluid is drained. Which of the following is the most likely cause of the bloody pericardial fluid in this patient?

    A. Trauma
    B. Malignancy
    C. Uremia
    D. Tuberculosis

240. A 50-year-old woman with a history of rheumatoid arthritis presents to the ICU with septic shock secondary to pneumonia. She is initiated on norepinephrine for vasopressor support and broad-spectrum antibiotics. After 72 hours, her blood cultures grow methicillin-resistant Staphylococcus aureus (MRSA). Which of the following antibiotics is most appropriate for the treatment of MRSA pneumonia in this patient?

    A. Vancomycin
    B. Linezolid
    C. Daptomycin
    D. Ceftaroline

241. A 58-year-old man with a history of hypertension and coronary artery disease is admitted to the ICU with new-onset atrial fibrillation with rapid ventricular response (RVR). His heart rate is 150 beats per minute, and his blood pressure is 80/40 mmHg. He has a history of COPD and heart failure with reduced ejection fraction (HFrEF). In addition to rate control, which of the following interventions should be prioritized in this patient?

    A. Anticoagulation
    B. Cardioversion
    C. Pulmonary artery catheter placement
    D. Renal replacement therapy

242. A 42-year-old woman with a history of systemic lupus erythematosus (SLE) presents to the ICU with altered mental status, seizures, and hypertension. A brain MRI reveals diffuse white matter lesions consistent with posterior reversible encephalopathy syndrome (PRES). Which of the following medications is most commonly associated with the development of PRES in SLE patients?

    A. Cyclophosphamide
    B. Mycophenolate mofetil
    C. Hydroxychloroquine
    D. Belimumab

243. A 75-year-old man with a history of chronic obstructive pulmonary disease (COPD) is admitted to the ICU with an acute exacerbation and hypercapnic respiratory failure. He is intubated and placed on mechanical ventilation. Which of the following is the most important factor to consider when adjusting the ventilator settings for this patient?

    A. Peak inspiratory pressure
    B. Plateau pressure
    C. PEEP
    D. Driving pressure

244. A 30-year-old woman with no significant medical history presents to the ICU with severe community-acquired pneumonia (CAP). She is intubated and mechanically ventilated. Despite appropriate antibiotic therapy and supportive care, her condition deteriorates, and she develops septic shock. Which of the following adjunctive therapies may be considered to modulate the inflammatory response in this patient?

    A. Vitamin C
    B. Thiamine
    C. Hydrocortisone
    D. All of the above

245. A 65-year-old man with a history of heart failure with reduced ejection fraction (HFrEF) is admitted to the ICU with cardiogenic shock. He is treated with inotropic and vasopressor support but remains hypotensive and oliguric. Which of the following interventions would be most appropriate to consider if he remains refractory to medical therapy and has a contraindication to other mechanical circulatory support devices?

    A. Extracorporeal membrane oxygenation (ECMO)
    B. Intra-aortic balloon pump (IABP)
    C. TandemHeart
    D. Cardiac transplantation

246. A 40-year-old man with a history of alcoholism is admitted to the ICU with acute pancreatitis. He develops acute kidney injury (AKI) due to acute tubular necrosis (ATN). Which of the following is the most appropriate initial management strategy for this patient?

    A. Aggressive fluid resuscitation
    B. Dopamine infusion
    C. Hemodialysis
    D. Renal biopsy

247. A 25-year-old woman with a history of asthma is admitted to the ICU with status asthmaticus. She is intubated and mechanically ventilated. Which of the following is a potential complication of prolonged neuromuscular blockade in this patient?

    A. Prolonged weakness
    B. Critical illness polyneuropathy
    C. Increased risk of ventilator-associated pneumonia (VAP)
    D. All of the above

248. A 55-year-old man with a history of hypertension and hyperlipidemia presents to the ICU with an acute Stanford type B aortic dissection. He is hemodynamically stable and is treated with medical therapy. Which of the following imaging modalities is most appropriate for follow-up assessment of his aortic dissection 6 months after initial presentation?

    A. Chest X-ray
    B. Computed tomography angiography (CTA) of the chest
    C. Transesophageal echocardiogram (TEE)
    D. Magnetic resonance imaging (MRI) of the chest

249. A 70-year-old woman with a history of chronic kidney disease (CKD) is admitted to the ICU with uremic pericarditis. She undergoes pericardiocentesis, and 500 mL of bloody fluid is drained. Which of the following is the most appropriate next step in the management of this patient?

    A. Continued observation
    B. Initiation of hemodialysis
    C. Administration of corticosteroids
    D. Pericardial window placement

250. A 50-year-old woman with a history of rheumatoid arthritis presents to the ICU with septic shock secondary to pneumonia. She is initiated on norepinephrine for vasopressor support and broad-spectrum antibiotics. After 72 hours, her blood cultures grow methicillin-resistant Staphylococcus aureus (MRSA). Which of the following is the most appropriate duration of antibiotic therapy for MRSA pneumonia in this patient?

A. 7 days
B. 14 days
C. 21 days
D. 28 days

251. A 65-year-old woman with a history of hypertension and type 2 diabetes mellitus presents to the ICU with new-onset atrial fibrillation with rapid ventricular response (RVR). Her heart rate is 150 beats per minute and blood pressure is 100/60 mmHg. She has a history of chronic kidney disease (CKD) with an estimated glomerular filtration rate (eGFR) of 30 mL/min/1.73 m2. Which of the following medications is the most appropriate for initial rate control in this patient?

A. Diltiazem
B. Metoprolol
C. Digoxin
D. Amiodarone

252. A 38-year-old male with a history of IV drug abuse presents with fever, chills, and a new murmur. Echocardiography reveals a mobile vegetation on the aortic valve. Blood cultures grow methicillin-sensitive Staphylococcus aureus (MSSA). What is the most appropriate empiric antibiotic therapy for this patient?

A. Vancomycin and gentamicin
B. Nafcillin and gentamicin
C. Daptomycin
D. Ceftaroline

253. A 75-year-old woman with a history of COPD is admitted to the ICU with acute respiratory failure. She is intubated and placed on mechanical ventilation. Which of the following strategies is most likely to reduce her risk of ventilator-induced lung injury (VILI)?

    A. High tidal volume ventilation (10-12 mL/kg of predicted body weight)
    B. Low respiratory rate (8-10 breaths/min)
    C. High PEEP (15-20 cm H2O)
    D. Lung-protective ventilation with low tidal volumes (6-8 mL/kg of predicted body weight) and PEEP titrated to maintain driving pressure < 15 cm H2O

254. A 30-year-old woman with a history of systemic lupus erythematosus (SLE) is admitted to the ICU with lupus nephritis and significant proteinuria. Which of the following medications is most effective in reducing proteinuria in this patient?

    A. Mycophenolate mofetil (MMF)
    B. Hydroxychloroquine
    C. Cyclophosphamide
    D. Belimumab

255. A 65-year-old man with a history of heart failure with reduced ejection fraction (HFrEF) is admitted to the ICU with cardiogenic shock after an acute myocardial infarction. Despite optimal medical therapy, he remains hypotensive and oliguric. Which of the following mechanical circulatory support devices is contraindicated in this patient if he has severe aortic insufficiency?

    A. Impella
    B. Intra-aortic balloon pump (IABP)
    C. TandemHeart
    D. Extracorporeal membrane oxygenation (ECMO)

256. A 40-year-old man with a history of alcoholism is admitted to the ICU with severe acute pancreatitis complicated by pancreatic necrosis. Which of the following interventions is most appropriate for the management of infected pancreatic necrosis?

A. Percutaneous drainage
B. Endoscopic drainage
C. Surgical necrosectomy
D. Antibiotics alone

257. A 25-year-old woman with no significant medical history is admitted to the ICU with severe sepsis due to community-acquired pneumonia. She is intubated and mechanically ventilated. Which of the following is the most appropriate target for central venous oxygen saturation (ScvO2) in this patient?

A. ScvO2 > 50%
B. ScvO2 > 60%
C. ScvO2 > 70%
D. ScvO2 > 80%

258. A 55-year-old man with a history of hypertension and hyperlipidemia presents to the ICU with an acute Stanford type A aortic dissection. He undergoes successful surgical repair of the dissection. Which of the following postoperative complications is most common in patients undergoing aortic dissection repair?

A. Stroke
B. Renal failure
C. Spinal cord ischemia
D. Myocardial infarction

259. A 70-year-old woman with a history of chronic kidney disease (CKD) is admitted to the ICU with uremic encephalopathy. Which of the following is the most appropriate treatment for this condition?

A. Hemodialysis
B. Peritoneal dialysis
C. Intravenous mannitol
D. Intravenous hypertonic saline

260. A 50-year-old woman with a history of rheumatoid arthritis presents to the ICU with septic shock secondary to pneumonia. She is initiated on norepinephrine for vasopressor support and broad-spectrum antibiotics. After 72 hours, her blood cultures remain negative, and her clinical status has not improved. Which of the following should be considered in the management of this patient?

    A. Add antifungal therapy
    B. Change to a different class of antibiotics
    C. Search for a non-infectious cause of her symptoms
    D. All of the above

261. A 68-year-old woman with a history of hypertension, type 2 diabetes mellitus, and atrial fibrillation presents to the ICU with new-onset left-sided weakness and facial droop. A head CT scan is negative for hemorrhage. When is it most appropriate to administer intravenous tissue plasminogen activator (tPA) in this patient?

    A. Within 3 hours of symptom onset
    B. Within 4.5 hours of symptom onset
    C. Within 6 hours of symptom onset
    D. Within 24 hours of symptom onset

262. A 45-year-old man with a history of intravenous drug use is admitted to the ICU with infective endocarditis complicated by a perivalvular abscess. He undergoes successful surgical valve replacement and debridement of the abscess. Which of the following is the most important factor in determining the duration of antibiotic therapy for this patient?

    A. The type of organism isolated from blood cultures
    B. The presence of complications, such as heart failure or embolic events
    C. The patient's immune status
    D. All of the above

263. A 75-year-old man with a history of chronic obstructive pulmonary disease (COPD) is admitted to the ICU with an acute exacerbation. He is intubated and placed on mechanical ventilation. After 72 hours, his sputum culture grows Pseudomonas aeruginosa. Which of the following antibiotics is most appropriate for the treatment of Pseudomonas aeruginosa pneumonia if the patient has a history of anaphylaxis to penicillin?

    A. Piperacillin/tazobactam
    B. Cefepime
    C. Meropenem
    D. Aztreonam

264. A 30-year-old woman with no significant medical history presents to the ICU with septic shock secondary to a pelvic abscess. She is initiated on norepinephrine for vasopressor support. Which of the following is the most appropriate target for mean arterial pressure (MAP) in this patient if she has a history of chronic hypertension?

    A. MAP > 60 mmHg
    B. MAP > 65 mmHg
    C. MAP > 70 mmHg
    D. MAP > 75 mmHg

265. A 65-year-old woman with a history of heart failure with preserved ejection fraction (HFpEF) is admitted to the ICU with acute decompensated heart failure. She is treated with intravenous diuretics, but her urine output remains low. Which of the following interventions should be considered next to improve her diuresis if she has a history of renal insufficiency?

    A. Continuous renal replacement therapy (CRRT)
    B. Ultrafiltration
    C. Low-dose dopamine infusion
    D. Metolazone

266. A 40-year-old man with a history of alcoholism is admitted to the ICU with alcoholic hepatitis and acute liver failure. He develops hepatorenal syndrome (HRS). Which of the following medications is most likely to improve renal function and survival in this patient?

    A. Octreotide
    B. Midodrine
    C. Terlipressin
    D. Albumin

267. A 25-year-old woman with a history of asthma is admitted to the ICU with status asthmaticus. She is intubated and mechanically ventilated. Which of the following weaning strategies is most appropriate for this patient?

    A. Once-daily spontaneous breathing trial (SBT)
    B. Intermittent mandatory ventilation (IMV)
    C. Pressure support ventilation (PSV)
    D. T-piece trials

268. A 55-year-old man with a history of hypertension and hyperlipidemia presents to the ICU with an acute Stanford type B aortic dissection. He is hemodynamically stable and is treated with medical therapy. Which of the following medications should be avoided in this patient due to the risk of worsening aortic wall stress?

    A. Beta-blockers
    B. Calcium channel blockers
    C. Hydralazine
    D. Nitroprusside

269. A 70-year-old woman with a history of chronic kidney disease (CKD) is admitted to the ICU with uremic pericarditis. She undergoes pericardiocentesis, and 500 mL of bloody fluid is drained. Which of the following is the most appropriate next step in the management of this patient if she continues to have symptoms of cardiac tamponade?

    A. Repeat pericardiocentesis
    B. Pericardial window placement
    C. Pericardiectomy
    D. Initiation of hemodialysis

270. A 50-year-old woman with a history of rheumatoid arthritis presents to the ICU with septic shock secondary to pneumonia. She is initiated on norepinephrine for vasopressor support and broad-spectrum antibiotics. After 72 hours, her blood cultures grow methicillin-resistant Staphylococcus aureus (MRSA). Which of the following is the most appropriate duration of antibiotic therapy for MRSA pneumonia in this patient if she has a complicated course with persistent bacteremia?

    A. 7 days
    B. 14 days
    C. 21 days
    D. 4-6 weeks

271. A 78-year-old woman with a history of hypertension and coronary artery disease presents to the ICU with new-onset chest pain and ST-segment depressions in leads V1-V4 on her electrocardiogram (ECG). She is diagnosed with non-ST-elevation myocardial infarction (NSTEMI). During her hospital course, she develops acute limb ischemia. Which of the following diagnostic tests is most appropriate to confirm the suspected diagnosis of cholesterol embolism?

    A. Doppler ultrasound of the lower extremities
    B. Computed tomography angiography (CTA) of the lower extremities
    C. Magnetic resonance angiography (MRA) of the lower extremities
    D. Skin biopsy of the affected limb

272. A 45-year-old man with a history of intravenous drug use is admitted to the ICU with infective endocarditis complicated by a perivalvular abscess. He undergoes successful surgical valve replacement and debridement of the abscess. Which of the following is the most common cause of prosthetic valve endocarditis within the first year after surgery?

    A. Staphylococcus aureus
    B. Staphylococcus epidermidis
    C. Streptococcus species
    D. Enterococcus species

273. A 75-year-old man with a history of chronic obstructive pulmonary disease (COPD) is admitted to the ICU with an acute exacerbation. He is intubated and placed on mechanical ventilation. Which of the following interventions is most likely to reduce his risk of ventilator-induced diaphragm dysfunction (VIDD)?

    A. Daily interruption of sedation
    B. Early mobilization
    C. Neuromuscular electrical stimulation (NMES)
    D. All of the above

274. A 30-year-old woman with no significant medical history presents to the ICU with septic shock secondary to a pelvic abscess. She is initiated on norepinephrine for vasopressor support. Which of the following is the most appropriate target for central venous oxygen saturation (ScvO2) in this patient?

    A. ScvO2 > 50%
    B. ScvO2 > 60%
    C. ScvO2 > 70%
    D. ScvO2 > 80%

275. A 65-year-old woman with a history of heart failure with preserved ejection fraction (HFpEF) is admitted to the ICU with acute decompensated heart failure. She is treated with intravenous diuretics, but her urine output remains low. Which of the following interventions should be considered next to improve her diuresis if she has a history of renal insufficiency and is not responding to high-dose loop diuretics?

    A. Continuous renal replacement therapy (CRRT)
    B. Ultrafiltration
    C. Low-dose dopamine infusion
    D. Metolazone

276. A 40-year-old man with a history of alcoholism is admitted to the ICU with alcoholic hepatitis and acute liver failure. He develops hepatorenal syndrome (HRS). Which of the following is the most important prognostic factor for survival in HRS?

    A. Serum creatinine level
    B. Serum bilirubin level
    C. Model for End-Stage Liver Disease (MELD) score
    D. Response to treatment with terlipressin

277. A 25-year-old woman with a history of asthma is admitted to the ICU with status asthmaticus. She is intubated and mechanically ventilated. Which of the following complications is most commonly associated with the use of neuromuscular blocking agents in patients with status asthmaticus?

    A. Prolonged weakness
    B. Myopathy
    C. Hyperkalemia
    D. All of the above

278. A 55-year-old man with a history of hypertension and hyperlipidemia presents to the ICU with an acute Stanford type B aortic dissection. He is hemodynamically stable and is treated with medical therapy. Which of the following is the most common long-term complication of type B aortic dissection?

    A. Aortic aneurysm formation
    B. Aortic rupture
    C. Stroke
    D. Renal failure

279. A 70-year-old woman with a history of chronic kidney disease (CKD) is admitted to the ICU with uremic pericarditis. She undergoes pericardiocentesis, and 500 mL of bloody fluid is drained. Which of the following laboratory tests is most helpful in differentiating uremic pericarditis from other causes of pericarditis?

    A. Pericardial fluid culture
    B. Pericardial fluid cytology
    C. Pericardial fluid triglyceride level
    D. Pericardial fluid adenosine deaminase (ADA) level

280. A 50-year-old woman with a history of rheumatoid arthritis presents to the ICU with septic shock secondary to pneumonia. She is initiated on norepinephrine for vasopressor support and broad-spectrum antibiotics. After 72 hours, her blood cultures grow methicillin-resistant Staphylococcus aureus (MRSA). Which of the following is the most appropriate duration of antibiotic therapy for MRSA pneumonia in this patient if she has a complicated course with persistent bacteremia and metastatic infection?

    A. 7 days
    B. 14 days
    C. 21 days
    D. 4-6 weeks

281. A 72-year-old woman with a history of hypertension and coronary artery disease is admitted to the ICU with new-onset chest pain and ST-segment depressions in leads V1-V4 on her electrocardiogram (ECG). She is diagnosed with non-ST-elevation myocardial infarction (NSTEMI). During her hospital course, she develops acute limb ischemia. If a skin biopsy of the affected limb reveals cholesterol crystals in the small arteries, which of the following interventions is most appropriate?

    A. Systemic anticoagulation with heparin
    B. Thrombolytic therapy with tissue plasminogen activator (tPA)
    C. Surgical revascularization
    D. Supportive care and statin therapy

282. A 45-year-old man with a history of intravenous drug use is admitted to the ICU with infective endocarditis complicated by a perivalvular abscess. He undergoes successful surgical valve replacement and debridement of the abscess. Which of the following factors is most predictive of a favorable outcome after surgery?

    A. Younger age
    B. Absence of prosthetic valve
    C. Early surgical intervention
    D. All of the above

283. A 75-year-old man with a history of chronic obstructive pulmonary disease (COPD) is admitted to the ICU with an acute exacerbation. He is intubated and placed on mechanical ventilation. Which of the following weaning parameters is most predictive of successful extubation in this patient?

    A. Rapid shallow breathing index (RSBI) less than 105
    B. Negative inspiratory force (NIF) greater than -20 cmH2O
    C. Vital capacity (VC) greater than 10 mL/kg
    D. All of the above

284. A 30-year-old woman with no significant medical history presents to the ICU with septic shock secondary to a pelvic abscess. She is initiated on norepinephrine for vasopressor support. Which of the following hemodynamic parameters is most indicative of adequate fluid resuscitation in this patient?

    A. Central venous pressure (CVP) greater than 8 mmHg
    B. Pulmonary capillary wedge pressure (PCWP) greater than 12 mmHg
    C. Mean arterial pressure (MAP) greater than 65 mmHg
    D. Passive leg raise test resulting in an increase in stroke volume or pulse pressure

285. A 65-year-old woman with a history of heart failure with preserved ejection fraction (HFpEF) is admitted to the ICU with acute decompensated heart failure. She is treated with intravenous diuretics, but her urine output remains low. Which of the following interventions should be considered next to improve her diuresis if she has a history of renal insufficiency and has failed to respond to metolazone?

  A. Tolvaptan
  B. Conivaptan
  C. Chlorothiazide
  D. Ultrafiltration

286. A 40-year-old man with a history of alcoholism is admitted to the ICU with alcoholic hepatitis and acute liver failure. He develops hepatorenal syndrome (HRS). Which of the following is the most common type of HRS?

  A. Type 1 HRS
  B. Type 2 HRS
  C. Type 3 HRS
  D. Type 4 HRS

287. A 25-year-old woman with a history of asthma is admitted to the ICU with status asthmaticus. She is intubated and mechanically ventilated. Which of the following is the most important factor to consider when weaning this patient from mechanical ventilation?

  A. Peak expiratory flow rate (PEFR)
  B. Forced expiratory volume in 1 second (FEV1)
  C. Airway responsiveness
  D. All of the above

288. A 55-year-old man with a history of hypertension and hyperlipidemia presents to the ICU with an acute Stanford type B aortic dissection. He is hemodynamically stable and is treated with medical therapy. Which of the following imaging modalities is most appropriate for follow-up assessment of his aortic dissection 1 year after initial presentation?

A. Chest X-ray
B. Computed tomography angiography (CTA) of the chest
C. Transesophageal echocardiogram (TEE)
D. Magnetic resonance imaging (MRI) of the chest

289. A 70-year-old woman with a history of chronic kidney disease (CKD) is admitted to the ICU with uremic pericarditis. She undergoes pericardiocentesis, and 500 mL of bloody fluid is drained. Which of the following is the most common complication of pericardiocentesis?

A. Pneumothorax
B. Cardiac perforation
C. Coronary artery laceration
D. Infection

290. A 50-year-old woman with a history of rheumatoid arthritis presents to the ICU with septic shock secondary to pneumonia. She is initiated on norepinephrine for vasopressor support and broad-spectrum antibiotics. After 72 hours, her blood cultures grow methicillin-resistant Staphylococcus aureus (MRSA). Which of the following is the most appropriate duration of antibiotic therapy for MRSA pneumonia in this patient if she has a complicated course with persistent bacteremia and metastatic infection to the spine?

A. 4-6 weeks
B. 6-8 weeks
C. 8-12 weeks
D. 12-16 weeks

291. A 35-year-old woman with a history of systemic lupus erythematosus (SLE) presents to the ICU with new-onset seizures and altered mental status. Her blood pressure is 180/110 mmHg, and she has proteinuria and hematuria. Which of the following is the most likely cause of her neurological symptoms?

    A. Posterior reversible encephalopathy syndrome (PRES)
    B. Lupus cerebritis
    C. Cerebral vasculitis
    D. Central nervous system (CNS) infection

292. A 65-year-old man with a history of coronary artery disease presents to the ICU with cardiogenic shock after an acute myocardial infarction (MI). He is on multiple inotropic and vasopressor agents, but his cardiac index remains low. Which of the following mechanical circulatory support devices would be most appropriate for this patient if he has severe peripheral arterial disease?

    A. Impella
    B. Intra-aortic balloon pump (IABP)
    C. TandemHeart
    D. Extracorporeal membrane oxygenation (ECMO)

293. A 48-year-old woman with a history of obesity and obstructive sleep apnea (OSA) is admitted to the ICU following bariatric surgery. On postoperative day 3, she develops tachycardia, tachypnea, and hypoxia. Which of the following is the most likely cause of her symptoms?

    A. Pulmonary embolism
    B. Pneumonia
    C. Anastomotic leak
    D. Acute respiratory distress syndrome (ARDS)

294. A 75-year-old man with a history of chronic obstructive pulmonary disease (COPD) is admitted to the ICU with an acute exacerbation and hypercapnic respiratory failure. He is intubated and placed on mechanical ventilation. Which of the following arterial blood gas (ABG) findings would be most concerning for this patient?

    A. pH 7.35, PaCO2 55 mmHg, PaO2 60 mmHg
    B. pH 7.25, PaCO2 80 mmHg, PaO2 50 mmHg
    C. pH 7.45, PaCO2 35 mmHg, PaO2 80 mmHg
    D. pH 7.30, PaCO2 40 mmHg, PaO2 70 mmHg

295. A 30-year-old woman with no significant medical history presents to the ICU with septic shock secondary to pyelonephritis. Despite adequate fluid resuscitation and norepinephrine, her lactate level remains elevated.Which of the following laboratory tests is most helpful in guiding further resuscitation efforts in this patient?

    A. Central venous oxygen saturation (ScvO2)
    B. Mixed venous oxygen saturation (SvO2)
    C. Arterial lactate
    D. Base deficit

296. A 65-year-old man with a history of heart failure with reduced ejection fraction (HFrEF) is admitted to the ICU with cardiogenic shock. He is treated with inotropic and vasopressor support but remains hypotensive and oliguric. Which of the following is the most common cause of right ventricular (RV) failure in the setting of left ventricular (LV) failure?

    A. Pulmonary embolism
    B. RV infarction
    C. Increased pulmonary vascular resistance
    D. Tricuspid regurgitation

297. A 40-year-old man with a history of alcoholism is admitted to the ICU with alcoholic hepatitis and acute liver failure. He develops hepatorenal syndrome (HRS). Which of the following is the most common precipitating factor for HRS in patients with cirrhosis?

A. Spontaneous bacterial peritonitis (SBP)
B. Gastrointestinal bleeding
C. Large-volume paracentesis
D. Diuretic therapy

298. A 25-year-old woman with a history of asthma is admitted to the ICU with status asthmaticus. She is intubated and mechanically ventilated. Which of the following adjunctive therapies is most effective in reducing airway inflammation and improving bronchodilation in this patient?

A. Magnesium sulfate
B. Ketamine
C. Heliox
D. Inhaled corticosteroids

299. A 55-year-old man with a history of hypertension and hyperlipidemia presents to the ICU with an acute Stanford type B aortic dissection. He is hemodynamically stable and is treated with medical therapy. Which of the following antihypertensive medications is preferred for the initial management of blood pressure in this patient?

A. Labetalol
B. Esmolol
C. Nitroprusside
D. Nicardipine

300. A 70-year-old woman with a history of chronic kidney disease (CKD) is admitted to the ICU with uremic pericarditis. She undergoes pericardiocentesis, and 500 mL of bloody fluid is drained. Which of the following findings on pericardial fluid analysis is most suggestive of uremic pericarditis?

A. High protein content
B. Low glucose concentration
C. Elevated lactate dehydrogenase (LDH) level
D. All of the above

301. A 55-year-old male presents to the ICU with acute respiratory distress syndrome (ARDS) secondary to severe sepsis. He is intubated and mechanically ventilated with a PaO2/FiO2 ratio of 100. Which of the following interventions would be most appropriate to improve oxygenation in this patient?

    A. Increase PEEP
    B. Initiate neuromuscular blockade
    C. Start inhaled nitric oxide therapy
    D. Administer prone positioning

302. A 68-year-old woman with a history of hypertension and type 2 diabetes mellitus is admitted to the ICU with diabetic ketoacidosis (DKA). Her initial laboratory values reveal a serum potassium of 2.8 mEq/L. Which of the following is the most appropriate next step in her management?

    A. Start an insulin drip at 0.1 units/kg/hour
    B. Administer intravenous potassium chloride
    C. Administer intravenous bicarbonate
    D. Start an isotonic saline infusion

303. A 45-year-old man with a history of alcohol abuse presents to the ICU with acute pancreatitis. He develops acute kidney injury (AKI) with oliguria. Which of the following is the most likely mechanism of AKI in this patient?

    A. Prerenal azotemia
    B. Acute tubular necrosis
    C. Interstitial nephritis
    D. Glomerulonephritis

304. A 75-year-old woman with a history of atrial fibrillation and chronic kidney disease is admitted to the ICU with an ischemic stroke. She is not a candidate for thrombolysis or thrombectomy. Which of the following medications is the most appropriate for secondary stroke prevention in this patient?

    A. Aspirin
    B. Clopidogrel
    C. Warfarin
    D. Apixaban

305. A 30-year-old woman with a history of systemic lupus erythematosus (SLE) is admitted to the ICU with acute lupus pneumonitis. Which of the following is the most common presenting symptom of lupus pneumonitis?

   A. Pleuritic chest pain
   B. Cough
   C. Dyspnea
   D. Hemoptysis

306. A 65-year-old man with a history of coronary artery disease presents to the ICU with cardiogenic shock after an acute myocardial infarction. He is on multiple inotropic and vasopressor agents, but his cardiac index remains low. Which of the following mechanical circulatory support devices would be most appropriate for this patient if he has severe peripheral arterial disease and is not a candidate for ECMO?

   A. Impella
   B. Intra-aortic balloon pump (IABP)
   C. TandemHeart
   D. Ventricular assist device (VAD)

307. A 40-year-old man with a history of alcoholism is admitted to the ICU with severe alcoholic hepatitis and encephalopathy. Which of the following medications is most effective in reducing ammonia levels in this patient?

   A. Lactulose
   B. Rifaximin
   C. Neomycin
   D. L-ornithine L-aspartate (LOLA)

308. A 25-year-old woman with a history of asthma is admitted to the ICU with status asthmaticus. She is intubated and mechanically ventilated. Which of the following interventions is most likely to reduce her risk of ventilator-induced lung injury (VILI) and barotrauma?

   A. High tidal volume ventilation
   B. High plateau pressure
   C. Permissive hypercapnia
   D. High respiratory rate

309. A 55-year-old man with a history of hypertension and hyperlipidemia presents to the ICU with an acute Stanford type B aortic dissection. He is hemodynamically stable and is treated with medical therapy. Which of the following is the most important factor in determining the long-term prognosis of this patient?

    A. Age
    B. Extent of the dissection
    C. Presence of complications
    D. Blood pressure control

310. A 70-year-old woman with a history of chronic kidney disease (CKD) is admitted to the ICU with uremic pericarditis. She undergoes pericardiocentesis, and 500 mL of bloody fluid is drained. Which of the following is the most appropriate next step in the management of this patient if she has recurrent cardiac tamponade?

    A. Repeat pericardiocentesis
    B. Pericardial window placement
    C. Pericardiectomy
    D. Initiation of hemodialysis

311. A 72-year-old woman presents to the ICU with altered mental status, agitation, and visual hallucinations. She is tachycardic and hypertensive. Her medication list includes atorvastatin, metformin, lisinopril, and a recent prescription for diphenhydramine for seasonal allergies. Which of the following is the most likely cause of her symptoms?

    A. Delirium due to anticholinergic toxicity
    B. Acute stroke
    C. Sepsis
    D. Worsening dementia

312. A 45-year-old man with a history of end-stage renal disease on hemodialysis is admitted to the ICU with fever, chills, and a swollen, erythematous arteriovenous fistula (AVF). Which of the following organisms is the most likely cause of his infection?

    A. Staphylococcus aureus
    B. Streptococcus viridans
    C. Pseudomonas aeruginosa
    D. Candida albicans

313. A 75-year-old man with a history of chronic obstructive pulmonary disease (COPD) and obesity hypoventilation syndrome is admitted to the ICU with hypercapnic respiratory failure. He is intubated and placed on mechanical ventilation. Which of the following ventilation modes is most appropriate for this patient?

    A. Assist-control ventilation (ACV)
    B. Pressure-controlled ventilation (PCV)
    C. Synchronized intermittent mandatory ventilation (SIMV)
    D. Pressure support ventilation (PSV)

314. A 30-year-old woman with no significant medical history presents to the ICU with septic shock secondary to community-acquired pneumonia. She is intubated and mechanically ventilated with a PaO2/FiO2 ratio of 80. Which of the following interventions should be considered to improve oxygenation in this patient?

    A. Increase PEEP
    B. Initiate neuromuscular blockade
    C. Start inhaled nitric oxide therapy
    D. Administer prone positioning

315. A 65-year-old man with a history of coronary artery disease presents to the ICU with cardiogenic shock after an acute myocardial infarction. He is treated with inotropic and vasopressor support, but his cardiac index remains low. Which of the following complications of cardiogenic shock is associated with the highest mortality rate?

    A. Acute kidney injury (AKI)
    B. Multi-organ failure
    C. Ventricular arrhythmias
    D. Stroke

316. A 40-year-old man with a history of alcoholism is admitted to the ICU with alcoholic hepatitis and acute liver failure. He develops hepatic encephalopathy. Which of the following is the most important factor in the pathogenesis of hepatic encephalopathy?

    A. Elevated ammonia levels
    B. Increased inflammatory cytokines
    C. Cerebral edema
    D. Oxidative stress

317. A 25-year-old woman with a history of cystic fibrosis is admitted to the ICU with a pulmonary exacerbation. Which of the following antibiotics is most appropriate for the treatment of Pseudomonas aeruginosa infection in this patient?

    A. Cefepime
    B. Meropenem
    C. Piperacillin/tazobactam
    D. Ciprofloxacin

318. A 55-year-old man with a history of hypertension and hyperlipidemia presents to the ICU with an acute Stanford type A aortic dissection. He undergoes successful surgical repair of the dissection. Which of the following postoperative complications is most specific to aortic dissection repair?

    A. Stroke
    B. Renal failure
    C. Spinal cord ischemia
    D. Postoperative delirium

319. A 70-year-old woman with a history of chronic kidney disease (CKD) is admitted to the ICU with uremic pericarditis. Which of the following findings on echocardiography would be most consistent with the diagnosis of uremic pericarditis?

    A. Pericardial effusion
    B. Left ventricular hypertrophy
    C. Mitral valve prolapse
    D. Aortic stenosis

320. A 50-year-old woman with a history of rheumatoid arthritis presents to the ICU with septic shock secondary to pneumonia. She is initiated on norepinephrine for vasopressor support and broad-spectrum antibiotics. After 72 hours, her blood cultures remain negative, and her clinical status has not improved. Which of the following diagnostic tests should be considered to identify a potential source of ongoing infection?

    A. Computed tomography (CT) scan of the abdomen and pelvis
    B. Transthoracic echocardiogram (TTE)
    C. Magnetic resonance imaging (MRI) of the spine
    D. All of the above

321. A 72-year-old man with a history of hypertension and coronary artery disease presents to the ICU with new-onset atrial fibrillation with rapid ventricular response (RVR). His heart rate is 150 beats per minute, and his blood pressure is 80/40 mmHg. He has a history of COPD and heart failure with reduced ejection fraction (HFrEF). In addition to rate control, which of the following should be prioritized in this patient's management?

    A. Anticoagulation with warfarin
    B. Immediate electrical cardioversion
    C. Initiation of amiodarone for rhythm control
    D. Assessment of reversible causes of atrial fibrillation

322. A 42-year-old woman with a history of systemic lupus erythematosus (SLE) presents to the ICU with altered mental status, seizures, and hypertension. A brain MRI reveals diffuse white matter lesions consistent with posterior reversible encephalopathy syndrome (PRES). Which of the following medications is most likely to be held or discontinued in this patient to facilitate recovery from PRES?

    A. Hydroxychloroquine
    B. Belimumab
    C. Mycophenolate mofetil
    D. Cyclophosphamide

323. A 75-year-old man with a history of chronic obstructive pulmonary disease (COPD) is admitted to the ICU with an acute exacerbation and hypercapnic respiratory failure. He is intubated and placed on mechanical ventilation. Which of the following parameters should be monitored closely to assess the effectiveness of ventilation and guide adjustments in ventilator settings?

    A. End-tidal carbon dioxide (EtCO2)
    B. Arterial blood gas (ABG)
    C. Peak inspiratory pressure (PIP)
    D. All of the above

324. A 30-year-old woman with no significant medical history presents to the ICU with septic shock secondary to community-acquired pneumonia. She is intubated and mechanically ventilated with a PaO2/FiO2 ratio of 80. Which of the following interventions may be considered to recruit collapsed alveoli and improve oxygenation in this patient?

    A. Increasing PEEP
    B. Prone positioning
    C. Recruitment maneuvers
    D. All of the above

325. A 65-year-old man with a history of heart failure with reduced ejection fraction (HFrEF) is admitted to the ICU with cardiogenic shock. He is treated with inotropic and vasopressor support but remains hypotensive and oliguric. Which of the following laboratory findings is most indicative of end-organ hypoperfusion in this patient?

  A. Elevated serum creatinine
  B. Elevated lactate levels
  C. Decreased urine output
  D. All of the above

326. A 40-year-old man with a history of alcoholism is admitted to the ICU with alcoholic hepatitis and acute liver failure. He develops hepatorenal syndrome (HRS). Which of the following medications is considered the first-line therapy for type 1 HRS?

  A. Terlipressin
  B. Midodrine
  C. Octreotide
  D. Albumin

327. A 25-year-old woman with a history of asthma is admitted to the ICU with status asthmaticus. She is intubated and mechanically ventilated. Which of the following adjunctive therapies may be considered to reduce airway inflammation and improve bronchodilation in this patient if she does not respond to standard therapy?

  A. Ketamine infusion
  B. Inhaled helium-oxygen mixture (heliox)
  C. Bronchial thermoplasty
  D. Extracorporeal membrane oxygenation (ECMO)

328. A 55-year-old man with a history of hypertension and hyperlipidemia presents to the ICU with an acute Stanford type B aortic dissection. He is hemodynamically stable and is treated with medical therapy. Which of the following is the most important lifestyle modification to recommend to this patient to reduce the risk of aortic dissection progression?

    A. Smoking cessation
    B. Weight loss
    C. Dietary sodium restriction
    D. Exercise

329. A 70-year-old woman with a history of chronic kidney disease (CKD) is admitted to the ICU with uremic pericarditis. She undergoes pericardiocentesis, and 500 mL of bloody fluid is drained. Which of the following microorganisms is most commonly associated with purulent pericarditis?

    A. Staphylococcus aureus
    B. Streptococcus pneumoniae
    C. Haemophilus influenzae
    D. Escherichia coli

330. A 50-year-old woman with a history of rheumatoid arthritis presents to the ICU with septic shock secondary to pneumonia. She is initiated on norepinephrine for vasopressor support and broad-spectrum antibiotics. After 72 hours, her blood cultures remain negative, and her clinical status has not improved. Which of the following should be considered in the management of this patient if a non-infectious cause of her symptoms is suspected?

    A. Discontinuation of antibiotics
    B. Initiation of immunosuppressive therapy
    C. Evaluation for underlying malignancy
    D. All of the above

331. A 62-year-old man with a history of hypertension and type 2 diabetes mellitus is admitted to the ICU with septic shock secondary to urosepsis. Which of the following is the most appropriate empiric antibiotic regimen for this patient?

    A. Vancomycin and piperacillin-tazobactam
    B. Cefepime and metronidazole
    C. Meropenem and vancomycin
    D. Ceftriaxone and azithromycin

332. A 35-year-old woman with a history of systemic lupus erythematosus (SLE) presents to the ICU with new-onset fever, chest pain, and friction rub on auscultation. An echocardiogram reveals a small pericardial effusion. Which of the following is the most likely diagnosis?

    A. Acute myocardial infarction (MI)
    B. Lupus pericarditis
    C. Dressler's syndrome
    D. Pulmonary embolism (PE)

333. A 75-year-old man with a history of chronic obstructive pulmonary disease (COPD) is admitted to the ICU with an acute exacerbation and hypercapnic respiratory failure. He is intubated and placed on mechanical ventilation. Which of the following strategies is most likely to improve his chances of successful extubation?

    A. Early mobilization and physical therapy
    B. Daily spontaneous awakening trial (SAT) and spontaneous breathing trial (SBT)
    C. Use of noninvasive ventilation (NIV) as a bridge to extubation
    D. All of the above

334. A 30-year-old woman with no significant medical history presents to the ICU with severe community-acquired pneumonia (CAP) and septic shock. She is initiated on norepinephrine for vasopressor support. Which of the following parameters should be used to guide the titration of norepinephrine in this patient?

    A. Mean arterial pressure (MAP)
    B. Central venous pressure (CVP)
    C. Cardiac index (CI)
    D. Systemic vascular resistance (SVR)

335. A 65-year-old woman with a history of heart failure with preserved ejection fraction (HFpEF) is admitted to the ICU with acute decompensated heart failure. She is treated with intravenous diuretics, but her urine output remains low. Which of the following adjunctive therapies may be considered to enhance diuresis in this patient?

    A. Low-dose dopamine
    B. Nesiritide
    C. Tolvaptan
    D. Conivaptan

336. A 40-year-old man with a history of alcoholism is admitted to the ICU with alcoholic hepatitis and acute liver failure. He develops hepatorenal syndrome (HRS) and is initiated on terlipressin. Which of the following laboratory parameters should be monitored closely to assess the response to therapy?

    A. Serum creatinine
    B. Urine output
    C. Serum sodium
    D. All of the above

337. A 25-year-old woman with a history of asthma is admitted to the ICU with status asthmaticus. She is intubated and mechanically ventilated. Despite aggressive bronchodilator therapy, her peak airway pressures remain high, and her oxygenation is worsening. Which of the following interventions should be considered next?

    A. Inhaled helium-oxygen mixture (heliox)
    B. Intravenous ketamine
    C. Bronchial thermoplasty
    D. Extracorporeal membrane oxygenation (ECMO)

338. A 55-year-old man with a history of hypertension and hyperlipidemia presents to the ICU with an acute Stanford type B aortic dissection. He is hemodynamically stable and is treated with medical therapy. Which of the following is the most important factor in determining the need for surgical or endovascular repair in this patient?

    A. Age of the patient
    B. Size of the aortic aneurysm
    C. Presence of complications, such as malperfusion or impending rupture
    D. Patient's preference

339. A 70-year-old woman with a history of chronic kidney disease (CKD) is admitted to the ICU with uremic pericarditis. Which of the following complications of uremic pericarditis should be monitored closely in this patient?

    A. Cardiac tamponade
    B. Pericardial constriction
    C. Pericardial effusion
    D. All of the above

340. A 50-year-old woman with a history of rheumatoid arthritis presents to the ICU with septic shock secondary to pneumonia. She is initiated on norepinephrine for vasopressor support and broad-spectrum antibiotics. After 72 hours, her blood cultures remain negative, and her clinical status has not improved. Which of the following diagnostic tests should be considered to evaluate for a non-infectious cause of her symptoms?

    A. Autoantibody testing
    B. Bone marrow biopsy
    C. Abdominal ultrasound
    D. All of the above

341. A 58-year-old man with a history of hypertension and alcoholic cirrhosis is admitted to the ICU with hematemesis and melena. His vital signs are stable, and he is hemodynamically stable. What is the next most appropriate step in management?

    A. Transfuse packed red blood cells (PRBCs)
    B. Initiate octreotide infusion
    C. Perform upper endoscopy
    D. Administer intravenous proton pump inhibitor (PPI)

342. A 35-year-old woman with a history of systemic lupus erythematosus (SLE) is admitted to the ICU with acute kidney injury (AKI) and new-onset thrombocytopenia. Which of the following laboratory tests is most important to evaluate for the potential diagnosis of thrombotic thrombocytopenic purpura (TTP)?

    A. Anti-nuclear antibody (ANA) titer
    B. Anti-dsDNA antibody titer
    C. ADAMTS13 activity
    D. Complement levels (C3 and C4)

343. A 75-year-old man with a history of chronic obstructive pulmonary disease (COPD) is admitted to the ICU with an acute exacerbation and hypercapnic respiratory failure. Despite optimal medical management, his respiratory status continues to deteriorate. Which of the following interventions is most likely to improve his survival?

    A. Inhaled corticosteroids
    B. Inhaled bronchodilators
    C. Noninvasive ventilation (NIV)
    D. Tracheostomy

344. A 30-year-old woman with no significant medical history presents to the ICU with septic shock secondary to community-acquired pneumonia. She is intubated and mechanically ventilated with a PaO2/FiO2 ratio of 80. Which of the following strategies is most likely to improve her oxygenation if conventional ventilation fails?

    A. High-frequency oscillatory ventilation (HFOV)
    B. Extracorporeal membrane oxygenation (ECMO)
    C. Inhaled nitric oxide
    D. Prone positioning

345. A 65-year-old man with a history of coronary artery disease presents to the ICU with cardiogenic shock after an acute myocardial infarction. He is on multiple inotropic and vasopressor agents, but his cardiac index remains low. Which of the following is the most important factor in determining the prognosis of cardiogenic shock?

    A. Age
    B. Extent of myocardial damage
    C. Presence of comorbidities
    D. Time to reperfusion therapy

346. A 40-year-old man with a history of alcoholism is admitted to the ICU with alcoholic hepatitis and acute liver failure. He develops hepatorenal syndrome (HRS). Which of the following is the most important prognostic factor for survival in HRS?

    A. Severity of liver disease
    B. Response to volume expansion
    C. Response to terlipressin therapy
    D. Baseline renal function

347. A 25-year-old woman with a history of asthma is admitted to the ICU with status asthmaticus. She is intubated and mechanically ventilated. Which of the following medications is most likely to improve her bronchodilation and reduce airway inflammation?

    A. Inhaled corticosteroids
    B. Intravenous magnesium sulfate
    C. Inhaled beta-agonists
    D. All of the above

348. A 55-year-old man with a history of hypertension and hyperlipidemia presents to the ICU with an acute Stanford type B aortic dissection. He is hemodynamically stable and is treated with medical therapy. Which of the following diagnostic tests is most appropriate for long-term surveillance of his aortic dissection?

    A. Computed tomography angiography (CTA) of the chest
    B. Transthoracic echocardiogram (TTE)
    C. Magnetic resonance imaging (MRI) of the chest
    D. Chest X-ray

349. A 70-year-old woman with a history of chronic kidney disease (CKD) is admitted to the ICU with uremic pericarditis. Which of the following is the most common ECG finding in uremic pericarditis?

    A. ST-segment elevation
    B. PR depression
    C. Electrical alternans
    D. Diffuse ST-segment depression and T-wave inversions

350. A 50-year-old woman with a history of rheumatoid arthritis presents to the ICU with septic shock secondary to pneumonia. She is initiated on norepinephrine for vasopressor support and broad-spectrum antibiotics. After 72 hours, her blood cultures remain negative, and her clinical status has not improved. Which of the following diagnostic tests should be considered to evaluate for a fungal infection?

   A. Serum galactomannan
   B. Beta-D-glucan
   C. Fungal blood cultures
   D. All of the above

351. A 72-year-old woman with a history of hypertension and coronary artery disease presents to the ICU with new-onset atrial fibrillation with rapid ventricular response (RVR). Her heart rate is 150 beats per minute and blood pressure is 100/60 mmHg. She has a history of chronic kidney disease (CKD) with an estimated glomerular filtration rate (eGFR) of 30 mL/min/1.73 m2. She is currently taking apixaban for stroke prevention in atrial fibrillation. What is the most appropriate initial management strategy for her RVR?

   A. Intravenous diltiazem
   B. Intravenous metoprolol
   C. Intravenous digoxin
   D. Electrical cardioversion

352. A 45-year-old man with a history of intravenous drug use is admitted to the ICU with infective endocarditis complicated by a perivalvular abscess. He undergoes successful surgical valve replacement and debridement of the abscess. Six weeks later, he presents with recurrent fevers, chills, and fatigue. Which of the following is the most likely cause of his symptoms?

   A. Recurrent infective endocarditis
   B. Postoperative infection
   C. Drug fever
   D. Deep vein thrombosis (DVT)

353. A 75-year-old man with a history of chronic obstructive pulmonary disease (COPD) is admitted to the ICU with an acute exacerbation and hypercapnic respiratory failure. He is intubated and placed on mechanical ventilation. Which of the following adjunctive therapies may be considered to improve his oxygenation and reduce ventilator-induced lung injury (VILI)?

    A. Inhaled nitric oxide
    B. High-frequency oscillatory ventilation (HFOV)
    C. Prone positioning
    D. All of the above

354. A 30-year-old woman with no significant medical history presents to the ICU with septic shock secondary to community-acquired pneumonia. She is intubated and mechanically ventilated with a PaO2/FiO2 ratio of 80. Which of the following ventilatory strategies is most likely to worsen her oxygenation?

    A. Lung-protective ventilation with low tidal volumes (6-8 mL/kg of predicted body weight)
    B. High PEEP (15-20 cm H2O)
    C. High tidal volume ventilation (10-12 mL/kg of predicted body weight)
    D. Recruitment maneuvers

355. A 65-year-old man with a history of heart failure with reduced ejection fraction (HFrEF) is admitted to the ICU with cardiogenic shock after an acute myocardial infarction. He is treated with inotropic and vasopressor support, but his cardiac index remains low. Which of the following biomarkers is most strongly associated with mortality in cardiogenic shock?

    A. Brain natriuretic peptide (BNP)
    B. Troponin I
    C. Lactate
    D. N-terminal pro-brain natriuretic peptide (NT-proBNP)

356. A 40-year-old man with a history of alcoholism is admitted to the ICU with alcoholic hepatitis and acute liver failure. He develops hepatorenal syndrome (HRS). Which of the following is the most important prognostic factor in determining the need for liver transplantation in this patient?

    A. MELD score
    B. Child-Pugh score
    C. Response to terlipressin therapy
    D. Presence of ascites

357. A 25-year-old woman with a history of asthma is admitted to the ICU with status asthmaticus. She is intubated and mechanically ventilated. Which of the following complications is most likely to occur in this patient due to prolonged mechanical ventilation?

    A. Pneumonia
    B. Barotrauma
    C. Diaphragmatic dysfunction
    D. All of the above

358. A 55-year-old man with a history of hypertension and hyperlipidemia presents to the ICU with an acute Stanford type B aortic dissection. He is hemodynamically stable and is treated with medical therapy. Which of the following medications is contraindicated in this patient due to the risk of worsening aortic wall stress?

    A. Beta-blockers
    B. Calcium channel blockers
    C. Hydralazine
    D. Nitroprusside

359. A 70-year-old woman with a history of chronic kidney disease (CKD) is admitted to the ICU with uremic pericarditis. She undergoes pericardiocentesis, and 500 mL of bloody fluid is drained. Which of the following is the most appropriate next step in the management of this patient if she has recurrent cardiac tamponade despite pericardiocentesis?

    A. Repeat pericardiocentesis
    B. Pericardial window placement
    C. Pericardiectomy
    D. Initiation of hemodialysis

360. A 50-year-old woman with a history of rheumatoid arthritis presents to the ICU with septic shock secondary to pneumonia. She is initiated on norepinephrine for vasopressor support and broad-spectrum antibiotics. After 72 hours, her blood cultures remain negative, and her clinical status has not improved. Which of the following alternative diagnoses should be considered in this patient?

    A. Macrophage activation syndrome (MAS)
    B. Drug-induced lupus
    C. Adult-onset Still's disease
    D. All of the above

361. A 78-year-old woman with a history of hypertension and coronary artery disease is admitted to the ICU with new-onset atrial fibrillation with rapid ventricular response (RVR). Her heart rate is 150 beats per minute and blood pressure is 100/60 mmHg. She has a history of chronic kidney disease (CKD) with an estimated glomerular filtration rate (eGFR) of 30 mL/min/1.73 m2. She is currently taking apixaban for stroke prevention in atrial fibrillation. In addition to rate control, what is the next most appropriate step in management?

    A. Perform electrical cardioversion
    B. Initiate amiodarone for rhythm control
    C. Assess and correct underlying causes of atrial fibrillation
    D. Start intravenous heparin infusion

362. A 45-year-old man with a history of intravenous drug use is admitted to the ICU with infective endocarditis complicated by a perivalvular abscess. He undergoes successful surgical valve replacement and debridement of the abscess. Six weeks later, he presents with recurrent fevers, chills, and fatigue. Blood cultures are negative. Which of the following diagnostic tests is most likely to reveal the source of his recurrent infection?

    A. Transthoracic echocardiogram (TTE)
    B. Transesophageal echocardiogram (TEE)
    C. 18F-FDG PET/CT scan
    D. Gallium scan

363. A 75-year-old man with a history of chronic obstructive pulmonary disease (COPD) is admitted to the ICU with an acute exacerbation and hypercapnic respiratory failure. He is intubated and placed on mechanical ventilation. After 72 hours, his sputum culture grows Pseudomonas aeruginosa. Which of the following antibiotics is most appropriate for the treatment of Pseudomonas aeruginosa pneumonia if the patient has a history of acute kidney injury (AKI)?

    A. Cefepime
    B. Meropenem
    C. Ceftazidime/avibactam
    D. Imipenem/cilastatin

364. A 30-year-old woman with no significant medical history presents to the ICU with septic shock secondary to a pelvic abscess. She is initiated on norepinephrine for vasopressor support. Which of the following hemodynamic parameters is the most reliable indicator of adequate fluid resuscitation in this patient?

    A. Central venous pressure (CVP)
    B. Pulmonary capillary wedge pressure (PCWP)
    C. Mean arterial pressure (MAP)
    D. Stroke volume variation (SVV)

365. A 65-year-old woman with a history of heart failure with preserved ejection fraction (HFpEF) is admitted to the ICU with acute decompensated heart failure. She is treated with intravenous diuretics, but her urine output remains low. Which of the following adjunctive therapies is contraindicated in this patient if she has a history of anuria?

    A. Continuous renal replacement therapy (CRRT)
    B. Ultrafiltration
    C. Low-dose dopamine infusion
    D. Metolazone

366. A 40-year-old man with a history of alcoholism is admitted to the ICU with alcoholic hepatitis and acute liver failure. He develops hepatic encephalopathy. Which of the following interventions is most effective in preventing recurrent episodes of hepatic encephalopathy in this patient?

    A. Lactulose
    B. Rifaximin
    C. Neomycin
    D. Dietary protein restriction

367. A 25-year-old woman with a history of asthma is admitted to the ICU with status asthmaticus. She is intubated and mechanically ventilated. Which of the following adjunctive therapies may be considered to reduce airway inflammation in this patient if she does not respond to standard therapy?

    A. Intravenous magnesium sulfate
    B. Inhaled helium-oxygen mixture (heliox)
    C. Bronchial thermoplasty
    D. Extracorporeal membrane oxygenation (ECMO)

368. A 55-year-old man with a history of hypertension and hyperlipidemia presents to the ICU with an acute Stanford type B aortic dissection. He is hemodynamically stable and is treated with medical therapy. Which of the following medications is most likely to be used for long-term blood pressure control in this patient if he has a history of reactive airway disease?

    A. Beta-blocker
    B. Calcium channel blocker
    C. Angiotensin-converting enzyme (ACE) inhibitor
    D. Angiotensin II receptor blocker (ARB)

369. A 70-year-old woman with a history of chronic kidney disease (CKD) is admitted to the ICU with uremic pericarditis. She undergoes pericardiocentesis, and 500 mL of bloody fluid is drained. Which of the following is the most appropriate next step in the management of this patient if she develops purulent pericarditis?

    A. Repeat pericardiocentesis
    B. Pericardial window placement
    C. Pericardiectomy
    D. Initiation of antibiotic therapy

370. A 50-year-old woman with a history of rheumatoid arthritis presents to the ICU with septic shock secondary to pneumonia. She is initiated on norepinephrine for vasopressor support and broad-spectrum antibiotics. After 72 hours, her blood cultures remain negative, and her clinical status has not improved. Which of the following additional diagnostic tests should be considered in this patient if she has a history of recent travel to an area endemic for fungal infections?

    A. Fungal blood cultures
    B. Serum galactomannan
    C. Beta-D-glucan
    D. All of the above

371. A 62-year-old woman with a history of end-stage renal disease (ESR**D.** on hemodialysis presents to the ICU with altered mental status, hypotension, and bradycardia. Her electrocardiogram (ECG) shows peaked T waves and a prolonged PR interval. Which of the following electrolyte abnormalities is the most likely cause of her symptoms?

    A. Hyperkalemia
    B. Hypokalemia
    C. Hypercalcemia
    D. Hypocalcemia

372. A 45-year-old man with a history of HIV infection presents to the ICU with fever, cough, and shortness of breath. Chest X-ray reveals bilateral interstitial infiltrates. Which of the following opportunistic infections is the most likely diagnosis?

    A. Pneumocystis pneumonia (PCP)
    B. Mycobacterium avium complex (MAC)
    C. Cytomegalovirus (CMV) pneumonia
    D. Histoplasmosis

373. A 75-year-old man with a history of chronic obstructive pulmonary disease (COPD) is admitted to the ICU with an acute exacerbation and hypercapnic respiratory failure. Despite optimal medical management and noninvasive ventilation (NIV), his respiratory status continues to deteriorate. Which of the following is the most appropriate next step in management?

    A. Tracheostomy
    B. High-frequency oscillatory ventilation (HFOV)
    C. Inhaled nitric oxide
    D. Intubation and mechanical ventilation

374. A 30-year-old woman with no significant medical history presents to the ICU with septic shock secondary to community-acquired pneumonia. She is intubated and mechanically ventilated with a PaO2/FiO2 ratio of 80. Which of the following is the most common cause of refractory hypoxemia in ARDS?

    A. Pulmonary embolism
    B. Pneumothorax
    C. Shunt
    D. Dead space ventilation

375. A 65-year-old man with a history of heart failure with reduced ejection fraction (HFrEF) is admitted to the ICU with cardiogenic shock. He is treated with inotropic and vasopressor support, but his lactate levels remain elevated.Which of the following interventions may be considered to improve tissue perfusion in this patient?

    A. Increase inotropic support
    B. Increase vasopressor support
    C. Inhaled pulmonary vasodilators (e.g., nitric oxide)
    D. All of the above

376. A 40-year-old man with a history of alcoholism is admitted to the ICU with alcoholic hepatitis and acute liver failure. He develops hepatorenal syndrome (HRS) and is initiated on terlipressin. Which of the following parameters should be monitored closely to assess the effectiveness of terlipressin therapy?

    A. Serum creatinine
    B. Urine output
    C. Serum sodium
    D. All of the above

377. A 25-year-old woman with a history of asthma is admitted to the ICU with status asthmaticus. She is intubated and mechanically ventilated. Which of the following ventilator settings is most likely to reduce the risk of dynamic hyperinflation in this patient?

    A. Low tidal volume
    B. Low respiratory rate
    C. High inspiratory flow rate
    D. Short expiratory time

378. A 55-year-old man with a history of hypertension and hyperlipidemia presents to the ICU with an acute Stanford type B aortic dissection. He is hemodynamically stable and is treated with medical therapy. Which of the following imaging modalities is most appropriate for follow-up assessment of his aortic dissection 1 year after initial presentation?

    A. Chest X-ray
    B. Computed tomography angiography (CTA) of the chest
    C. Transesophageal echocardiogram (TEE)
    D. Magnetic resonance imaging (MRI) of the chest

379. A 70-year-old woman with a history of chronic kidney disease (CKD) is admitted to the ICU with uremic pericarditis. Which of the following is the most common electrocardiogram (ECG) finding in uremic pericarditis?

    A. ST-segment elevation
    B. PR depression
    C. Electrical alternans
    D. Diffuse ST-segment depression and T-wave flattening

380. A 50-year-old woman with a history of rheumatoid arthritis presents to the ICU with septic shock secondary to pneumonia. She is initiated on norepinephrine for vasopressor support and broad-spectrum antibiotics. After 72 hours, her blood cultures remain negative, and her clinical status has not improved. Which of the following should be considered in the management of this patient if a non-infectious cause of her symptoms is suspected?

    A. Discontinuation of antibiotics
    B. Initiation of immunosuppressive therapy
    C. Evaluation for underlying malignancy
    D. All of the above

381. A 65-year-old man with a history of hypertension and diabetes presents with chest pain radiating to his left arm and jaw. His ECG shows ST-segment elevation in leads II, III, and aVF. Which of the following is the most likely culprit artery?

    A. Left anterior descending artery (LAD)
    B. Left circumflex artery (LCx)
    C. Right coronary artery (RCA)
    D. Left main coronary artery (LMCA)

382. A 48-year-old woman with a history of systemic lupus erythematosus (SLE) is admitted to the ICU with altered mental status, fever, and rash. Her blood pressure is 80/40 mmHg, and she has elevated creatinine and decreased urine output. Which of the following is the most appropriate initial intervention?

    A. Broad-spectrum antibiotics
    B. Intravenous corticosteroids
    C. Fluid resuscitation with crystalloids
    D. Dialysis

383. A 75-year-old man with a history of chronic obstructive pulmonary disease (COPD) is admitted to the ICU with acute respiratory failure. He is intubated and placed on mechanical ventilation. Which of the following ventilator strategies is most appropriate to prevent ventilator-induced lung injury (VILI)?

    A. High tidal volume ventilation (Vt)
    B. High respiratory rate (RR)
    C. High positive end-expiratory pressure (PEEP)
    D. Low Vt ventilation

384. A 30-year-old woman with no significant medical history is admitted to the ICU with septic shock secondary to pyelonephritis. Despite fluid resuscitation and vasopressor therapy, she remains hypotensive and has cool extremities. Which of the following is the most appropriate next step in management?

    A. Increase norepinephrine dose
    B. Start vasopressin infusion
    C. Administer hydrocortisone
    D. Start epinephrine infusion

385. A 65-year-old man with a history of heart failure with reduced ejection fraction (HFrEF) is admitted to the ICU with cardiogenic shock after an acute myocardial infarction. He is on multiple inotropic and vasopressor agents, but his cardiac index remains low. Which of the following is a contraindication for intra-aortic balloon pump (IABP) placement in this patient?

  A. Aortic regurgitation
  B. Peripheral arterial disease
  C. Severe aortic atherosclerosis
  D. All of the above

386. A 40-year-old man with a history of alcoholism is admitted to the ICU with alcoholic hepatitis and acute liver failure. He develops hepatorenal syndrome (HRS). Which of the following medications is most likely to improve short-term survival in this patient?

  A. Terlipressin
  B. Midodrine
  C. Octreotide
  D. Albumin

387. A 25-year-old woman with a history of asthma is admitted to the ICU with status asthmaticus. She is intubated and mechanically ventilated. Which of the following is a potential complication of high-dose inhaled beta-agonist therapy in this patient?

  A. Hypokalemia
  B. Hyperkalemia
  C. Hypoglycemia
  D. Hyperglycemia

388. A 55-year-old man with a history of hypertension and hyperlipidemia presents to the ICU with an acute Stanford type B aortic dissection. He is hemodynamically stable and is treated with medical therapy. Which of the following is the most common long-term complication of type B aortic dissection?

   A. Aortic aneurysm formation
   B. Aortic rupture
   C. Stroke
   D. Renal failure

389. A 70-year-old woman with a history of chronic kidney disease (CKD) is admitted to the ICU with uremic pericarditis. Which of the following is the most definitive treatment for uremic pericarditis with persistent or recurrent cardiac tamponade?

   A. Hemodialysis
   B. Pericardiocentesis
   C. Pericardial window
   D. Pericardiectomy

390. A 50-year-old woman with a history of rheumatoid arthritis presents to the ICU with septic shock secondary to pneumonia. She is initiated on norepinephrine for vasopressor support and broad-spectrum antibiotics. After 72 hours, her blood cultures remain negative, and her clinical status has not improved. Which of the following is the most likely diagnosis if she has a history of recent travel to the southwestern United States?

   A. Histoplasmosis
   B. Coccidioidomycosis
   C. Blastomycosis
   D. Aspergillosis

391. A 68-year-old woman with a history of hypertension and coronary artery disease presents to the ICU with new-onset atrial fibrillation with rapid ventricular response (RVR). Her heart rate is 150 beats per minute and blood pressure is 100/60 mmHg. She has a history of chronic kidney disease (CKD) with an estimated glomerular filtration rate (eGFR) of 30 mL/min/1.73 m2. She is currently taking apixaban for stroke prevention in atrial fibrillation. In addition to rate control, what is the next most appropriate step in management if she is hemodynamically unstable?

   A. Perform electrical cardioversion
   B. Initiate amiodarone for rhythm control
   C. Assess and correct underlying causes of atrial fibrillation
   D. Start intravenous heparin infusion

392. A 45-year-old man with a history of intravenous drug use is admitted to the ICU with infective endocarditis complicated by a perivalvular abscess. He undergoes successful surgical valve replacement and debridement of the abscess. Six weeks later, he presents with recurrent fevers, chills, and fatigue. Blood cultures are negative. Which of the following diagnostic tests is most likely to reveal the source of his recurrent infection if the TEE is negative?

   A. 18F-FDG PET/CT scan
   B. Gallium scan
   C. Indium-111-labeled white blood cell scan
   D. Computed tomography (CT) scan of the chest

393. A 75-year-old man with a history of chronic obstructive pulmonary disease (COPD) is admitted to the ICU with an acute exacerbation and hypercapnic respiratory failure. He is intubated and placed on mechanical ventilation. After 72 hours, his sputum culture grows Pseudomonas aeruginosa. Which of the following antibiotics is most appropriate for the treatment of Pseudomonas aeruginosa pneumonia if the patient has a history of acute kidney injury (AKI) and is on continuous renal replacement therapy (CRRT)?

   A. Cefepime with extended interval dosing
   B. Meropenem with dose adjustment based on CRRT clearance
   C. Ceftazidime/avibactam with dose adjustment based on CRRT clearance
   D. Imipenem/cilastatin with dose adjustment based on CRRT clearance

394. A 30-year-old woman with no significant medical history presents to the ICU with septic shock secondary to a pelvic abscess. She is initiated on norepinephrine for vasopressor support. Which of the following interventions is most likely to improve her cardiac output if she remains hypotensive despite adequate fluid resuscitation and norepinephrine?

    A. Dobutamine infusion
    B. Increase in norepinephrine dose
    C. Vasopressin infusion
    D. Epinephrine infusion

395. A 65-year-old woman with a history of heart failure with preserved ejection fraction (HFpEF) is admitted to the ICU with acute decompensated heart failure. She is treated with intravenous diuretics, but her urine output remains low. Which of the following adjunctive therapies may be considered to enhance diuresis in this patient if she has a history of renal insufficiency and is not responding to high-dose loop diuretics or metolazone?

    A. Chlorothiazide
    B. Acetazolamide
    C. Low-dose dopamine
    D. Tolvaptan or conivaptan

396. A 40-year-old man with a history of alcoholism is admitted to the ICU with alcoholic hepatitis and acute liver failure. He develops hepatorenal syndrome (HRS). Which of the following is the most appropriate duration of terlipressin therapy for this patient?

    A. 3 days
    B. 7 days
    C. 14 days
    D. Until renal function improves

397. A 25-year-old woman with a history of asthma is admitted to the ICU with status asthmaticus. She is intubated and mechanically ventilated. Which of the following adjunctive therapies may be considered to facilitate extubation in this patient if she fails a spontaneous breathing trial (SBT)?

A. Noninvasive ventilation (NIV)
B. Heliox
C. Methylxanthines
D. Inhaled anesthetics

398. A 55-year-old man with a history of hypertension and hyperlipidemia presents to the ICU with an acute Stanford type B aortic dissection. He is hemodynamically stable and is treated with medical therapy. Which of the following imaging modalities is most appropriate for follow-up assessment of his aortic dissection 5 years after initial presentation?

A. Chest X-ray
B. Computed tomography angiography (CTA) of the chest
C. Transesophageal echocardiogram (TEE)
D. Magnetic resonance imaging (MRI) of the chest

399. A 70-year-old woman with a history of chronic kidney disease (CKD) is admitted to the ICU with uremic pericarditis. She undergoes pericardiocentesis, and 500 mL of bloody fluid is drained. Which of the following laboratory tests on the pericardial fluid is most helpful in differentiating uremic pericarditis from other causes of pericarditis?

A. Pericardial fluid culture
B. Pericardial fluid cytology
C. Pericardial fluid glucose
D. Pericardial fluid creatinine

400. A 50-year-old woman with a history of rheumatoid arthritis presents to the ICU with septic shock secondary to pneumonia. She is initiated on norepinephrine for vasopressor support and broad-spectrum antibiotics. After 72 hours, her blood cultures remain negative, and her clinical status has not improved. Which of the following should be considered in the management of this patient if a non-infectious cause of her symptoms is suspected and she has a high ferritin level?

A. Macrophage activation syndrome (MAS)
B. Drug-induced lupus
C. Adult-onset Still's disease
D. All of the above

401. A 68-year-old woman with a history of hypertension and coronary artery disease is admitted to the ICU with new-onset atrial fibrillation with rapid ventricular response (RVR). Her heart rate is 150 beats per minute and blood pressure is 100/60 mmHg. She has a history of chronic kidney disease (CKD) with an estimated glomerular filtration rate (eGFR) of 30 mL/min/1.73 m2. She is currently taking apixaban for stroke prevention in atrial fibrillation. In addition to rate control, what is the next most appropriate step in management if she has new-onset chest pain and ECG changes concerning for acute myocardial ischemia?

A. Perform emergent electrical cardioversion
B. Initiate amiodarone for rhythm control
C. Perform coronary angiography with possible percutaneous coronary intervention (PCI)
D. Start intravenous heparin infusion

402. A 45-year-old man with a history of intravenous drug use is admitted to the ICU with infective endocarditis complicated by a perivalvular abscess. He undergoes successful surgical valve replacement and debridement of the abscess. Six weeks later, he presents with recurrent fevers, chills, and fatigue. Blood cultures are negative. After ruling out other infectious sources, which of the following is the most appropriate next step in management?

A. Empiric antibiotic therapy for prosthetic valve endocarditis
B. Repeat surgical intervention
C. Continue observation and supportive care
D. Initiate antifungal therapy

403. A 75-year-old man with a history of chronic obstructive pulmonary disease (COPD) is admitted to the ICU with an acute exacerbation and hypercapnic respiratory failure. He is intubated and placed on mechanical ventilation. After 72 hours, his sputum culture grows Pseudomonas aeruginosa. Which of the following antibiotics is most appropriate for the treatment of Pseudomonas aeruginosa pneumonia if the patient has a history of anaphylaxis to both penicillins and cephalosporins?

    A. Cefepime
    B. Meropenem
    C. Ceftazidime/avibactam
    D. Aztreonam

404. A 30-year-old woman with no significant medical history presents to the ICU with septic shock secondary to a pelvic abscess. She is initiated on norepinephrine for vasopressor support. Which of the following is the most appropriate goal for central venous oxygen saturation (ScvO2) in this patient if she is not responding to initial resuscitation?

    A. ScvO2 > 50%
    B. ScvO2 > 60%
    C. ScvO2 > 70%
    D. ScvO2 > 80%

405. A 65-year-old woman with a history of heart failure with preserved ejection fraction (HFpEF) is admitted to the ICU with acute decompensated heart failure. She is treated with intravenous diuretics, but her urine output remains low. Which of the following adjunctive therapies may be considered to enhance diuresis in this patient if she has a history of renal insufficiency and has failed to respond to high-dose loop diuretics, metolazone, or tolvaptan/conivaptan?

    A. Low-dose dopamine
    B. Nesiritide
    C. Milrinone
    D. Continuous renal replacement therapy (CRRT)

406. A 40-year-old man with a history of alcoholism is admitted to the ICU with alcoholic hepatitis and acute liver failure. He develops hepatorenal syndrome (HRS). Which of the following interventions is most likely to improve survival in this patient?

    A. Liver transplantation
    B. Terlipressin
    C. Midodrine and octreotide
    D. Albumin

407. A 25-year-old woman with a history of asthma is admitted to the ICU with status asthmaticus. She is intubated and mechanically ventilated. Which of the following adjunctive therapies may be considered to reduce airway hyperresponsiveness and inflammation in this patient if she does not respond to standard therapy?

    A. Ketamine infusion
    B. Inhaled helium-oxygen mixture (heliox)
    C. Magnesium sulfate
    D. Bronchial thermoplasty

408. A 55-year-old man with a history of hypertension and hyperlipidemia presents to the ICU with an acute Stanford type B aortic dissection. He is hemodynamically stable and is treated with medical therapy. Which of the following imaging modalities is most appropriate for assessing the response to medical therapy and the need for potential intervention in this patient?

    A. Chest X-ray
    B. Computed tomography angiography (CTA) of the chest
    C. Transesophageal echocardiogram (TEE)
    D. Magnetic resonance imaging (MRI) of the chest

409. A 70-year-old woman with a history of chronic kidney disease (CKD) is admitted to the ICU with uremic pericarditis. Which of the following laboratory findings is most specific for uremic pericarditis?

    A. Elevated C-reactive protein (CRP)
    B. Elevated erythrocyte sedimentation rate (ESR)
    C. Pericardial fluid with high urea and creatinine levels
    D. Pericardial fluid with positive bacterial culture

410. A 50-year-old woman with a history of rheumatoid arthritis presents to the ICU with septic shock secondary to pneumonia. She is initiated on norepinephrine for vasopressor support and broad-spectrum antibiotics. After 72 hours, her blood cultures remain negative, and her clinical status has not improved. Which of the following should be considered in the management of this patient if a non-infectious cause of her symptoms is suspected and she has a high ferritin level?

    A. Hemophagocytic lymphohistiocytosis (HLH)
    B. Systemic mastocytosis
    C. Castleman disease
    D. All of the above

411. A 78-year-old woman with a history of hypertension and coronary artery disease is admitted to the ICU with new-onset atrial fibrillation with rapid ventricular response (RVR). Her heart rate is 150 beats per minute and blood pressure is 100/60 mmHg. She has a history of chronic kidney disease (CKD) with an estimated glomerular filtration rate (eGFR) of 30 mL/min/1.73 m2. She is currently taking apixaban for stroke prevention in atrial fibrillation. In addition to rate control, what is the next most appropriate step in management if she has new-onset chest pain and ECG changes concerning for acute myocardial ischemia and her CHA2DS2-VASc score is 5?

    A. Perform emergent electrical cardioversion
    B. Initiate amiodarone for rhythm control
    C. Perform coronary angiography with possible percutaneous coronary intervention (PCI)
    D. Perform transesophageal echocardiogram (TEE) to assess for left atrial appendage thrombus before cardioversion

412. A 45-year-old man with a history of intravenous drug use is admitted to the ICU with infective endocarditis complicated by a perivalvular abscess. He undergoes successful surgical valve replacement and debridement of the abscess. Six weeks later, he presents with recurrent fevers, chills, and fatigue. Blood cultures are negative. After ruling out other infectious sources and a negative TEE, which of the following is the most appropriate next step in management?

    A. Repeat TEE
    B. 18F-FDG PET/CT scan
    C. Gallium scan
    D. Indium-111-labeled white blood cell scan

413. A 75-year-old man with a history of chronic obstructive pulmonary disease (COPD) is admitted to the ICU with an acute exacerbation and hypercapnic respiratory failure. He is intubated and placed on mechanical ventilation. After 72 hours, his sputum culture grows Pseudomonas aeruginosa. Which of the following antibiotics is most appropriate for the treatment of Pseudomonas aeruginosa pneumonia if the patient has a history of acute kidney injury (AKI) and is on continuous renal replacement therapy (CRRT) and has a penicillin allergy?

    A. Cefepime with extended interval dosing
    B. Meropenem with dose adjustment based on CRRT clearance
    C. Ceftazidime/avibactam with dose adjustment based on CRRT clearance
    D. Levofloxacin

414. A 30-year-old woman with no significant medical history presents to the ICU with septic shock secondary to a pelvic abscess. She is initiated on norepinephrine for vasopressor support. Which of the following is the most appropriate goal for mixed venous oxygen saturation (SvO2) in this patient if she is not responding to initial resuscitation?

    A. SvO2 > 50%
    B. SvO2 > 60%
    C. SvO2 > 70%
    D. SvO2 > 80%

415. A 65-year-old woman with a history of heart failure with preserved ejection fraction (HFpEF) is admitted to the ICU with acute decompensated heart failure. She is treated with intravenous diuretics, but her urine output remains low. Which of the following adjunctive therapies may be considered to enhance diuresis in this patient if she has a history of renal insufficiency and has failed to respond to high-dose loop diuretics, metolazone, or tolvaptan/conivaptan? In addition, she has a history of hyperkalemia.

    A. Chlorothiazide
    B. Acetazolamide
    C. Low-dose dopamine
    D. Milrinone

416. A 40-year-old man with a history of alcoholism is admitted to the ICU with alcoholic hepatitis and acute liver failure. He develops hepatorenal syndrome (HRS). Which of the following is the most common electrolyte abnormality seen in patients with HRS?

    A. Hyponatremia
    B. Hypernatremia
    C. Hypokalemia
    D. Hyperkalemia

417. A 25-year-old woman with a history of asthma is admitted to the ICU with status asthmaticus. She is intubated and mechanically ventilated. Which of the following adjunctive therapies may be considered to decrease airway inflammation and improve bronchodilation in this patient if she does not respond to standard therapy and has elevated eosinophil count?

    A. Ketamine infusion
    B. Inhaled helium-oxygen mixture (heliox)
    C. Magnesium sulfate
    D. Bronchial thermoplasty

418. A 55-year-old man with a history of hypertension and hyperlipidemia presents to the ICU with an acute Stanford type B aortic dissection. He is hemodynamically stable and is treated with medical therapy. Which of the following imaging modalities is most appropriate for assessing the response to medical therapy and the need for potential intervention in this patient after 1 year of initial presentation?

    A. Chest X-ray
    B. Computed tomography angiography (CTA) of the chest
    C. Transesophageal echocardiogram (TEE)
    D. Magnetic resonance imaging (MRI) of the chest

419. A 70-year-old woman with a history of chronic kidney disease (CKD) is admitted to the ICU with uremic pericarditis. Which of the following is the most common complication of uremic pericarditis?

    A. Pericardial effusion
    B. Cardiac tamponade
    C. Constrictive pericarditis
    D. Pericardial calcification

420. A 50-year-old woman with a history of rheumatoid arthritis presents to the ICU with septic shock secondary to pneumonia. She is initiated on norepinephrine for vasopressor support and broad-spectrum antibiotics. After 72 hours, her blood cultures remain negative, and her clinical status has not improved. Which of the following should be considered in the management of this patient if a non-infectious cause of her symptoms is suspected and she has a high ferritin level, cytopenias, and hepatosplenomegaly?

    A. Macrophage activation syndrome (MAS)
    B. Drug-induced lupus
    C. Adult-onset Still's disease
    D. Systemic vasculitis

421. A 62-year-old male presents to the ICU with new-onset atrial fibrillation with rapid ventricular response (RVR). His heart rate is 150 beats per minute, and his blood pressure is 80/40 mmHg. He has a history of COPD and heart failure with reduced ejection fraction (HFrEF). In addition to rate control, what is the next most appropriate step in management if he has new-onset chest pain and ECG changes concerning for acute myocardial ischemia and his CHA2DS2-VASc score is 0?

    A. Perform emergent electrical cardioversion
    B. Initiate amiodarone for rhythm control
    C. Perform coronary angiography with possible percutaneous coronary intervention (PCI)
    D. Perform transesophageal echocardiogram (TEE) to assess for left atrial appendage thrombus before cardioversion

422. A 45-year-old man with a history of intravenous drug use is admitted to the ICU with infective endocarditis complicated by a perivalvular abscess. He undergoes successful surgical valve replacement and debridement of the abscess. Six weeks later, he presents with recurrent fevers, chills, and fatigue. Blood cultures are negative. After ruling out other infectious sources and a negative TEE, which of the following is the most appropriate next step in management to rule out prosthetic valve endocarditis (PVE) if other imaging modalities are negative?

    A. Repeat TEE
    B. 18F-FDG PET/CT scan
    C. Gallium scan
    D. Empirical antibiotic therapy for PVE

423. A 75-year-old man with a history of chronic obstructive pulmonary disease (COPD) is admitted to the ICU with an acute exacerbation and hypercapnic respiratory failure. He is intubated and placed on mechanical ventilation. After 72 hours, his sputum culture grows Pseudomonas aeruginosa. Which of the following antibiotics is most appropriate for the treatment of Pseudomonas aeruginosa pneumonia if the patient has a history of acute kidney injury (AKI) and is on continuous renal replacement therapy (CRRT), has a penicillin allergy, and is also colonized with methicillin-resistant Staphylococcus aureus (MRSA)?

A. Cefepime with extended interval dosing and vancomycin
B. Meropenem with dose adjustment based on CRRT clearance and vancomycin
C. Ceftazidime/avibactam with dose adjustment based on CRRT clearance and vancomycin
D. Levofloxacin and vancomycin

424. A 30-year-old woman with no significant medical history presents to the ICU with septic shock secondary to a pelvic abscess. She is initiated on norepinephrine for vasopressor support. Which of the following is the most appropriate goal for lactate clearance in this patient if she is not responding to initial resuscitation?

A. Lactate clearance > 10%
B. Lactate clearance > 20%
C. Lactate clearance > 30%
D. Lactate clearance > 40%

425. A 65-year-old woman with a history of heart failure with preserved ejection fraction (HFpEF) is admitted to the ICU with acute decompensated heart failure. She is treated with intravenous diuretics, but her urine output remains low. Which of the following adjunctive therapies may be considered to enhance diuresis in this patient if she has a history of renal insufficiency and is not responding to high-dose loop diuretics, metolazone, or tolvaptan/conivaptan? In addition, she has a history of hyperkalemia and hyponatremia.

A. Chlorothiazide
B. Acetazolamide
C. Low-dose dopamine
D. Hypertonic saline with furosemide

426. A 40-year-old man with a history of alcoholism is admitted to the ICU with alcoholic hepatitis and acute liver failure. He develops hepatorenal syndrome (HRS). Which of the following is the most important factor in determining the need for liver transplantation in this patient if he has type 1 HRS that is refractory to medical therapy?

    A. MELD score
    B. Child-Pugh score
    C. Presence of ascites
    D. Age

427. A 25-year-old woman with a history of asthma is admitted to the ICU with status asthmaticus. She is intubated and mechanically ventilated. Which of the following adjunctive therapies may be considered to decrease airway hyperresponsiveness and inflammation in this patient if she does not respond to standard therapy and has elevated eosinophil count and has already received magnesium sulfate?

    A. Ketamine infusion
    B. Inhaled helium-oxygen mixture (heliox)
    C. Leukotriene modifiers (e.g., montelukast)
    D. Bronchial thermoplasty

428. A 55-year-old man with a history of hypertension and hyperlipidemia presents to the ICU with an acute Stanford type B aortic dissection. He is hemodynamically stable and is treated with medical therapy. Which of the following is the most important factor to monitor closely in this patient to assess the risk of aortic rupture?

    A. Blood pressure
    B. Heart rate
    C. Aortic diameter
    D. Pain intensity

429. A 70-year-old woman with a history of chronic kidney disease (CKD) is admitted to the ICU with uremic pericarditis. She undergoes pericardiocentesis, and 500 mL of bloody fluid is drained. Which of the following is the most appropriate next step in the management of this patient if she has purulent pericarditis and is hemodynamically unstable?

    A. Repeat pericardiocentesis
    B. Pericardial window placement
    C. Pericardiectomy
    D. Initiation of antibiotic therapy

430. A 50-year-old woman with a history of rheumatoid arthritis presents to the ICU with septic shock secondary to pneumonia. She is initiated on norepinephrine for vasopressor support and broad-spectrum antibiotics. After 72 hours, her blood cultures remain negative, and her clinical status has not improved. Which of the following should be considered in the management of this patient if a non-infectious cause of her symptoms is suspected and she has a high ferritin level, cytopenias, hepatosplenomegaly, and hemophagocytosis on bone marrow biopsy?

    A. Macrophage activation syndrome (MAS)
    B. Drug-induced lupus
    C. Adult-onset Still's disease
    D. Systemic vasculitis

431. A 65-year-old male with a history of alcohol abuse presents with confusion, ataxia, and ophthalmoplegia. What is the most likely diagnosis and appropriate treatment?

    A. Wernicke encephalopathy, thiamine replacement
    B. Korsakoff syndrome, glucose infusion
    C. Delirium tremens, benzodiazepines
    D. Alcoholic hepatitis, corticosteroids

432. A patient in the ICU develops acute respiratory distress syndrome (ARDS) after a severe pneumonia. Which of the following ventilator settings is most appropriate for this patient?

A. High tidal volumes, low PEEP
B. Low tidal volumes, high PEEP
C. High respiratory rate, low inspiratory flow
D. Low respiratory rate, high inspiratory flow

433. A 78-year-old female with a history of heart failure is admitted with worsening dyspnea, orthopnea, and peripheral edema. Which medication is most likely to exacerbate her symptoms?

A. Furosemide
B. Metoprolol
C. Lisinopril
D. NSAIDs

434. A 50-year-old male presents to the ED with severe abdominal pain radiating to the back, nausea, and vomiting. His lipase is elevated.What is the most likely diagnosis and priority intervention?

A. Acute pancreatitis, pain management and fluid resuscitation
B. Cholecystitis, antibiotics and laparoscopic cholecystectomy
C. Peptic ulcer disease, proton pump inhibitors and endoscopy
D. Appendicitis, antibiotics and appendectomy

435. A patient with sepsis is experiencing hypotension and tachycardia despite adequate fluid resuscitation. Which vasopressor is most appropriate for this patient?

A. Dobutamine
B. Norepinephrine
C. Phenylephrine
D. Epinephrine

436. A 60-year-old male with a history of type 2 diabetes mellitus presents with acute onset of right-sided weakness and facial droop. Which diagnostic test is most important to determine the cause of his symptoms?

   A. Electrocardiogram (ECG)
   B. Head CT scan
   C. Carotid ultrasound
   D. Transthoracic echocardiogram

437. A patient with a history of chronic kidney disease is admitted with hyperkalemia. Which of the following interventions is most effective in shifting potassium intracellularly?

   A. Calcium gluconate
   B. Insulin and glucose
   C. Sodium polystyrene sulfonate (Kayexalate)
   D. Hemodialysis

438. A patient with a suspected pulmonary embolism undergoes a CT pulmonary angiogram, which confirms the diagnosis. What is the most appropriate initial treatment for this patient?

   A. Unfractionated heparin
   B. Low molecular weight heparin
   C. Warfarin
   D. Thrombolytic therapy

439. A 75-year-old female with a history of osteoporosis presents with a sudden onset of severe back pain after lifting a heavy object. What is the most likely diagnosis and appropriate imaging study?

   A. Spinal cord compression, MRI
   B. Vertebral compression fracture, X-ray
   C. Herniated disc, CT scan
   D. Spinal stenosis, myelogram

440. A patient with acute decompensated heart failure is receiving intravenous diuretics. Which electrolyte abnormality is most important to monitor for in this patient?

    A. Hypokalemia
    B. Hyperkalemia
    C. Hyponatremia
    D. Hypernatremia

441. A 35-year-old female with a history of intravenous drug use presents with fever, chills, and a new heart murmur. Which of the following is the most likely diagnosis?

    A. Acute pericarditis
    B. Infective endocarditis
    C. Myocarditis
    D. Rheumatic heart disease

442. A 70-year-old male with a history of hypertension and hyperlipidemia presents with sudden onset of severe chest pain radiating to the back. His blood pressure is 200/120 mmHg. Which of the following diagnostic tests is most likely to confirm the diagnosis of aortic dissection?

    A. Chest X-ray
    B. Electrocardiogram (ECG)
    C. Computed tomography angiography (CTA) of the chest
    D. Transesophageal echocardiogram (TEE)

443. A 55-year-old female with a history of cirrhosis presents with hematemesis and melena. Which of the following is the most likely source of bleeding?

    A. Mallory-Weiss tear
    B. Esophageal varices
    C. Gastric ulcer
    D. Duodenal ulcer

444. A 40-year-old male with a history of asthma presents with acute exacerbation. Which of the following is the most appropriate initial treatment?

    A. Inhaled corticosteroids
    B. Short-acting beta-agonists
    C. Long-acting beta-agonists
    D. Leukotriene modifiers

445. A 65-year-old female with a history of diabetes mellitus presents with acute onset of right lower quadrant pain, fever, and leukocytosis. Which of the following is the most likely diagnosis?

    A. Appendicitis
    B. Diverticulitis
    C. Cholecystitis
    D. Pancreatitis

446. A 50-year-old male with a history of chronic kidney disease presents with hyperkalemia. Which of the following medications is most likely to worsen his hyperkalemia?

    A. Furosemide
    B. Hydrochlorothiazide
    C. Spironolactone
    D. Acetazolamide

447. A 75-year-old female with a history of atrial fibrillation presents with sudden onset of left-sided weakness and aphasi**A.** Which of the following is the most appropriate initial intervention?

    A. Aspirin
    B. Tissue plasminogen activator (tPA)
    C. Warfarin
    D. Heparin

448. A 60-year-old male with a history of smoking presents with hoarseness, dysphagia, and weight loss. Which of the following is the most likely diagnosis?

    A. Laryngeal cancer
    B. Esophageal cancer
    C. Lung cancer
    D. Thyroid cancer

449. A 45-year-old female with a history of systemic lupus erythematosus (SLE) presents with fatigue, fever, and malar rash. Which of the following laboratory tests is most likely to be positive?

    A. Antinuclear antibodies (ANA)
    B. Anti-dsDNA antibodies
    C. Anti-Smith antibodies
    D. All of the above

450. A 30-year-old male presents with a painless testicular mass. Which of the following is the most likely diagnosis?

    A. Testicular torsion
    B. Epididymitis
    C. Testicular cancer
    D. Hydrocele

451. A 25-year-old male presents with a severe headache, stiff neck, and photophobi**A.** Which of the following diagnostic tests is most appropriate to rule out meningitis?

    A. Complete blood count (CBC)
    B. Lumbar puncture (LP)
    C. Computed tomography (CT) scan of the head
    D. Magnetic resonance imaging (MRI) of the brain

452. A 68-year-old female with a history of atrial fibrillation is admitted with acute decompensated heart failure. Which of the following medications would be most appropriate to control her ventricular rate?

　　A. Digoxin
　　B. Amiodarone
　　C. Diltiazem
　　D. Metoprolol

453. A 32-year-old male presents with sudden onset of right flank pain radiating to the groin. Which of the following diagnostic tests is most likely to confirm a diagnosis of nephrolithiasis?

　　A. Abdominal ultrasound
　　B. Non-contrast computed tomography (CT) of the abdomen and pelvis
　　C. Intravenous pyelogram (IVP)
　　D. Kidney, ureter, and bladder (KUB) X-ray

454. A 58-year-old male with a history of chronic alcoholism presents with confusion, ataxia, and nystagmus. Which of the following vitamin deficiencies is most likely responsible for his symptoms?

　　A. Vitamin B1 (thiamine)
　　B. Vitamin B12 (cobalamin)
　　C. Vitamin C (ascorbic acid)
　　D. Vitamin D (calciferol)

455. A 45-year-old female with a history of type 2 diabetes mellitus presents with a non-healing foot ulcer. Which of the following diagnostic tests is most important to assess for osteomyelitis?

　　A. X-ray of the foot
　　B. Magnetic resonance imaging (MRI) of the foot
　　C. Bone scan
　　D. Wound culture

456. A 70-year-old male with a history of hypertension and hyperlipidemia presents with acute onset of left-sided weakness and slurred speech. Which of the following interventions is the most time-sensitive in this scenario?

A. Administer aspirin
B. Administer tissue plasminogen activator (tPA)
C. Initiate intravenous heparin
D. Start antihypertensive therapy

457. A 28-year-old female with a history of asthma presents with an acute exacerbation. Which of the following arterial blood gas (ABG) findings would be most consistent with respiratory alkalosis?

A. pH 7.30, PaCO2 50 mmHg, HCO3- 24 mEq/L
B. pH 7.48, PaCO2 30 mmHg, HCO3- 22 mEq/L
C. pH 7.35, PaCO2 40 mmHg, HCO3- 28 mEq/L
D. pH 7.25, PaCO2 60 mmHg, HCO3- 26 mEq/L

458. A 55-year-old male with a history of chronic obstructive pulmonary disease (COPD) is admitted with an exacerbation. Which of the following findings on pulmonary function tests (PFTs) would be most consistent with this diagnosis?

A. Decreased forced expiratory volume in 1 second (FEV1)/forced vital capacity (FVC) ratio
B. Increased FEV1/FVC ratio
C. Normal FEV1/FVC ratio
D. Increased total lung capacity (TLC)

459. A 65-year-old female with a history of heart failure presents with worsening dyspnea, orthopnea, and peripheral edema. Which of the following laboratory tests is most important to monitor in this patient?

A. Serum creatinine
B. Brain natriuretic peptide (BNP)
C. Troponin
D. Complete blood count (CBC)

460. A 35-year-old male with a history of ulcerative colitis presents with abdominal pain, bloody diarrhea, and fever. Which of the following medications is most likely to be used for induction of remission in this patient?

A. Mesalamine
B. Sulfasalazine
C. Infliximab
D. Prednisone

DETAILED ANSWER EXPLAINATION

1. Correct Answer: C. CT angiography of the chest

Explanation:

Pulmonary embolism (PE) is the most likely diagnosis given the patient's presentation of acute chest pain, dyspnea, hemoptysis, history of DVT, and recent immobilization. These are classic risk factors and symptoms for PE.

CT angiography of the chest is the most appropriate diagnostic test in this case because:

- **Direct visualization of pulmonary arteries:** It provides a clear image of the pulmonary arteries, allowing for the identification of any blood clots (pulmonary emboli).
- **Rapid and accurate:** CT angiography is a quick and reliable test that can be performed in the emergency department.
- **High sensitivity and specificity:** It has excellent diagnostic accuracy in detecting or excluding PE.

Why other options are incorrect:

- **D-dimer:** While elevated D-dimer levels can suggest the possibility of a blood clot, it is a non-specific test and can be elevated in many other conditions. It is not diagnostic of PE, especially in older patients where D-dimer levels may be naturally elevated.
- **Troponin I:** This test is used to diagnose myocardial injury, not pulmonary embolism. Chest pain can be a symptom of both PE and myocardial infarction, so it's important to differentiate between the two.
- **Ventilation/perfusion (V/Q) scan:** This test was previously used for diagnosing PE, but it has been largely replaced by CT angiography due to its lower sensitivity and specificity, especially in patients with underlying lung disease.

Case Study:

A 78-year-old male with a history of DVT and recent hip surgery presents to the emergency department with sudden onset of shortness of breath, chest pain, and coughing up blood. A CT angiography is ordered and reveals a large pulmonary embolism in the right pulmonary artery. The patient is immediately started on anticoagulant therapy and is admitted to the intensive care unit for monitoring and further management.

In this case, CT angiography was essential for confirming the diagnosis of PE, allowing for prompt treatment and preventing potentially fatal complications.

2. Correct Answer: D. Administer a 30 mL/kg bolus of crystalloid solution
Explanation:

The patient presents with septic shock secondary to pneumonia, a life-threatening condition characterized by persistent hypotension despite adequate fluid resuscitation. The primary goal of initial management is to rapidly restore intravascular volume and improve tissue perfusion.

A 30 mL/kg bolus of crystalloid solution is the most appropriate initial step for several reasons:

- **Rapid volume expansion:** Crystalloids are readily available, inexpensive, and effectively increase intravascular volume.
- **Evidence-based:** The Surviving Sepsis Campaign guidelines recommend early goal-directed therapy, including a 30 mL/kg fluid bolus within the first three hours of resuscitation.
- **Improves hemodynamics:** Adequate fluid resuscitation can improve blood pressure, cardiac output, and tissue perfusion.

Why other options are incorrect:

- **Administer a 500 mL bolus of 0.9% normal saline:** While this may provide some volume expansion, it is not sufficient to address the severe fluid deficit in septic shock. A larger volume is needed to rapidly improve hemodynamics.
- **Initiate norepinephrine infusion:** Vasopressors are indicated for persistent hypotension after adequate fluid resuscitation. They should not be the first-line treatment.
- **Start hydrocortisone 50 mg IV every 6 hours:** Corticosteroids have a role in the management of septic shock, but they are not the initial treatment. Fluid resuscitation takes priority.

Case Study:

A 65-year-old woman with hypertension and type 2 diabetes mellitus is admitted to the ICU with septic shock secondary to pneumonia. Her blood pressure is 80/40 mmHg, heart rate is 120 beats/min, and respiratory rate is 30 breaths/min. She is confused and oliguric. The medical team immediately administers a 30 mL/kg bolus of crystalloid solution. After the fluid bolus, her blood pressure improves to 90/60 mmHg, and her mentation becomes clearer.

The patient continues to require vasopressor support and other supportive measures.

In this case, rapid fluid resuscitation with a crystalloid bolus was essential in stabilizing the patient and preventing further deterioration.

3. Correct Answer: A. Elevated serum lipase and amylase
Explanation:

Elevated serum lipase and amylase are the hallmark laboratory findings in acute pancreatitis. These enzymes are produced by the pancreas and are released into the bloodstream when the pancreas becomes inflamed.

- **Lipase** is generally considered more specific for pancreatitis than amylase.
- **Amylase** can be elevated in other conditions, such as salivary gland inflammation or macroamylasemia.

Why other options are incorrect:

- **Decreased serum calcium:** While hypocalcemia can occur in severe pancreatitis due to fat necrosis and saponification, it's a complication rather than an early diagnostic marker.
- **Elevated serum ALT and AST:** These enzymes are primarily associated with liver injury. While pancreatitis can sometimes cause liver involvement, it's not the primary abnormality in this condition.
- **All of the above:** While hypocalcemia and elevated liver enzymes can occur in severe pancreatitis, they are not consistent findings and are not the primary diagnostic markers.

Case Study:

A 50-year-old male with a history of alcoholism presents with severe abdominal pain radiating to the back, nausea, vomiting, and fever. Laboratory tests reveal an elevated serum lipase of 10 times the normal range and an elevated serum amylase of 5 times the normal range. These findings, in conjunction with the patient's clinical presentation, strongly support the diagnosis of acute pancreatitis.

4. Correct Answer: C. Synchronized intermittent mandatory ventilation (SIMV) mode, tidal volume of 6 mL/kg, PEEP of 10 cmH2O

Explanation:

A 72-year-old female with COPD experiencing acute respiratory failure requires specific ventilator settings to optimize oxygenation and minimize ventilator-induced lung injury (VILI).

Synchronized intermittent mandatory ventilation (SIMV) is the most appropriate mode for this patient because:

- **Combines controlled and spontaneous breathing:** It allows for patient-initiated breaths, which helps maintain respiratory muscle strength and reduce ventilator-induced muscle weakness.
- **Tidal volume of 6 mL/kg:** This lower tidal volume helps prevent VILI, a common complication in patients with COPD.
- **PEEP of 10 cmH2O:** Positive end-expiratory pressure (PEEP) helps to improve oxygenation by preventing alveolar collapse and increasing functional residual capacity.

Why other options are incorrect:

- **Assist control mode:** This mode provides full ventilator support and can lead to overventilation and VILI in patients with COPD.
- **Pressure control mode:** This mode can be used in certain situations, but it's generally not the first choice for patients with COPD due to the potential for overdistension.
- **Pressure support ventilation (PSV):** This mode relies heavily on patient effort and may not be adequate for a patient with acute respiratory failure.

Case Study:

A 72-year-old female with COPD is admitted to the ICU with acute respiratory failure and is intubated. She is placed on SIMV with a tidal volume of 6 mL/kg and PEEP of 10 cmH2O. Over time, her respiratory status improves, and she is gradually weaned from mechanical ventilation.

It's important to note that ventilator management is dynamic and requires frequent reassessment based on the patient's clinical condition and blood gas analysis.

5. Correct Answer: A. Cardiac tamponade

Explanation:

The classic triad of **hypotension, tachycardia, and decreased urine output** in a postoperative CABG patient is highly suggestive of **cardiac tamponade**. This occurs when fluid accumulates in the pericardial sac, compressing the heart and impairing its ability to pump effectively.

Why other options are incorrect:

- **Acute kidney injury (AKI):** While AKI can cause decreased urine output, it would typically not present with hypotension and tachycardia.
- **Pulmonary embolism (PE):** PE can cause dyspnea, chest pain, and tachypnea, but it's less likely to present with hypotension and decreased urine output in the early postoperative period.
- **Myocardial infarction (MI):** While an MI can occur post-CABG, it would typically present with chest pain and elevated cardiac markers, not the classic triad of cardiac tamponade.

Case Study:

A 60-year-old male undergoes CABG surgery and is admitted to the ICU. On postoperative day 2, he develops hypotension, tachycardia, and decreased urine output. A bedside echocardiogram reveals a large pericardial effusion with evidence of right ventricular collapse. The patient undergoes pericardiocentesis, and his symptoms improve dramatically.

In this case, rapid diagnosis and treatment of cardiac tamponade were crucial to prevent further deterioration and improve patient outcomes.

6. Correct Answer: B. Renal biopsy

Explanation:

A 45-year-old woman with a history of systemic lupus erythematosus (SLE) presenting with acute kidney injury (AKI) is highly suggestive of **lupus nephritis**. Given the complexity and potential implications of various types of lupus nephritis, a **renal biopsy** is the most appropriate initial diagnostic test to determine the specific type of kidney injury.

Why other options are incorrect:

- **Renal ultrasound:** While a renal ultrasound can provide information about kidney size, shape, and presence of obstruction, it cannot definitively diagnose the underlying cause of AKI in this patient.

- **Urine protein-to-creatinine ratio:** This test can help assess the severity of proteinuria, but it does not provide information about the specific type of kidney injury.
- **Anti-nuclear antibody (ANA) titer:** While ANA is a marker for SLE, it does not specifically diagnose lupus nephritis or its severity.

Case Study:

A 45-year-old woman with SLE presents with AKI. A renal biopsy is performed, revealing proliferative lupus nephritis with significant glomerular involvement. This diagnosis guides the treatment plan, which includes immunosuppressive therapy and close monitoring of kidney function.

A renal biopsy is essential in this case to determine the specific type of lupus nephritis, as different types of lupus nephritis require different treatment approaches.

7. Correct Answer: A. Maintain head of bed elevation at 30 degrees

Explanation:

Maintaining head of bed elevation at 30 degrees is a cornerstone of managing intracranial pressure (ICP) in patients with traumatic brain injury (TBI). This position promotes venous outflow from the brain, helping to reduce ICP.

Why other options are incorrect:

- **Hyperventilate to maintain PaCO2 between 25-30 mmHg:** While hyperventilation can temporarily decrease ICP by causing cerebral vasoconstriction, it is not a sustained or recommended strategy. Prolonged hyperventilation can lead to cerebral ischemia.
- **Administer mannitol to reduce intracranial pressure (ICP):** Mannitol is a valuable tool for acute management of elevated ICP, but it should be used judiciously and in combination with other interventions. It's not the initial or primary strategy.
- **Initiate therapeutic hypothermia:** Therapeutic hypothermia is used in specific circumstances, such as cardiac arrest or severe TBI with refractory intracranial hypertension. It's not a first-line intervention for all TBI patients.

Case Study:

A 35-year-old male is brought to the ICU after a motorcycle accident with severe head injury. To optimize intracranial pressure management, the healthcare team maintains the patient's head of bed at 30 degrees, administers appropriate sedation and analgesia, and closely monitors ICP. Mannitol and other interventions are reserved for refractory intracranial hypertension.

By consistently maintaining head of bed elevation, the healthcare team can help prevent secondary brain injury and improve patient outcomes.

8. Correct Answer: A. Octreotide

Explanation:

Octreotide is the most appropriate medication to reduce portal pressure and control bleeding in a patient with cirrhosis and acute variceal bleeding.

• **Reduces portal pressure:** Octreotide causes vasoconstriction of the splanchnic circulation, leading to a decrease in portal pressure.

• **Controls bleeding:** By reducing portal pressure, octreotide helps to control active bleeding from varices.

• **Rapid onset of action:** Octreotide works quickly, making it ideal for emergency situations.

Why other options are incorrect:

• **Propranolol:** While propranolol is used in the long-term management of portal hypertension to prevent variceal bleeding, it has a slower onset of action and is not as effective in acute bleeding.

• **Lactulose:** Lactulose is used to manage hepatic encephalopathy, not to control variceal bleeding.

• **Spironolactone:** Spironolactone is a diuretic used in the management of ascites, not for acute variceal bleeding.

Case Study:

A 55-year-old woman with cirrhosis presents to the emergency department with hematemesis. Endoscopy confirms active variceal bleeding. The patient is immediately started on octreotide infusion, and balloon tamponade is placed. The bleeding is controlled, and the patient is admitted to the ICU for further management.

In this case, octreotide was crucial in rapidly reducing portal pressure and controlling the acute variceal bleeding.

9. Correct Answer: B. Decreased cardiac index, increased systemic vascular resistance

Explanation:

Cardiogenic shock is a condition where the heart is unable to pump enough blood to meet the body's needs. This results in decreased cardiac output and tissue hypoperfusion.

- **Decreased cardiac index:** This indicates reduced cardiac output relative to body size, a hallmark of cardiogenic shock.
- **Increased systemic vascular resistance (SVR):** The body compensates for the decreased cardiac output by constricting blood vessels to maintain blood pressure. This increased SVR further exacerbates the problem as it increases the afterload on the heart.

Why other options are incorrect:

- **Increased cardiac index:** This would indicate increased cardiac output, which is opposite to what occurs in cardiogenic shock.
- **Decreased systemic vascular resistance:** This would indicate vasodilation, which is also opposite to the compensatory mechanisms in cardiogenic shock.
- **Combinations of increased or decreased cardiac index and SVR:** These combinations do not accurately reflect the hemodynamic profile of cardiogenic shock.

Understanding these hemodynamic parameters is crucial for guiding treatment strategies, such as inotropic support, vasodilators, and mechanical circulatory support.

10. Correct Answer: C. Lorazepam

Explanation:

Lorazepam is the most appropriate first-line treatment for status epilepticus.

- **Rapid onset of action:** It quickly terminates seizures, which is crucial in this life-threatening condition.
- **Predictable efficacy:** Lorazepam has a consistent response rate in terminating seizures.

Why other options are incorrect:

- **Phenytoin:** While effective in preventing seizures, it has a slower onset of action and is not the first-line treatment for status epilepticus.

- **Levetiracetam:** Primarily used as a maintenance anti-epileptic drug, it is not as effective as benzodiazepines in terminating acute seizures.
- **Valproic acid:** While effective in preventing seizures, it also has a slower onset of action and is not the first-line treatment for status epilepticus.

Case Study:

A 28-year-old male is brought to the ICU with ongoing seizure activity. Lorazepam is administered intravenously, and the seizure activity stops within minutes. The patient is monitored closely for seizure recurrence and additional anti-epileptic medications are considered for seizure prophylaxis.

11. Correct Answer: B. Marfan syndrome

Explanation:

A young, tall, and thin individual presenting with a spontaneous pneumothorax is highly suggestive of an underlying connective tissue disorder. **Marfan syndrome** is a genetic disorder affecting connective tissue, including the lungs. Patients with Marfan syndrome often have long, slender limbs and are at increased risk of developing spontaneous pneumothorax due to weakened lung tissue.

Why other options are incorrect:

- **Cystic fibrosis:** This is a genetic disorder primarily affecting the lungs and pancreas, but it typically presents with chronic respiratory symptoms, not acute pneumothorax.
- **Pulmonary embolism:** This is a blood clot in the lung artery, and its presentation typically includes dyspnea, chest pain, and tachypnea, without a specific association with tall and thin individuals.
- **Sarcoidosis:** This is an inflammatory condition that can affect multiple organs, including the lungs, but it doesn't have a specific association with spontaneous pneumothorax in tall, thin individuals.

In conclusion, the combination of a young, tall, thin patient with spontaneous pneumothorax strongly points to Marfan syndrome as the most likely underlying condition.

12. Correct Answer: A. Dobutamine
Explanation:
Dobutamine is the most appropriate medication to improve cardiac output in a patient with acute decompensated heart failure.

• **Increases cardiac contractility:** Dobutamine is a beta-adrenergic agonist that directly increases the force of heart muscle contractions, leading to improved cardiac output.

• **Improves short-term hemodynamics:** It provides a rapid and effective way to increase cardiac output in patients with acute decompensated heart failure.

Why other options are incorrect:

• **Nitroglycerin:** While nitroglycerin is a vasodilator that can reduce preload and afterload, it primarily helps to reduce pulmonary congestion rather than improving cardiac output.

• **Furosemide:** A loop diuretic, furosemide is used to reduce fluid overload and improve symptoms of heart failure, but it does not directly improve cardiac output.

• **Metoprolol:** A beta-blocker, metoprolol is used in the chronic management of heart failure but is not appropriate for acute decompensated heart failure as it can worsen cardiac output.

In conclusion, dobutamine is the most appropriate initial therapy to improve cardiac output in a patient with acute decompensated heart failure. However, it's important to note that this is often used in combination with other therapies, such as diuretics and vasodilators, to optimize patient management.

13. Correct Answer: D. All of the above
Explanation:
All of the listed physical exam findings are associated with infective endocarditis, though their occurrence varies in frequency.

• **Janeway lesions:** These are painless, erythematous macules on the palms and soles, caused by septic emboli.

• **Osler nodes:** These are painful, red nodules on the fingers and toes, also caused by septic emboli.

• **Roth spots:** These are retinal hemorrhages with pale centers, indicating embolization to the retina.

While not all patients with infective endocarditis will exhibit all of these findings, their presence is highly suggestive of the diagnosis, especially in a high-risk patient like a 48-year-old male with a history of intravenous drug use.

14. Correct Answer: D. Increase the positive end-expiratory pressure (PEEP)

Explanation:

Acute Respiratory Distress Syndrome (ARDS) is characterized by diffuse alveolar damage leading to hypoxemia refractory to oxygen therapy. The primary goal in managing ARDS is to improve oxygenation while minimizing lung injury.

- **Increasing PEEP** is the most appropriate initial intervention to improve oxygenation in this case. PEEP helps to recruit collapsed alveoli and prevent their collapse at the end of expiration, improving oxygenation.

Why other options are incorrect:

- **Increasing FiO2 to 100%:** While increasing FiO2 can temporarily improve oxygenation, it can lead to oxygen toxicity and should be used judiciously.
- **Initiating prone positioning:** Prone positioning can be very effective in improving oxygenation in ARDS patients, but it is typically implemented after initial stabilization and is not the first-line intervention.
- **Administering inhaled nitric oxide:** Inhaled nitric oxide can be beneficial in certain cases, but it is not the first-line treatment for ARDS and requires careful monitoring due to potential side effects.

Note: In addition to increasing PEEP, other management strategies for ARDS include protective lung ventilation (low tidal volumes, low respiratory rates), fluid management, and consideration of additional therapies like prone positioning and extracorporeal membrane oxygenation (ECMO) in severe cases.

15. Correct Answer: C. pH 7.25, PaCO2 60 mmHg, PaO2 55 mmHg, HCO3- 28 mEq/L

Explanation:

Status asthmaticus is a severe, life-threatening exacerbation of asthma that is unresponsive to standard therapy. It leads to progressive airway obstruction and respiratory failure.

The arterial blood gas (ABG) values in option C are most consistent with this condition:

- **pH 7.25:** Indicates respiratory acidosis, a hallmark of severe airway obstruction and impending respiratory failure.
- **PaCO2 60 mmHg:** Elevated PaCO2 confirms the respiratory acidosis and indicates worsening ventilation.
- **PaO2 55 mmHg:** Low PaO2 signifies hypoxemia, which is common in severe asthma.
- **HCO3- 28 mEq/L:** The bicarbonate level is compensatory for the respiratory acidosis but cannot fully correct the pH.

Why other options are incorrect:
- Options A and B represent milder degrees of respiratory distress with normal or compensated acid-base balance.
- Option D shows respiratory alkalosis, which is typically seen in the early stages of an asthma exacerbation, not status asthmaticus.

In conclusion, the ABG values in option C reflect the severe respiratory compromise characteristic of status asthmaticus.

16. Correct Answer: B. Blood glucose of 350 mg/dL, serum bicarbonate of 15 mEq/L, anion gap of 20

Explanation:

Diabetic ketoacidosis (DKA) is characterized by hyperglycemia, metabolic acidosis (indicated by low bicarbonate), and an increased anion gap due to the accumulation of ketone bodies.

- **Hyperglycemia:** A blood glucose level of 350 mg/dL is consistent with DKA.
- **Metabolic acidosis:** A serum bicarbonate of 15 mEq/L indicates metabolic acidosis, a hallmark of DKA.
- **Increased anion gap:** An anion gap of 20 is elevated and supports the diagnosis of DKA due to the accumulation of unmeasured anions (ketone bodies).

Why other options are incorrect:
- Options A and C have normal or near-normal bicarbonate levels, which are inconsistent with DKA.
- Option D has an excessively low bicarbonate level and a very high anion gap, which might indicate a more severe metabolic acidosis but is less likely to be the initial presentation of DKA.

In conclusion, the laboratory findings in option B are most consistent with the diagnosis of diabetic ketoacidosis.

17. Correct Answer: D. All of the above

Explanation:

A patient with subarachnoid hemorrhage (SAH) is at risk for several serious complications:

- **Vasospasm:** This is a narrowing of blood vessels in the brain, which can lead to decreased blood flow and ischemic injury.
- **Hydrocephalus:** This is an accumulation of cerebrospinal fluid (CSF) in the brain, which can increase intracranial pressure and cause brain damage.
- **Rebleeding:** This occurs when the aneurysm ruptures again, leading to further bleeding in the brain.

All of these complications are potentially life-threatening and require aggressive management.

18. Correct Answer: B. Prolonged prothrombin time (PT)

Explanation:

Acute liver failure results in impaired liver function, including the synthesis of clotting factors. A **prolonged prothrombin time (PT)** is a hallmark of liver failure due to the liver's inability to produce clotting factors.

Why other options are incorrect:

- **Elevated serum albumin:** Albumin is synthesized by the liver, and its levels tend to decrease in liver failure, not increase.
- **Decreased serum ammonia:** The liver plays a crucial role in converting ammonia to urea. In liver failure, ammonia levels increase, not decrease.
- **Normal serum bilirubin:** Bilirubin levels are typically elevated in liver failure due to impaired conjugation and excretion.

A prolonged PT, in conjunction with other clinical and laboratory findings, is a strong indicator of acute liver failure.

19. Correct Answer: A. Syndrome of inappropriate antidiuretic hormone secretion (SIADH)

Explanation:

Small cell lung cancer is notoriously associated with a variety of paraneoplastic syndromes, but the most common is the **Syndrome of Inappropriate Antidiuretic Hormone (SIADH)**. This occurs when the tumor produces or stimulates the release of antidiuretic hormone (ADH), leading to water retention, hyponatremia, and concentrated urine.

Why other options are incorrect:

- **Cushing syndrome** is more commonly associated with small cell lung cancer, but it's not the most common paraneoplastic syndrome.
- **Lambert-Eaton myasthenic syndrome** and **hypercalcemia** are more frequently associated with other types of lung cancer or other malignancies.

Therefore, in a patient with small cell lung cancer presenting with symptoms of water retention, hyponatremia, and concentrated urine, SIADH should be strongly suspected.

20. Correct Answer: D. All of the above
Explanation:

All of the listed interventions are crucial in managing an acute exacerbation of COPD:

- **Inhaled corticosteroids:** Help to reduce airway inflammation and improve lung function.
- **Inhaled bronchodilators:** Relax the airway muscles, improving airflow and reducing symptoms like wheezing and shortness of breath.
- **Noninvasive positive pressure ventilation (NIPPV):** Can be used to support ventilation and oxygenation in patients with worsening respiratory failure.

The specific combination and timing of these interventions will depend on the severity of the exacerbation and the patient's clinical status.

21. Correct Answer: B. Ceftriaxone plus azithromycin
Explanation:

The patient is a 40-year-old woman with rheumatoid arthritis presenting with community-acquired pneumonia (CAP). Given the patient's underlying immunosuppression due to rheumatoid arthritis, it is crucial to select an antibiotic regimen that covers atypical and typical pathogens.

Ceftriaxone plus azithromycin is the most appropriate choice for empiric treatment in this case because:

- **Ceftriaxone** provides coverage for typical respiratory pathogens like Streptococcus pneumoniae, Haemophilus influenzae, and Moraxella catarrhalis.

- **Azithromycin** covers atypical pathogens like Legionella pneumophila, Mycoplasma pneumoniae, and Chlamydia pneumoniae.

Why other options are incorrect:

- **Azithromycin:** While effective against atypical pathogens, it lacks coverage for common typical respiratory pathogens.
- **Moxifloxacin:** This is a respiratory fluoroquinolone with broad coverage, but it is generally reserved for patients with severe CAP or those who have failed initial therapy due to concerns about increasing antibiotic resistance.
- **Piperacillin/tazobactam:** This is a broad-spectrum antibiotic primarily used for severe infections, including hospital-acquired pneumonia, and is not typically the first-line choice for community-acquired pneumonia.

Case Study:

A 40-year-old woman with rheumatoid arthritis presents to the emergency department with fever, chills, productive cough, and right lower lobe consolidation on chest x-ray. She is started on intravenous ceftriaxone and oral azithromycin. Blood cultures are obtained, and sputum is sent for culture and sensitivity. After 48-72 hours, if the patient is clinically improving, the intravenous ceftriaxone can be switched to oral amoxicillin-clavulanate.

By combining ceftriaxone and azithromycin, we ensure broad-spectrum coverage for both typical and atypical pathogens in an immunocompromised patient with pneumonia.

22. Correct Answer: A. Esmolol

Explanation:

Aortic dissection is a life-threatening condition characterized by a tear in the aorta. The primary goal of initial management is to reduce aortic shear stress by decreasing blood pressure and heart rate.

Esmolol is the most appropriate medication for initial blood pressure management in this case because:

- **Rapid onset and short half-life:** Esmolol has a rapid onset of action and a very short half-life, allowing for precise blood pressure control. This is crucial in managing the dynamic hemodynamic changes associated with aortic dissection.
- **Selective beta-1 blocker:** Esmolol selectively blocks beta-1 receptors, reducing heart rate and myocardial contractility without significantly affecting

peripheral vascular resistance. This helps to decrease afterload while minimizing the risk of hypotension.

Why other options are incorrect:

- **Nitroprusside, Nicardipine, and Hydralazine:** While these are vasodilators and can lower blood pressure, they do not address the increased myocardial contractility and heart rate that contribute to aortic shear stress. Rapidly decreasing blood pressure without controlling heart rate can worsen the dissection.

Case Study:

A 55-year-old man presents with severe chest pain radiating to his back. A CT scan confirms an aortic dissection. The patient is immediately started on an esmolol infusion to rapidly reduce heart rate and blood pressure. Pain management with intravenous opioids is also initiated. The patient is monitored closely for hemodynamic stability and progression of the dissection.

By using esmolol as the initial treatment, we aim to quickly reduce aortic shear stress and stabilize the patient while awaiting further diagnostic and therapeutic interventions.

23. Correct Answer: C. Sacubitril/valsartan

Explanation:

A 65-year-old woman with heart failure with reduced ejection fraction (HFrEF) presenting with worsening dyspnea and peripheral edema, along with elevated BNP levels, indicates a worsening of her heart failure.

Sacubitril/valsartan is the most appropriate medication to add to her regimen in this case because:

- **Combination therapy:** It combines a neprilysin inhibitor (sacubitril) and an angiotensin receptor blocker (valsartan) in a single pill.
- **Reduces morbidity and mortality:** It has been shown to reduce the risk of cardiovascular death and hospitalization for heart failure compared to other treatments.
- **Improves symptoms:** It improves symptoms of heart failure, including dyspnea and fatigue.

Why other options are incorrect:

- **Spironolactone:** While spironolactone is a valuable medication for managing heart failure, it is typically added after optimizing other therapies, such as angiotensin-converting enzyme inhibitors (ACEIs) or angiotensin receptor blockers (ARBs).

- **Furosemide:** A loop diuretic like furosemide is useful for managing acute fluid overload and reducing symptoms, but it does not address the underlying pathophysiology of heart failure.
- **Digoxin:** While digoxin can be used for rate control in atrial fibrillation and may improve some symptoms of heart failure, it has a narrow therapeutic index and is not considered a first-line treatment for HFrEF.

Case Study:

A 65-year-old woman with HFrEF is admitted to the ICU with worsening dyspnea and peripheral edema. Despite optimal medical therapy with an ACE inhibitor, beta-blocker, and diuretic, her symptoms continue to worsen. A BNP level is elevated, confirming worsening heart failure. The patient is started on sacubitril/valsartan, and her symptoms gradually improve. She is discharged home with close follow-up and continues on the medication.

By adding sacubitril/valsartan to the patient's treatment regimen, we aim to improve her heart failure symptoms, reduce the risk of hospitalization, and improve overall prognosis.

24. Correct Answer: B. Bowel rest and nasogastric decompression
Explanation:

Toxic megacolon is a life-threatening complication of inflammatory bowel disease characterized by severe colonic dilation and inflammation. The primary goal of initial management is to decrease colonic distention and reduce the risk of colonic perforation.

Bowel rest and nasogastric decompression are the cornerstone of initial management because:

- **Decreases colonic distention:** By stopping oral intake and decompressing the stomach, we reduce the amount of intraluminal contents, allowing the colon to rest and potentially decrease inflammation.
- **Reduces risk of perforation:** Decompression helps to lower the intraluminal pressure, reducing the risk of colonic perforation.

Why other options are incorrect:

- **Intravenous corticosteroids:** While corticosteroids can be beneficial in managing severe ulcerative colitis, they are not the initial treatment for toxic megacolon.
- **Surgical colectomy:** Surgery is considered if medical management fails or if there is evidence of peritonitis or impending perforation. It is not the initial treatment.
- **Intravenous antibiotics and fluids:** While important for supportive care, they are not the primary intervention for managing toxic megacolon.

Case Study:

A 30-year-old man with ulcerative colitis presents with severe abdominal pain, bloody diarrhea, and fever. A CT scan confirms toxic megacolon. The patient is immediately placed on bowel rest with nasogastric decompression. Intravenous fluids and electrolytes are initiated, and broad-spectrum antibiotics are administered for suspected infection. The patient is closely monitored for signs of clinical deterioration or peritonitis, which would indicate the need for surgical intervention.

By implementing bowel rest and nasogastric decompression, we aim to reduce colonic distention, decrease the risk of perforation, and stabilize the patient while preparing for potential surgical intervention.

25. Correct Answer: B. Mechanical thrombectomy

Explanation:

A 70-year-old woman with atrial fibrillation presenting with a large left middle cerebral artery (MCA) occlusion is a classic indication for **mechanical thrombectomy**.

- **Large vessel occlusion (LVO):** A large MCA occlusion is a type of LVO, which has a high risk of disability or death.
- **Time-sensitive intervention:** Mechanical thrombectomy is a minimally invasive procedure that can rapidly remove the clot, restoring blood flow to the brain.
- **Improved outcomes:** Studies have shown that mechanical thrombectomy significantly improves functional outcomes compared to medical management alone.

Why other options are incorrect:

- **Intravenous tissue plasminogen activator (tPA):** While tPA is effective in some cases of ischemic stroke, it has limitations, including a narrow therapeutic window and increased risk of hemorrhagic transformation. For large vessel occlusions, mechanical thrombectomy is generally preferred.
- **Aspirin and clopidogrel:** These antiplatelet agents are used for stroke prevention but are not effective in acute stroke treatment.
- **Heparin drip:** Heparin is an anticoagulant used for prevention of deep vein thrombosis (DVT) but is not indicated for acute stroke treatment.

Case Study:

A 70-year-old woman with atrial fibrillation presents with acute onset of weakness and slurred speech. A CT scan shows no evidence of hemorrhage, and a CT angiography reveals a large left MCA occlusion. The patient is immediately taken to the interventional radiology suite for mechanical thrombectomy. The procedure is successful in removing the clot, and the patient shows significant improvement in neurological function.

By performing mechanical thrombectomy promptly, we can maximize the chances of a good outcome for the patient.

26. Correct Answer: A. Low tidal volume ventilation (6 mL/kg)

Explanation:

A patient with acute pancreatitis who develops ARDS requires specific ventilator settings to protect the lungs and improve oxygenation.

Low tidal volume ventilation (6 mL/kg) is the cornerstone of ARDS management. This strategy aims to minimize lung injury by reducing alveolar overdistension and preventing volutrauma.

Why other options are incorrect:

- **High positive end-expiratory pressure (PEEP):** While PEEP is important in ARDS management to improve oxygenation by preventing alveolar collapse, it should be titrated carefully to avoid overdistension. High PEEP can increase lung injury.
- **High respiratory rate:** Increasing respiratory rate can lead to increased tidal volumes, which can worsen lung injury. The focus should be on low tidal volumes with appropriate PEEP.

- **Prone positioning:** Prone positioning is a valuable adjunct therapy for ARDS, but it is not a primary ventilator setting. It is typically used in conjunction with low tidal volume ventilation and PEEP.

Case Study:

A 50-year-old man with acute pancreatitis develops ARDS requiring mechanical ventilation. The ventilator is set to low tidal volume (6 mL/kg) and PEEP is titrated to optimize oxygenation while minimizing lung injury. The patient is closely monitored for hemodynamic stability and oxygenation status. Prone positioning is considered if there is persistent hypoxemia despite optimal ventilator settings.

By using low tidal volume ventilation, we aim to protect the lungs from further injury and improve overall outcomes in this patient with ARDS.

27. Correct Answer: B. Cyclophosphamide

Explanation:

A 45-year-old woman with SLE presenting with lupus nephritis, significant proteinuria, and hematuria requires aggressive immunosuppression to induce remission.

Cyclophosphamide is the most appropriate choice for inducing remission in this case due to its potent immunosuppressive effects. It is effective in reducing proteinuria, hematuria, and preventing progression to end-stage renal disease.

Why other options are incorrect:

- **Mycophenolate mofetil:** While effective in maintaining remission, mycophenolate mofetil is generally used as a steroid-sparing agent or for less severe forms of lupus nephritis. It is not the first-line treatment for active, proliferative lupus nephritis.
- **Rituximab:** This is a B-cell depleting agent primarily used in refractory lupus nephritis or for patients with anti-neutrophil cytoplasmic antibody (ANCA)-associated glomerulonephritis. It is not the initial treatment for active lupus nephritis.
- **Hydroxychloroquine:** This is a first-line treatment for mild lupus but is not effective in inducing remission in patients with active lupus nephritis.

Case Study:

A 45-year-old woman with SLE presents with worsening renal function, significant proteinuria, and hematuria. A renal biopsy confirms active proliferative lupus nephritis. The patient is initiated on intravenous cyclophosphamide for induction therapy, followed by oral maintenance therapy with mycophenolate mofetil and corticosteroids. Close monitoring of renal function and complete blood count is essential to manage potential side effects.

By using cyclophosphamide as the induction therapy, we aim to rapidly induce remission of lupus nephritis and prevent progression to end-stage renal disease.

28. Correct Answer: B. Intravenous normal saline
Explanation:

Hyperosmolar hyperglycemic state (HHS) is a serious complication of type 2 diabetes characterized by severe hyperglycemia, dehydration, and hyperosmolarity. The primary goal of initial management is to correct severe dehydration.

Intravenous normal saline is the most appropriate intervention for initial management because:

• **Rapid volume expansion:** Intravenous fluids are essential to correct severe dehydration and restore intravascular volume.

• **Improved hemodynamics:** Volume expansion helps to improve blood pressure and organ perfusion.

• **Reduction of serum osmolality:** By correcting dehydration, we can gradually reduce the elevated serum osmolality.

Why other options are incorrect:

• **Intravenous insulin infusion:** While insulin is crucial for lowering blood glucose in HHS, it should be initiated after adequate fluid resuscitation. Administering insulin without adequate fluid replacement can worsen cellular dehydration.

• **Subcutaneous insulin:** Subcutaneous insulin is not effective in rapidly correcting hyperglycemia in HHS. Intravenous insulin is required.

• **Oral hypoglycemic agents:** Oral hypoglycemic agents are ineffective in the setting of severe hyperglycemia and dehydration.

Case Study:

A 60-year-old man with type 2 diabetes presents with altered mental status, polyuria, and polydipsia. Laboratory tests reveal a blood glucose of 1200 mg/dL and a serum osmolality of 350 mOsm/kg. The patient is immediately started on intravenous normal saline to correct dehydration. Once hemodynamic stability is achieved, an insulin infusion is initiated to gradually lower blood glucose levels.

By prioritizing fluid resuscitation with intravenous normal saline, we can prevent life-threatening complications associated with severe dehydration and improve the overall outcome for the patient.

29. Correct Answer: A. Intravenous magnesium sulfate

Explanation:

A 25-year-old woman with status asthmaticus who has failed to respond to inhaled bronchodilators and systemic corticosteroids is experiencing severe airway obstruction.

Intravenous magnesium sulfate is the most appropriate next step in management. It has bronchodilator properties and can help to relax airway smooth muscle, improve gas exchange, and reduce airway hyperresponsiveness.

Why other options are incorrect:

- **Inhaled heliox:** While heliox can improve gas exchange in some cases, it is not a primary treatment for severe status asthmaticus and is often used as an adjunct therapy.

- **Intravenous ketamine:** Ketamine is a sedative-hypnotic agent with some bronchodilator properties, but its role in the management of status asthmaticus is limited and not well-established.

- **Endotracheal intubation and mechanical ventilation:** These are considered when the patient is in respiratory failure and is not responding to maximal medical therapy. While this may be necessary in the future, it is not the most appropriate next step at this point.

Case Study:

A 25-year-old woman with status asthmaticus is admitted to the ICU and treated with inhaled bronchodilators and intravenous corticosteroids. Despite these measures, her respiratory status continues to deteriorate. Intravenous magnesium sulfate is administered, and there is a gradual improvement in her respiratory function. The patient is closely monitored, and additional therapies may be considered if necessary.

By administering intravenous magnesium sulfate, we aim to improve airway function and prevent further deterioration of respiratory status.

30. Correct Answer: C. Extracorporeal membrane oxygenation (ECMO)

Explanation:

A 75-year-old man with cardiogenic shock refractory to inotropic and vasopressor support, and presenting with oliguria, is in a critical condition. The patient is likely experiencing severe cardiac dysfunction and end-organ hypoperfusion.

Extracorporeal membrane oxygenation (ECMO) is the most appropriate intervention in this scenario. ECMO provides temporary circulatory and respiratory support by removing blood from the body, oxygenating it, and returning it to the body. This allows the heart and lungs to rest and recover.

Why other options are incorrect:

- **Intra-aortic balloon pump (IABP):** While IABP can improve coronary blood flow and reduce afterload, it is not sufficient for patients in refractory cardiogenic shock with severe hemodynamic instability.
- **Impella device:** This is a percutaneous left ventricular assist device that can improve cardiac output, but it may not be adequate for patients with severe cardiogenic shock and end-organ dysfunction.
- **Surgical revascularization:** While surgical revascularization may be considered as a definitive treatment for cardiogenic shock secondary to coronary artery disease, it is not the immediate intervention in this critically ill patient.

Case Study:

A 75-year-old man with a history of hypertension and coronary artery disease presents with cardiogenic shock refractory to inotropic and vasopressor support. Despite maximal medical therapy, the patient remains hypotensive and oliguric. Given the severity of the patient's condition, ECMO is initiated to provide temporary circulatory and respiratory support while awaiting further management options, such as cardiac transplantation or ventricular assist device implantation.

ECMO is a complex and high-risk therapy, but it can be lifesaving for patients with refractory cardiogenic shock.

31. Correct Answer: C. Dexmedetomidine

Explanation:

A 75-year-old man with Parkinson's disease who is intubated and agitated in the ICU requires careful medication selection.

Dexmedetomidine is the most appropriate choice for managing agitation and delirium in this patient because:

- **Sedative and analgesic properties:** Dexmedetomidine provides sedation and analgesia without the respiratory depressant effects of other sedatives.
- **Preservation of spontaneous breathing:** It allows for frequent sedation interruptions, which can help to assess the patient's readiness for weaning from mechanical ventilation.
- **Reduced risk of delirium:** Dexmedetomidine may have a lower risk of delirium compared to other sedatives.

Why other options are incorrect:

- **Haloperidol:** While haloperidol can be effective for managing agitation, it carries a risk of extrapyramidal side effects, which can be exacerbated in patients with Parkinson's disease.
- **Quetiapine:** This is an antipsychotic medication primarily used for psychosis, and its role in managing ICU delirium is less established. It also carries a risk of hypotension and QT prolongation.
- **Propofol:** While propofol is a potent sedative, it is primarily used for induction and maintenance of anesthesia. It is not ideal for long-term sedation in the ICU due to its potential for respiratory depression and propofol infusion syndrome.

Case Study:

A 75-year-old man with Parkinson's disease develops aspiration pneumonia requiring intubation and mechanical ventilation. He becomes agitated and delirious. Dexmedetomidine is initiated as a sedative, and the patient's agitation gradually subsides. Sedation is titrated to allow for frequent sedation interruptions to assess readiness for weaning.

By using dexmedetomidine, we aim to manage agitation and delirium while minimizing respiratory depression and preserving spontaneous breathing.

32. Correct Answer: B. Exploratory laparotomy with bowel resection and anastomosis

Explanation:

A 35-year-old woman with Crohn's disease presenting with severe abdominal pain, fever, and leukocytosis, and subsequently diagnosed with a perforated bowel, requires immediate surgical intervention.

Exploratory laparotomy with bowel resection and anastomosis is the most appropriate management in this case because:

- **Identification of the perforation:** Exploratory laparotomy allows for direct visualization of the abdomen to locate the perforation site.
- **Resection of diseased bowel:** The affected portion of the bowel, which is likely inflamed and necrotic, can be removed.
- **Restoration of bowel continuity:** Anastomosis reconnects the healthy ends of the bowel, preserving bowel function whenever possible.

Why other options are incorrect:

- **Laparoscopic appendectomy:** This procedure is indicated for appendicitis, not perforated bowel.
- **Hartmann's procedure:** This procedure involves a temporary colostomy and is typically reserved for cases of severe peritonitis or when primary anastomosis is not feasible.
- **Laparoscopic ileostomy:** An ileostomy is a permanent procedure creating an opening for stool to pass through the abdomen. It is not the initial treatment for a perforated bowel.

Case Study:

A 35-year-old woman with Crohn's disease presents with severe abdominal pain, fever, and leukocytosis. A CT scan confirms a perforated bowel. The patient is immediately taken to the operating room for exploratory laparotomy. The surgical team identifies a perforated segment of the ileum and resect the affected bowel. A primary anastomosis is performed, and a temporary ileostomy is created to protect the anastomosis.

By performing exploratory laparotomy with bowel resection and anastomosis, we aim to control the infection, prevent further complications, and preserve bowel function whenever possible.

33. Correct Answer: A. Hyperkalemia, hyperphosphatemia, hypocalcemia, hyperuricemia

Explanation:

Tumor lysis syndrome (TLS) is a rapid breakdown of tumor cells, leading to the release of intracellular contents into the bloodstream. This results in a characteristic electrolyte imbalance.

- **Hyperkalemia:** Increased potassium levels due to the release of intracellular potassium.
- **Hyperphosphatemia:** Increased phosphate levels due to the release of intracellular phosphate.
- **Hypocalcemia:** Calcium is bound to phosphate, leading to decreased ionized calcium levels.
- **Hyperuricemia:** Increased uric acid levels due to the breakdown of nucleic acids from tumor cells.

These electrolyte abnormalities can lead to life-threatening complications, such as cardiac arrhythmias, renal failure, and acute kidney injury.

Why other options are incorrect:

Options B, C, and D contain incorrect electrolyte imbalances that are not consistent with TLS.

34. Correct Answer: A. Pyridostigmine

Explanation:

A 45-year-old woman with multiple sclerosis (MS) experiencing acute respiratory failure secondary to a myasthenic crisis requires immediate intervention to improve respiratory function.

Pyridostigmine is a cholinesterase inhibitor that prolongs the action of acetylcholine, improving neuromuscular transmission. In patients with myasthenic crisis, it can significantly improve muscle strength, including respiratory muscles, and help to improve respiratory function.

Why other options are incorrect:

- **Edrophonium:** While edrophonium is a cholinesterase inhibitor, it has a shorter duration of action compared to pyridostigmine and is primarily used for diagnostic purposes in myasthenia gravis.
- **Neostigmine:** Similar to pyridostigmine, neostigmine is a cholinesterase inhibitor, but it has a higher risk of side effects, including gastrointestinal upset and increased muscarinic effects.
- **Plasmapheresis:** Plasmapheresis is a therapeutic procedure that removes antibodies from the blood and can be beneficial in managing myasthenic crisis. However, it is not a first-line treatment and requires time to take effect.

Case Study:

A 45-year-old woman with MS presents with rapidly worsening respiratory failure. A diagnosis of myasthenic crisis is made. The patient is intubated and placed on mechanical ventilation. Pyridostigmine is initiated intravenously to improve muscle strength and respiratory function. The patient's respiratory status is closely monitored, and additional therapies, such as plasmapheresis or intravenous immunoglobulins, may be considered if necessary.

By administering pyridostigmine, we aim to rapidly improve respiratory muscle strength and support the patient's respiratory function until the crisis is resolved.

35. Correct Answer: D. All of the above
Explanation:

Hepatic encephalopathy is a serious complication of liver disease characterized by impaired brain function due to the accumulation of ammonia in the blood. The goal of treatment is to reduce ammonia levels and improve mental status. All of the listed medications play a role in this process.

- **Lactulose:** This is a non-absorbable osmotic laxative that acidifies the colon, trapping ammonia and promoting its excretion in the stool.
- **Rifaximin:** This is a non-absorbable antibiotic that reduces intestinal bacteria, which are responsible for producing ammonia.
- **Neomycin:** Similar to rifaximin, neomycin is an antibiotic that decreases intestinal bacteria and ammonia production.

While all three medications contribute to reducing ammonia levels, they often work synergistically. The choice of specific medication may depend on factors such as patient tolerance, severity of hepatic encephalopathy, and underlying liver disease.

36. Correct Answer: A. Captopril
Explanation:

Scleroderma renal crisis is a rapidly progressive, potentially fatal complication of systemic sclerosis characterized by severe hypertension and acute kidney injury.

Captopril, an angiotensin-converting enzyme (ACE) inhibitor, is the cornerstone of treatment for scleroderma renal crisis. It effectively lowers blood pressure and improves renal perfusion.

Why other options are incorrect:

- **Losartan:** While an angiotensin receptor blocker (ARB), losartan is not as effective as ACE inhibitors in managing scleroderma renal crisis. ACE inhibitors have been shown to be more effective in reducing renal vascular resistance and improving renal blood flow.
- **Amlodipine:** A calcium channel blocker, amlodipine can lower blood pressure but does not specifically target the underlying pathophysiology of scleroderma renal crisis.
- **Hydralazine:** A vasodilator, hydralazine can lower blood pressure but is not as effective as ACE inhibitors in managing scleroderma renal crisis and has a higher risk of side effects, such as lupus-like syndrome.

Case Study:

A 30-year-old woman with systemic sclerosis presents with rapidly worsening hypertension and acute kidney injury. Scleroderma renal crisis is suspected. Captopril is initiated immediately to lower blood pressure and protect renal function. The patient is closely monitored for blood pressure and renal function, and additional antihypertensive agents may be added if needed.

Early and aggressive treatment with captopril is crucial in improving outcomes for patients with scleroderma renal crisis.

37. Correct Answer: A. Intravenous calcium gluconate

Explanation:

A patient with a serum potassium of 7.0 mEq/L and ECG changes (peaked T waves and widening QRS complex) is experiencing a medical emergency due to the risk of life-threatening cardiac arrhythmias.

Intravenous calcium gluconate is the most appropriate immediate intervention to stabilize the cardiac membrane. It directly counteracts the effects of hyperkalemia on the heart, protecting against lethal arrhythmias.

Why other options are incorrect:

- **Intravenous insulin and glucose:** While this is an effective way to shift potassium into the intracellular space, it takes longer to act compared to calcium gluconate and is not as immediate in protecting the heart.
- **Inhaled beta-agonist:** Beta-agonists can help shift potassium intracellularly, but their effect is less predictable and slower than calcium gluconate and insulin.

- **Hemodialysis:** While hemodialysis is a definitive treatment for hyperkalemia, it is not the immediate intervention needed to stabilize the cardiac membrane in this critical situation.

Case Study:

A 65-year-old man with CKD presents with acute hyperkalemia and ECG changes. Intravenous calcium gluconate is administered immediately to protect the heart. Simultaneously, other measures to lower potassium levels, such as insulin and glucose, as well as calcium carbonate and sodium polystyrene sulfonate, are initiated. The patient is closely monitored for cardiac rhythm disturbances and renal function.

By administering calcium gluconate first, we can quickly stabilize the cardiac membrane and prevent life-threatening arrhythmias.

38. Correct Answer: A. Propylthiouracil (PTU)

Explanation:

Thyroid storm is a life-threatening condition characterized by severe hyperthyroidism. The primary goal of treatment is to block the production of thyroid hormones.

Propylthiouracil (PTU) is the most appropriate medication to achieve this. It inhibits both thyroid peroxidase and peripheral conversion of T4 to T3, rapidly reducing thyroid hormone levels.

Why other options are incorrect:

- **Methimazole:** While also effective in blocking thyroid hormone synthesis, PTU is preferred in thyroid storm due to its additional ability to inhibit peripheral conversion of T4 to T3.
- **Propranolol:** A beta-blocker, propranolol helps manage the sympathetic symptoms of thyroid storm (tachycardia, hypertension), but it does not address the underlying hyperthyroidism.
- **Iodine:** Iodine can be used to block thyroid hormone release in preparation for surgery, but it is not the initial treatment for thyroid storm and can exacerbate the condition in the short term.

Case Study:

A 40-year-old woman with Graves' disease presents with severe tachycardia, hypertension, fever, and agitation consistent with thyroid storm. PTU is immediately administered intravenously to block thyroid hormone production.

Additional measures, such as beta-blockers (propranolol) and corticosteroids, are initiated to manage the hyperadrenergic state. The patient is closely monitored for hemodynamic stability and thyroid function.

By using PTU as the initial treatment, we aim to rapidly reduce thyroid hormone levels and prevent further deterioration of the patient's condition.

39. Correct Answer: A. Dobutamine

Explanation:

A 55-year-old man with a history of hypertension and coronary artery disease who develops cardiogenic shock post-STEMI requires a medication that can rapidly increase cardiac contractility.

Dobutamine is the most appropriate choice in this scenario because:

- **Increases cardiac contractility:** It directly stimulates beta-1 adrenergic receptors, leading to increased heart rate and contractility.
- **Improves cardiac output:** Increased contractility results in improved cardiac output, which is crucial in cardiogenic shock.
- **Rapid onset of action:** Dobutamine has a rapid onset of action, allowing for quick hemodynamic improvement.

Why other options are incorrect:

- **Milrinone:** While it also increases cardiac contractility, milrinone has a longer onset of action compared to dobutamine and is often used as a second-line agent.
- **Dopamine:** Dopamine has both inotropic and vasopressor effects, but at higher doses, it can cause vasoconstriction, which may worsen tissue perfusion in cardiogenic shock.
- **Norepinephrine:** Primarily a vasopressor, norepinephrine increases systemic vascular resistance but has limited inotropic effects. It is more suitable for maintaining blood pressure rather than improving cardiac output.

Case Study:

A 55-year-old man with STEMI develops cardiogenic shock despite PCI. Dobutamine is initiated as an infusion to improve cardiac contractility and increase cardiac output. The patient is closely monitored for hemodynamic response and potential side effects.

By using dobutamine, we aim to rapidly improve cardiac function and support tissue perfusion in the setting of cardiogenic shock.

40. Correct Answer: A. Norepinephrine
Explanation:
A 25-year-old woman with septic shock secondary to a UTI who remains hypotensive and tachycardic despite fluid resuscitation and antibiotics requires vasopressor support.

Norepinephrine is the first-line vasopressor for septic shock. It has both alpha and beta-adrenergic effects, leading to vasoconstriction and increased heart rate, which effectively raises blood pressure and improves tissue perfusion.

Why other options are incorrect:

• **Vasopressin:** While vasopressin can be used as a second-line agent in septic shock, it is generally reserved for patients who do not respond to norepinephrine. It can cause vasoconstriction, leading to decreased blood flow to the kidneys and other organs.

• **Hydrocortisone:** Corticosteroids have a role in the management of septic shock but are not first-line therapy for hypotension. They are typically used in patients with persistent hypotension despite adequate fluid resuscitation and vasopressor support.

• **All of the above:** While all of these medications may have a role in the management of septic shock, norepinephrine is the initial vasopressor of choice.

Case Study:

A 25-year-old woman presents with septic shock secondary to a UTI. Despite fluid resuscitation and antibiotics, she remains hypotensive and tachycardic. Norepinephrine is initiated as a vasopressor infusion to improve blood pressure and tissue perfusion. The patient is closely monitored for hemodynamic response and potential side effects.

By using norepinephrine, we aim to rapidly stabilize the patient's blood pressure and improve organ perfusion in the setting of septic shock.

41. Correct Answer: B. Nitroglycerin
Explanation:
Nitroglycerin is the most appropriate medication to reduce cardiac preload in a patient with acute decompensated heart failure (ADHF). It is a potent vasodilator that primarily affects venous capacitance, leading to a decrease in preload. This reduces the amount of blood returning to the heart, decreasing ventricular filling pressures and improving symptoms of congestion.

Why other options are incorrect:

- **Milrinone:** This is an inotropic agent that increases cardiac contractility, which can actually increase preload.
- **Dobutamine:** Similar to milrinone, dobutamine is an inotropic agent that increases cardiac contractility and can elevate preload.
- **Dopamine:** Primarily a vasoconstrictor, dopamine would increase afterload and worsen congestion in a patient with ADHF.

By reducing preload with nitroglycerin, we aim to alleviate pulmonary congestion and improve the patient's dyspnea.

42. Correct Answer: A. Staphylococcus aureus

Explanation:

Staphylococcus aureus is the most likely cause of infective endocarditis in a 30-year-old man with a history of intravenous drug use.

- **Intravenous drug use (IVDU):** This is a significant risk factor for endocarditis caused by Staphylococcus aureus.
- **Rapid onset:** Staphylococcus aureus often leads to a more aggressive and rapidly progressive form of endocarditis compared to other organisms.
- **High mortality rate:** Infections caused by Staphylococcus aureus are associated with higher rates of complications and mortality.

Why other options are incorrect:

- **Streptococcus pneumoniae:** This organism is more commonly associated with pneumonia.
- **Enterococcus faecalis:** While enterococci can cause endocarditis, they are more commonly associated with nosocomial infections and patients with underlying comorbidities.
- **Pseudomonas aeruginosa:** This organism is often associated with hospital-acquired infections and is less likely to be the cause of community-acquired endocarditis.

In conclusion, the patient's history of intravenous drug use, along with the presentation of fever, chills, and a new heart murmur, strongly suggests Staphylococcus aureus as the most likely causative organism.

43. Correct Answer: D. All of the above
Explanation:
Acute kidney injury (AKI) in the setting of acute pancreatitis is a complex issue with multiple potential causes. In this patient with a history of alcohol abuse, all three types of AKI can potentially contribute to the renal dysfunction:
- **Prerenal AKI:** Hypovolemia due to fluid shifts, vomiting, and decreased oral intake can lead to reduced renal perfusion and AKI.
- **Intrinsic AKI:** Direct damage to the kidneys from pancreatic enzymes, inflammatory mediators, and ischemia can cause acute tubular necrosis (ATN).
- **Postrenal AKI:** While less common, obstruction of the urinary tract due to factors such as kidney stones or retroperitoneal fibrosis can contribute to AKI.

It's important to note that these factors often interact and contribute to AKI in a synergistic manner. Therefore, a combination of these mechanisms is likely responsible for the AKI in this patient.

44. Correct Answer: A. Cyclophosphamide
Explanation:
Diffuse alveolar hemorrhage (DAH) in a patient with systemic lupus erythematosus (SLE) is a life-threatening condition. It requires aggressive immunosuppression to control the underlying inflammatory process.

Cyclophosphamide is the most appropriate medication for this condition due to its potent immunosuppressive effects. It has been shown to be effective in inducing remission of DAH and improving survival rates.

Why other options are incorrect:
- **Azathioprine:** While azathioprine is an immunosuppressant, it has a slower onset of action compared to cyclophosphamide and is generally less effective in rapidly controlling severe inflammation like DAH.
- **Mycophenolate mofetil:** This is a immunosuppressive agent, but it is not as potent as cyclophosphamide and is often used as a maintenance therapy rather than for induction of remission in severe cases like DAH.
- **Rituximab:** While rituximab is effective in certain autoimmune conditions, it is not the first-line treatment for DAH. It may be considered in refractory cases or for patients with specific autoantibody profiles.

Case Study:

A 45-year-old woman with SLE presents with acute respiratory failure and is diagnosed with DAH. She is immediately started on high-dose intravenous cyclophosphamide to induce remission of the underlying inflammatory process. Supportive measures, such as blood transfusions and plasmapheresis, may also be required to manage the acute phase of the illness.

By using cyclophosphamide, we aim to rapidly control the underlying inflammation, stop the bleeding, and improve the patient's respiratory function.

45. Correct Answer: C. Synchronized intermittent mandatory ventilation (SIMV)

Explanation:

A 70-year-old man with COPD experiencing an acute exacerbation requiring intubation and mechanical ventilation needs a ventilator mode that balances support with patient-driven breathing.

Synchronized intermittent mandatory ventilation (SIMV) is the most appropriate choice for this patient because:

• **Combines controlled and spontaneous breathing:** It allows for a set number of mandatory breaths delivered by the ventilator (mandatory breaths) and spontaneous breaths initiated by the patient.

• **Preserves respiratory muscle function:** By allowing spontaneous breaths, SIMV helps maintain respiratory muscle strength and reduces the risk of ventilator-induced muscle weakness.

• **Facilitates weaning:** As the patient improves, the number of mandatory breaths can be gradually reduced, promoting weaning from the ventilator.

Why other options are incorrect:

• **Assist control (AC):** This mode provides full ventilator support and may lead to overventilation and muscle weakness in COPD patients.

• **Pressure control (PC):** While PC can be used in certain situations, it may not be the best choice for COPD patients due to the potential for overdistension.

• **Pressure support ventilation (PSV):** This mode relies heavily on patient effort and may not be adequate for a patient with acute respiratory failure.

By using SIMV, we aim to optimize oxygenation, minimize ventilator-induced lung injury, and facilitate weaning from mechanical ventilation in a patient with COPD exacerbation.

46. Correct Answer: D. Endotracheal intubation and mechanical ventilation
Explanation:

A patient with status asthmaticus who has failed to respond to maximal medical therapy, including inhaled bronchodilators, systemic corticosteroids, and intravenous magnesium sulfate, is experiencing severe respiratory failure.

Endotracheal intubation and mechanical ventilation are indicated to protect the airway, improve oxygenation, and prevent respiratory muscle fatigue.

Why other options are incorrect:

• **Intravenous ketamine:** While ketamine has some bronchodilator properties, it is not a primary treatment for severe status asthmaticus and is not indicated at this stage.

• **Inhaled heliox:** While heliox can improve gas exchange in some cases, it is not a substitute for mechanical ventilation when the patient is in respiratory failure.

• **Noninvasive positive pressure ventilation (NIPPV):** NIPPV can be effective in some cases of acute respiratory failure, but it is often insufficient in patients with severe status asthmaticus who require invasive ventilation.

By initiating endotracheal intubation and mechanical ventilation, we can provide the necessary respiratory support to stabilize the patient and prevent further deterioration.

47. Correct Answer: A. Nimodipine
Explanation:

Nimodipine is the standard of care for preventing and treating cerebral vasospasm after subarachnoid hemorrhage (SAH). It is a calcium channel blocker that specifically targets cerebral arteries, helping to prevent and reduce the severity of vasospasm.

Why other options are incorrect:

• **Nicardipine, Verapamil, and Diltiazem:** While these are also calcium channel blockers, they primarily affect peripheral blood vessels and have not been shown to be as effective in preventing cerebral vasospasm as nimodipine.

By administering nimodipine early in the course of SAH, we aim to reduce the risk of delayed ischemic neurological deficits (DIND) caused by cerebral vasospasm.

48. Correct Answer: A. Intravenous potassium chloride

Explanation:

Hypokalemia is a common complication of diabetic ketoacidosis (DKA) due to several factors including osmotic diuresis, insulin-mediated cellular potassium shift, and vomiting. It is crucial to correct hypokalemia promptly to prevent serious cardiac arrhythmias.

- **Intravenous potassium chloride** is the most appropriate and rapid method to correct severe hypokalemia in this setting. It allows for immediate and controlled potassium replacement.

Why other options are incorrect:

- **Oral potassium chloride:** Oral potassium would be too slow to correct severe hypokalemia and is not suitable in this acute setting.
- **Discontinue insulin infusion:** Discontinuing insulin would worsen hyperglycemia and exacerbate the underlying metabolic imbalance.
- **Administer kayexalate:** Kayexalate is used for the treatment of hyperkalemia, not hypokalemia. It is a cation-exchange resin that binds potassium in the gastrointestinal tract for excretion.

By administering intravenous potassium chloride, we can rapidly correct the hypokalemia and prevent potentially fatal cardiac arrhythmias.

49. Correct Answer: A. Propranolol

Explanation:

Propranolol is the most commonly used beta-blocker for the prevention of variceal rebleeding in patients with cirrhosis. It reduces portal pressure by decreasing cardiac output and reducing hepatic blood flow.

Why other options are incorrect:

- **Nadolol and Carvedilol:** While these are also beta-blockers, propranolol is the most extensively studied and recommended for the prevention of variceal rebleeding.

By using propranolol, we aim to reduce the risk of recurrent variceal bleeding and improve the overall prognosis for patients with cirrhosis.

50. Correct Answer: D. Apixaban

Explanation:

A 75-year-old woman with atrial fibrillation who has experienced an ischemic stroke despite not being a candidate for reperfusion therapy requires effective anticoagulation to prevent recurrent stroke.

Apixaban is the most appropriate choice in this case. It is a direct oral anticoagulant (DOAC) that has been shown to be more effective than warfarin in preventing stroke in patients with atrial fibrillation. It also has the advantage of not requiring regular INR monitoring.

Why other options are incorrect:

• **Aspirin:** While aspirin can reduce the risk of stroke, it is less effective than anticoagulants in preventing stroke in patients with atrial fibrillation.

• **Clopidogrel:** This is an antiplatelet agent primarily used for preventing coronary artery disease events, not for stroke prevention in patients with atrial fibrillation.

• **Warfarin:** While warfarin was the standard of care for stroke prevention in atrial fibrillation, DOACs like apixaban are now preferred due to their superior efficacy and safety profile.

By using apixaban, we aim to significantly reduce the risk of recurrent stroke in this patient while minimizing the risk of bleeding complications.

51. Correct Answer: B. Cyclophosphamide

Explanation:

Cyclophosphamide is the standard of care for induction therapy in patients with diffuse proliferative lupus nephritis (Class IV). It is a highly effective immunosuppressant that rapidly reduces disease activity and prevents progression to end-stage renal disease.

Why other options are incorrect:

• **Mycophenolate mofetil (MMF):** While MMF is used for maintenance therapy in lupus nephritis, it is not as potent as cyclophosphamide for induction therapy, especially in severe cases like Class IV.

• **Rituximab:** Rituximab is primarily used in refractory lupus nephritis or for patients with anti-neutrophil cytoplasmic antibody (ANCA)-associated glomerulonephritis.

- **Hydroxychloroquine:** This is a first-line treatment for mild lupus but is not effective in inducing remission in patients with active lupus nephritis, especially in severe cases like Class IV.

Therefore, cyclophosphamide is the most appropriate choice for induction therapy in this patient with severe lupus nephritis.

52. Correct Answer: C. Computed tomography angiography (CTA) of the chest

Explanation:

The patient's presentation of severe tearing chest pain radiating to the back, along with hypertension and tachycardia, is highly suggestive of an aortic dissection.

Computed tomography angiography (CTA) of the chest is the most appropriate diagnostic test to confirm this diagnosis. It provides a rapid and accurate visualization of the aorta, allowing for the identification of an aortic dissection.

Why other options are incorrect:

- **Chest X-ray:** While it can show mediastinal widening suggestive of aortic dissection, it is not as specific as CTA.
- **Electrocardiogram (ECG):** An ECG can rule out myocardial infarction, but it is not diagnostic for aortic dissection.
- **Transthoracic echocardiogram (TTE):** While it can detect some aortic dissections, it is limited in its ability to visualize the entire thoracic aorta.

A CTA of the chest is the gold standard for diagnosing aortic dissection and is essential for guiding immediate management.

53. Correct Answer: A. Norepinephrine

Explanation:

The patient is presenting with hypotension and tachycardia despite adequate fluid resuscitation, which are classic signs of septic shock, even in the absence of an obvious infection.

Norepinephrine is the first-line vasopressor for septic shock. It has both alpha and beta-adrenergic effects, leading to vasoconstriction and increased heart rate, which effectively raises blood pressure and improves tissue perfusion.

Why other options are incorrect:

- **Dobutamine:** Primarily increases cardiac contractility, which may not be the primary issue in this patient.
- **Milrinone:** Also primarily inotropic, and may not be the best choice for initial management of hypotension in septic shock.
- **Vasopressin:** Used as a second-line agent for septic shock, typically after inadequate response to norepinephrine.

By using norepinephrine, we aim to rapidly stabilize the patient's blood pressure and improve organ perfusion in the setting of suspected septic shock.

54. Correct Answer: D. Lung-protective ventilation with low tidal volumes and appropriate PEEP

Explanation:

Acute Respiratory Distress Syndrome (ARDS) requires a specific approach to ventilation to prevent further lung injury.

- **Lung-protective ventilation** with **low tidal volumes** and **appropriate PEEP** is the cornerstone of ARDS management. This strategy aims to minimize alveolar overdistension (volutrauma) and prevent alveolar collapse (atelectasis).
- **Low tidal volumes** reduce the amount of air delivered to the lungs with each breath, preventing excessive pressure on the delicate alveolar structures.
- **Positive end-expiratory pressure (PEEP)** helps to keep the alveoli open, preventing collapse and improving oxygenation.

Why other options are incorrect:

- **High tidal volume ventilation:** This can lead to volutrauma and worsen lung injury in ARDS patients.
- **Low PEEP:** Insufficient PEEP can lead to alveolar collapse and decreased oxygenation.
- **High respiratory rate:** Increasing respiratory rate can increase tidal volume, which is detrimental in ARDS.

By implementing lung-protective ventilation, we aim to improve oxygenation while minimizing further lung injury in patients with ARDS.

55. Correct Answer: B. Decreased fibrinogen level

Explanation:

Disseminated Intravascular Coagulation (DIC) is a complex disorder characterized by widespread activation of the clotting cascade, leading to both thrombosis and bleeding.

- **Decreased fibrinogen level:** Fibrinogen is consumed in the clotting process. Thus, a decreased fibrinogen level is a hallmark of DIC.

Why other options are incorrect:

- **Elevated platelet count:** Platelets are actually consumed in DIC, leading to thrombocytopenia.
- **Normal prothrombin time (PT):** PT would be prolonged in DIC due to the consumption of clotting factors.
- **Decreased D-dimer level:** D-dimer is a marker of fibrinolysis, and it would be elevated in DIC, not decreased.

Therefore, a decreased fibrinogen level is the most consistent laboratory finding with DIC.

56. Correct Answer: B. Intravenous insulin and glucose

Explanation:

To shift potassium intracellularly and rapidly lower serum potassium levels, the combination of **intravenous insulin and glucose** is the most effective intervention.

- **Insulin** stimulates the sodium-potassium pump, driving potassium into the cells.
- **Glucose** is administered to prevent hypoglycemia induced by insulin.

Why other options are incorrect:

- **Intravenous calcium gluconate:** While essential for stabilizing cardiac membranes in hyperkalemia, it does not shift potassium intracellularly.
- **Oral sodium polystyrene sulfonate (Kayexalate):** This is used for long-term management of hyperkalemia, but it has a slow onset of action and is not suitable for acute hyperkalemia with ECG changes.
- **Hemodialysis:** This is a definitive treatment for hyperkalemia but is not the first-line therapy for acute management.

By administering intravenous insulin and glucose, we can quickly lower serum potassium levels and reduce the risk of life-threatening cardiac arrhythmias.

57. Correct Answer: D. All of the above

Explanation:

All of the listed hemodynamic goals are important during the initial resuscitation phase of septic shock:

- **Mean arterial pressure (MAP) > 65 mmHg:** Adequate blood pressure is essential to maintain organ perfusion.
- **Central venous pressure (CVP) 8-12 mmHg:** CVP is a surrogate marker for intravascular volume status. A CVP within this range generally indicates adequate fluid resuscitation.
- **Urine output > 0.5 mL/kg/hour:** Urine output is a marker of renal perfusion and is a crucial indicator of tissue perfusion.

Achieving these hemodynamic goals is part of the early goal-directed therapy (EGDT) approach to managing septic shock. It's important to note that these are initial targets and may need to be adjusted based on the patient's response to treatment and ongoing assessment.

58. Answer: A. Aspirin

Explanation:

Aspirin is the most appropriate medication to prevent recurrent stroke in this patient.

- **Reasoning:**
  o The patient has a history of atrial fibrillation, a known risk factor for ischemic stroke.
  o He has experienced an acute ischemic stroke, indicating a high risk of recurrence.
  o He is ineligible for reperfusion therapy, limiting other treatment options.
  o Aspirin is a platelet inhibitor that reduces the risk of clot formation, thereby decreasing the likelihood of another ischemic stroke.

Why other options are incorrect:

- **Clopidogrel:** While also a platelet inhibitor, it is generally preferred after percutaneous coronary intervention (PCI) or in patients with aspirin intolerance.
- **Warfarin:** This anticoagulant is indicated for patients with non-valvular atrial fibrillation but carries a higher risk of bleeding compared to newer anticoagulants. Given the patient's recent stroke and being in the ICU, the risk of bleeding is increased.

- **Apixaban:** This is a newer anticoagulant with a better bleeding profile than warfarin. However, it is generally reserved for patients with atrial fibrillation who are not candidates for aspirin or other antiplatelet agents. In this case, aspirin is the more appropriate choice.

Case Study:

Mr. Johnson, a 70-year-old man with a history of atrial fibrillation, is admitted to the ICU after experiencing an ischemic stroke. Due to the timing of the stroke, he is not eligible for reperfusion therapy. Given his risk factors and the nature of his stroke, the decision is made to start aspirin therapy to reduce the risk of another stroke.

By understanding the patient's specific condition and the mechanisms of action of different medications, the healthcare provider can select the most appropriate treatment to prevent recurrent stroke.

59. A. Hypoglycemia

Explanation:

High-dose intravenous corticosteroids are a common treatment for lupus nephritis, but they can lead to several metabolic side effects. Among the options provided, **hypoglycemia** is the most likely complication.

- **Reasoning:**
  o Corticosteroids can increase blood sugar levels (hyperglycemia), a well-known side effect. However, paradoxically, when started at high doses, they can cause a temporary drop in blood sugar, leading to hypoglycemia.
  o This is often seen in patients with underlying conditions like diabetes or those who are fasting or have poor nutritional intake.

Why other options are incorrect:

- **Hyperkalemia:** This is more commonly associated with conditions like kidney failure or the use of potassium-sparing diuretics. Corticosteroids tend to cause hypokalemia, not hyperkalemia.
- **Hypernatremia:** Corticosteroids can actually lead to hyponatremia (low sodium levels), not hypernatremia.
- **Hypercalcemia:** This is more associated with conditions like hyperparathyroidism or certain types of cancer. Corticosteroids do not typically cause hypercalcemia.

Case Study:

A 35-year-old woman with SLE is admitted to the ICU for lupus nephritis. Despite her normal blood sugar levels before starting high-dose corticosteroids, she develops hypoglycemia within the first 24 hours of treatment. This is managed by close monitoring of blood glucose levels and administration of glucose as needed.

It's crucial for healthcare providers to be aware of the potential for hypoglycemia when initiating high-dose corticosteroid therapy, especially in at-risk patients, to prevent severe complications.

60. A. Ciprofloxacin

Explanation:

Prophylactic antibiotics are often used in patients with cirrhosis and variceal bleeding to prevent spontaneous bacterial peritonitis (SBP). Among the options given, **ciprofloxacin** is the most commonly used and recommended antibiotic for this purpose.

- **Reasoning:**
  - Ciprofloxacin is a broad-spectrum antibiotic that effectively covers the most common bacteria responsible for SBP, such as *Escherichia coli* and the *Enterobacteriaceae* family.
  - It has good oral bioavailability, allowing for continued prophylaxis after discharge from the ICU.

Why other options are incorrect:

- **Ceftriaxone:** While effective against gram-negative bacteria, it has a narrower spectrum compared to ciprofloxacin and requires parenteral administration.
- **Trimethoprim-sulfamethoxazole (TMP-SMX):** This antibiotic is effective against a wide range of bacteria, but it is not the first-line choice for SBP prophylaxis.
- **Amoxicillin-clavulanate:** This antibiotic is primarily used for infections caused by beta-lactamase-producing bacteria, which are not typically the predominant pathogens in SBP.

Case Study:

A 50-year-old man with a history of alcoholism is admitted to the ICU with acute variceal bleeding. After successful endoscopic variceal ligation and initiation of octreotide, the patient is started on prophylactic ciprofloxacin to reduce the risk of developing spontaneous bacterial peritonitis. Regular monitoring of liver function and abdominal examinations are performed to assess for early signs of SBP.

By using prophylactic antibiotics like ciprofloxacin, the risk of SBP can be significantly reduced in patients with cirrhosis and variceal bleeding.

61. D. Intravenous antibiotics and fluids

Explanation:

Acute cholangitis is a serious infection of the bile ducts, characterized by the Charcot's triad: fever, right upper quadrant pain, and jaundice. The initial management focuses on stabilizing the patient and controlling the infection.

- **Reasoning:**

o Intravenous antibiotics are essential to combat the underlying infection and prevent sepsis. Broad-spectrum antibiotics are typically initiated based on local resistance patterns.

o Intravenous fluids are necessary to correct dehydration and maintain hemodynamic stability.

Why other options are incorrect:

- **Laparoscopic cholecystectomy:** While definitive management of acute cholangitis often involves cholecystectomy, it is not the initial intervention. The patient's condition needs to be stabilized first.

- **Endoscopic retrograde cholangiopancreatography (ERCP):** This is a diagnostic and therapeutic procedure used to visualize the bile ducts and treat biliary obstruction. However, it is not the first-line treatment for acute cholangitis and carries risks of pancreatitis.

- **Percutaneous transhepatic cholangiography (PTC):** Similar to ERCP, PTC is a diagnostic and therapeutic procedure used to visualize the bile ducts. It is not the initial management for acute cholangitis.

Case Study:

A 55-year-old woman presents to the emergency department with fever, chills, and right upper quadrant abdominal pain. Blood tests reveal elevated liver enzymes and an elevated white blood cell count, consistent with acute cholangitis. The patient is immediately started on intravenous antibiotics and fluids. Once the patient is stabilized, further diagnostic tests and interventions, such as ERCP or PTC, can be considered.

By promptly initiating appropriate antibiotic and fluid therapy, the risk of complications from acute cholangitis can be significantly reduced.

62. B. Intra-aortic balloon pump (IABP)

Explanation:

In a patient with STEMI undergoing emergent PCI, an **intra-aortic balloon pump (IABP)** is often considered to improve outcomes.

- **Reasoning:**
  o An IABP provides temporary circulatory support by increasing coronary and cerebral perfusion, reducing afterload, and augmenting cardiac output.
  o It is particularly beneficial in patients with severe heart failure or cardiogenic shock following STEMI.

Why other options are incorrect:

- **Therapeutic hypothermia:** This is indicated primarily in patients with post-cardiac arrest refractory ventricular fibrillation.
- **Glycoprotein IIb/IIIa inhibitors:** These are antiplatelet agents used during PCI to prevent stent thrombosis, but they are not considered adjunctive therapy to improve overall outcomes in this setting.
- **Thrombolytic therapy:** This is the preferred treatment for STEMI patients who cannot access PCI within a timely manner. In this case, the patient is undergoing PCI, so thrombolytics are not indicated.

Case Study:

A 65-year-old man with a history of hypertension and diabetes mellitus presents to the ICU with STEMI. Despite successful PCI, the patient develops cardiogenic shock. An IABP is inserted to improve cardiac output and reduce afterload, leading to improved hemodynamic stability.

The judicious use of IABP in patients with STEMI and cardiogenic shock can significantly improve outcomes by providing temporary circulatory support until the heart can recover or other interventions are implemented.

63. A. Interstitial Lung Disease (ILD)

Explanation:

- **Interstitial Lung Disease (ILD)** is the most likely diagnosis given the patient's history of systemic sclerosis (scleroderma), worsening dyspnea, hypoxemia, and the characteristic HRCT findings of ground-glass opacities and honeycombing.

- **Systemic sclerosis** is a connective tissue disease that often involves the lungs, leading to ILD.
- **Ground-glass opacities** and **honeycombing** on HRCT are classic findings of interstitial lung disease.

Why other options are incorrect:

- **Pulmonary embolism (PE):** While PE can cause dyspnea and hypoxemia, the HRCT findings are not consistent with PE. PE typically presents with perfusion defects on CT angiography.
- **Pulmonary hypertension (PH):** While PH can occur in patients with scleroderma, it typically doesn't present with ground-glass opacities and honeycombing on HRCT.
- **Pneumonia:** Pneumonia can cause dyspnea, hypoxemia, and ground-glass opacities on HRCT, but it typically presents with fever, cough, and other inflammatory markers. Additionally, the patient's history of scleroderma and the characteristic honeycombing pattern are not consistent with pneumonia.

Case Study:

A 40-year-old woman with known systemic sclerosis presents with worsening shortness of breath and decreased oxygen saturation. An HRCT scan reveals bilateral ground-glass opacities and honeycombing, consistent with interstitial lung disease. The patient is started on supportive care, including oxygen therapy, and is referred to a pulmonologist for further evaluation and management.

Understanding the association between systemic sclerosis and ILD is crucial for early diagnosis and management of respiratory complications in these patients.

Would you like to proceed to the next question?

64. **D. All of the above**

Explanation:

All of the listed interventions are commonly used to decrease intracranial pressure (ICP) in patients with traumatic brain injury (TBI).

- **Mannitol infusion:** This osmotic diuretic helps to reduce cerebral edema by drawing fluid from the brain tissue into the bloodstream.
- **Hyperventilation:** Lowering the partial pressure of carbon dioxide ($PaCO_2$) through controlled hyperventilation causes vasoconstriction of cerebral blood vessels, reducing intracranial blood volume.

- **Head-of-bed elevation to 30 degrees:** This position promotes venous drainage from the brain, helping to decrease ICP.

While these interventions are effective in reducing ICP, it's crucial to monitor for potential side effects and complications, such as hypotension, electrolyte imbalances, and cerebral ischemia.

65. B. Uremic acidosis

Explanation:

The patient is a 70-year-old woman with a history of chronic kidney disease (CKD) presenting with metabolic acidosis. The ABG results (pH 7.25, PaCO2 30 mmHg, HCO3- 15 mEq/L) confirm a metabolic acidosis with respiratory compensation (decreased PaCO2).

- **Uremic acidosis** is the most likely cause in this patient due to her underlying CKD. The kidneys are responsible for acid-base balance, and when they are impaired, they cannot effectively excrete acid, leading to metabolic acidosis.

Why other options are incorrect:

- **Diabetic ketoacidosis (DKA):** While DKA can cause metabolic acidosis, it is more common in patients with type 1 diabetes and is characterized by hyperglycemia, ketonuria, and an anion gap metabolic acidosis.
- **Lactic acidosis:** This is often associated with tissue hypoxia or shock and is characterized by an elevated lactate level. There is no indication of these conditions in the patient's history or presentation.
- **Salicylate toxicity:** This can cause metabolic acidosis, but it is usually accompanied by other symptoms such as tinnitus, hyperventilation, and fever. There is no evidence of salicylate ingestion in the patient's history.

Case Study:

A 70-year-old woman with a history of CKD is admitted to the ICU with worsening fatigue and shortness of breath. Laboratory tests reveal elevated creatinine and blood urea nitrogen (BUN) levels, consistent with worsening kidney function. An ABG is obtained, confirming metabolic acidosis. The patient is initiated on dialysis to correct the acid-base imbalance and manage the underlying CKD.

Understanding the relationship between CKD and metabolic acidosis is crucial for timely diagnosis and management of this complication.

66. D. All of the above
Explanation:
Hepatic encephalopathy is a complex condition resulting from the accumulation of toxins in the blood due to liver dysfunction. The management often involves a multi-faceted approach to reduce the ammonia levels and improve brain function.

- **Lactulose:** This is a non-absorbable sugar that acidifies the colon, trapping ammonia and converting it to ammonium ions, which are less readily absorbed.
- **Rifaximin:** This is a non-absorbable antibiotic that reduces intestinal bacteria, which are responsible for ammonia production.
- **Neomycin:** Similar to rifaximin, neomycin is an antibiotic that decreases intestinal bacteria and ammonia production.

All three medications work synergistically to improve mental status in patients with hepatic encephalopathy by targeting different aspects of ammonia metabolism.

67. A. Metronidazole
Explanation:
Metronidazole is the most appropriate treatment for amebic liver abscess. It is a potent antiprotozoal agent that effectively kills the Entamoeba histolytica parasite responsible for the infection.

Why other options are incorrect:
- **Chloroquine:** While used for other protozoal infections, it is not effective against Entamoeba histolytica.
- **Praziquantel:** This drug is used for treating infections caused by flatworms, not amebiasis.
- **Albendazole:** Effective against intestinal parasites, albendazole is not the first-line treatment for amebic liver abscess.

Case Study:
A 30-year-old woman with a history of intravenous drug use presents with fever, chills, and right upper quadrant pain. Ultrasound reveals a liver abscess. Given her risk factors and symptoms, amebic liver abscess is suspected. Metronidazole is initiated immediately to treat the infection. The patient's symptoms improve, and the abscess gradually resolves.

Early and appropriate treatment with metronidazole is crucial for the successful management of amebic liver abscess and preventing complications.

68. D. ACE inhibitor

Explanation:

ACE inhibitors are the most appropriate choice to reduce the risk of ventricular remodeling in a patient with STEMI who is not a candidate for reperfusion therapy.

- **Reasoning:**
  - Ventricular remodeling is the process by which the heart changes its structure and function after a heart attack. ACE inhibitors help prevent this by reducing left ventricular afterload, decreasing blood pressure, and inhibiting the renin-angiotensin-aldosterone system (RAAS).
  - By blocking the RAAS, ACE inhibitors help to reduce myocardial fibrosis and improve cardiac function.

Why other options are incorrect:

- **Aspirin and Clopidogrel:** These are antiplatelet agents used to prevent blood clot formation and are crucial in the acute management of STEMI, but they do not directly impact ventricular remodeling.
- **Beta-blocker:** While beta-blockers are essential in the management of STEMI for reducing heart rate and myocardial oxygen demand, their primary role is in reducing myocardial ischemia, not specifically targeting ventricular remodeling.

Case Study:

A 65-year-old man with hypertension and diabetes mellitus presents with STEMI. Due to delayed presentation, he is not eligible for reperfusion therapy. In addition to standard treatment, an ACE inhibitor is initiated to help prevent adverse ventricular remodeling and improve long-term outcomes.

By starting ACE inhibitor therapy early in the course of STEMI, healthcare providers can significantly reduce the risk of heart failure and improve the patient's quality of life.

69. B. Computed tomography (CT) scan of the abdomen

Explanation:

A CT scan of the abdomen is the most appropriate imaging modality to confirm a diagnosis of toxic megacolon.

- **Reasoning:**

o CT scan provides detailed images of the abdomen, allowing for accurate assessment of colon dilation, bowel wall thickening, presence of free air (indicating perforation), and other complications.

o It can also help identify other potential causes of the patient's symptoms, such as abscesses or ileus.

Why other options are incorrect:

• **Abdominal X-ray:** While it can show colonic distention, it is less sensitive and specific than CT for evaluating the bowel wall, identifying complications, and assessing other abdominal organs.

• **Magnetic resonance imaging (MRI):** Although MRI can provide excellent soft tissue detail, it is not the first-line imaging for acute conditions like toxic megacolon. It is also more time-consuming and expensive than CT.

• **Ultrasound of the abdomen:** While useful for evaluating other abdominal organs, ultrasound is limited in its ability to assess the entire colon and identify complications of toxic megacolon.

Case Study:

A 40-year-old woman with a history of ulcerative colitis presents to the ICU with abdominal pain, distention, and fever. A CT scan of the abdomen reveals massive colonic dilation, bowel wall thickening, and evidence of peritonitis, confirming the diagnosis of toxic megacolon. The patient is immediately taken to surgery for colectomy.

Early diagnosis and prompt management are crucial for improving outcomes in patients with toxic megacolon.

70. C. Noninvasive positive pressure ventilation (NIPPV)

Explanation:

Noninvasive positive pressure ventilation (NIPPV) is the most appropriate adjunctive therapy for this patient with refractory status asthmaticus.

• **Reasoning:**

o NIPPV can improve oxygenation, reduce the work of breathing, and decrease the risk of intubation in patients with severe respiratory failure due to asthma.

o It helps to maintain alveolar ventilation, improve gas exchange, and reduce hyperinflation.

Why other options are incorrect:

- **Heliox:** While it can improve gas flow in airways, it is generally not as effective as NIPPV in improving oxygenation and reducing respiratory distress in severe asthma.
- **Ketamine:** This is a sedative-analgesic agent primarily used for procedural sedation or pain management. It does not directly address the underlying respiratory failure in status asthmaticus.
- **Extracorporeal membrane oxygenation (ECMO):** This is a highly invasive and complex therapy reserved for patients with severe refractory respiratory failure who are unresponsive to other interventions. It is not typically the first-line treatment for status asthmaticus.

Case Study:

A 25-year-old man with asthma presents to the ICU with severe respiratory distress despite maximal medical therapy. NIPPV is initiated, leading to improvement in oxygenation and a decrease in respiratory rate. The patient's condition stabilizes, and he is successfully weaned off NIPPV.

Early initiation of NIPPV in patients with severe asthma can improve outcomes and reduce the need for invasive mechanical ventilation.

71. D. All of the above

Explanation:

Hypocalcemia in patients with end-stage renal disease (ESRD) is a complex issue with multiple contributing factors.

- **Decreased parathyroid hormone (PTH) production:** The kidneys are essential for activating vitamin D, which is necessary for PTH production. In ESRD, decreased PTH production leads to impaired calcium absorption from the gut and bone resorption.
- **Vitamin D deficiency:** As mentioned, the kidneys play a crucial role in activating vitamin D, and their dysfunction leads to vitamin D deficiency, further contributing to hypocalcemia.
- **Hyperphosphatemia:** In ESRD, the kidneys cannot effectively eliminate phosphate, leading to elevated phosphate levels. This can bind to calcium, forming insoluble calcium phosphate, reducing the amount of free calcium available in the bloodstream.

All three factors are interconnected and contribute to the development of hypocalcemia in patients with ESRD.

72. A. Plasma exchange

Explanation:

Plasma exchange is the most appropriate initial treatment for thrombotic thrombocytopenic purpura (TTP) in a patient with systemic lupus erythematosus (SLE).

Why plasma exchange?

• TTP is characterized by the formation of small blood clots that block small blood vessels throughout the body. This is primarily due to a deficiency or abnormality of ADAMTS13, an enzyme that breaks down von Willebrand factor (vWF).

• Plasma exchange removes the harmful antibodies that inhibit ADAMTS13 and replaces them with healthy plasma containing normal ADAMTS13. This helps to restore normal clotting function and prevent further clot formation.

Why other options are incorrect:

• **Corticosteroids:** While often used as adjunctive therapy, corticosteroids alone are not sufficient for treating acute TTP. They can help reduce inflammation but do not address the underlying problem of ADAMTS13 deficiency.

• **Rituximab:** This is a B-cell depleting agent primarily used in refractory or relapsing TTP. It is not the first-line treatment for acute TTP.

• **Splenectomy:** Splenectomy is considered in patients with chronic TTP who do not respond to other treatments or have recurrent disease. It is not the initial management for acute TTP.

Case Study:

A 35-year-old woman with a history of SLE presents to the ICU with fever, confusion, and petechiae. Laboratory tests reveal thrombocytopenia, microangiopathic hemolytic anemia, and elevated LDH. A diagnosis of TTP is made. The patient is immediately started on plasma exchange, which leads to improvement in her symptoms and laboratory values within a few days.

By understanding the pathophysiology of TTP and the mechanism of action of different treatment options, it is clear that plasma exchange is the most effective treatment for this patient.

73. D. Lung-protective ventilation with low tidal volumes and appropriate PEEP

Explanation:

Lung-protective ventilation is the cornerstone of managing patients with Acute Respiratory Distress Syndrome (ARDS). It involves using low tidal volumes and appropriate positive end-expiratory pressure (PEEP).

Why lung-protective ventilation?

- ARDS is characterized by diffuse alveolar damage leading to decreased lung compliance and increased risk of ventilator-induced lung injury (VILI).
- High tidal volumes can increase lung injury by overdistending alveoli and causing shear stress.
- Low tidal volumes, typically 6-8 mL/kg of predicted body weight, minimize alveolar overdistension.
- PEEP helps to recruit collapsed alveoli and improve oxygenation without excessive pressure.

Why other options are incorrect:

- **High tidal volume ventilation:** This strategy is outdated and harmful, as it increases the risk of VILI.
- **Low PEEP:** Insufficient PEEP can lead to alveolar collapse and decreased oxygenation.
- **High respiratory rate:** Increasing respiratory rate can lead to increased dead space ventilation and worsening hypercapnia.

Case Study:

A 60-year-old man is admitted to the ICU with ARDS following a motor vehicle accident. He is intubated and placed on mechanical ventilation. The ventilator settings are adjusted to a low tidal volume of 6 mL/kg and a PEEP of 8 cm H2O. Regular assessment of lung mechanics and blood gases is performed to optimize ventilation and minimize lung injury.

By implementing lung-protective ventilation strategies, the risk of VILI is reduced, and the patient's chances of recovery are improved.

74. B. Humoral hypercalcemia of malignancy

Explanation:

Humoral hypercalcemia of malignancy (HHM) is the most likely cause of hypercalcemia in a patient with a history of breast cancer presenting with severe hypercalcemia, altered mental status, polyuria, and polydipsia.

Why HHM?

- Breast cancer is a common malignancy associated with HHM.
- HHM occurs when tumor cells produce substances (e.g., parathyroid hormone-related protein) that mimic the effects of parathyroid hormone, leading to increased bone resorption and elevated calcium levels.
- Severe hypercalcemia, as seen in this case, is characteristic of HHM.

Why other options are incorrect:

- **Primary hyperparathyroidism:** While it can cause hypercalcemia, it is less likely in a patient with a known malignancy and severe hypercalcemic symptoms.
- **Vitamin D intoxication:** This usually presents with hypercalcemia, but without the severe symptoms and rapid onset seen in this case.
- **Milk-alkali syndrome:** This is typically seen in patients with excessive calcium and alkali intake, which is not the case here.

Case Study:

A 50-year-old woman with a history of breast cancer presents to the ICU with severe confusion, excessive urination, and thirst. Laboratory tests reveal a serum calcium level of 15 mg/dL. A bone scan shows multiple lytic bone lesions, suggesting metastatic bone disease. The diagnosis of HHM is confirmed. The patient is treated with aggressive hydration, calcitonin, and bisphosphonates to lower calcium levels.

Understanding the clinical presentation, associated malignancies, and pathophysiology of HHM is crucial for accurate diagnosis and timely management.

75. A. Ceftriaxone and azithromycin

Explanation:

Ceftriaxone and azithromycin is the most appropriate empiric antibiotic regimen for a young, previously healthy patient with severe community-acquired pneumonia (CAP) requiring mechanical ventilation.

Why this combination?

- **Ceftriaxone:** A third-generation cephalosporin with broad-spectrum coverage against common CAP pathogens, including *Streptococcus pneumoniae*.
- **Azithromycin:** A macrolide with excellent tissue penetration and activity against atypical pathogens like *Legionella* and *Mycoplasma*, which can cause severe pneumonia.

Why other options are incorrect:

- **Piperacillin/tazobactam and vancomycin:** This combination is overly broad-spectrum and reserved for patients with suspected or confirmed multidrug-resistant organisms (MDRO) or severe sepsis. It is not necessary for empiric therapy in a young, healthy patient without risk factors for MDRO.
- **Meropenem and vancomycin:** Similar to option B, this combination is too aggressive and should be reserved for patients with severe infections caused by highly resistant organisms.
- **Levofloxacin and azithromycin:** While both drugs have activity against common CAP pathogens, the combination is not typically recommended as first-line therapy due to potential increased risk of adverse effects and development of resistance.

Case Study:

A 25-year-old previously healthy man is admitted to the ICU with severe CAP requiring mechanical ventilation. Blood cultures are obtained, and empiric therapy with ceftriaxone and azithromycin is initiated. Within 48 hours, the patient shows clinical improvement, and blood cultures are negative. The antibiotics are continued for a total of 7-10 days based on clinical response and culture results.

By selecting an appropriate empiric antibiotic regimen, the risk of treatment failure and development of complications is reduced.

76. **A. Furosemide**

Explanation:

Furosemide is the most likely medication to improve symptoms in a patient with acute decompensated heart failure (ADHF) and preserved ejection fraction (HFpEF).

Why furosemide?

- HFpEF is characterized by fluid congestion despite preserved ejection fraction.

- Diuretics, such as furosemide, are the cornerstone of treatment for ADHF as they rapidly reduce fluid overload and improve symptoms like shortness of breath, edema, and congestion.

Why other options are incorrect:

- **Spironolactone:** While a valuable medication for HFpEF, its effects are slower in onset and primarily focus on long-term symptom management and reducing hospitalizations. It is not the first-line treatment for acute decompensation.
- **Sacubitril/valsartan:** This medication is primarily beneficial for patients with heart failure with reduced ejection fraction (HFrEF). Its effects on HFpEF are less established and it would not be the first choice for acute decompensation.
- **Digoxin:** While traditionally used in heart failure, its role is limited in modern management, especially in HFpEF. It has a narrow therapeutic index and carries risks of toxicity.

Case Study:

A 70-year-old woman with a history of HFpEF presents to the ICU with worsening shortness of breath, orthopnea, and peripheral edema. Her echocardiogram confirms preserved ejection fraction but shows evidence of increased left ventricular filling pressures. Intravenous furosemide is initiated, resulting in rapid diuresis and improvement in her symptoms.

By promptly addressing fluid overload with a potent diuretic like furosemide, the patient's comfort and overall condition can be significantly improved.

77. D. All of the above

Explanation:

Hepatorenal syndrome (HRS) is a severe complication of liver disease characterized by rapidly progressing kidney failure without intrinsic kidney damage. Treatment typically involves a combination of therapies aimed at improving renal perfusion and volume status.

- **Terlipressin:** A synthetic analogue of vasopressin, terlipressin causes vasoconstriction, improving renal perfusion and reducing portal pressure.
- **Midodrine and octreotide:** Midodrine is an alpha-adrenergic agonist that increases peripheral vascular resistance, while octreotide reduces splanchnic blood flow, both contributing to improved renal perfusion.
- **Albumin:** This colloid solution expands plasma volume, increasing intravascular volume and renal perfusion.

Why all are important?

The combination of these therapies has been shown to improve renal function and survival in patients with HRS. It's essential to note that HRS is a complex condition, and individual patient responses may vary. Therefore, careful monitoring of renal function and hemodynamic parameters is crucial during treatment.

Case Study:

A 45-year-old man with alcoholic hepatitis develops rapidly worsening renal function. Diagnosis of HRS is confirmed. Treatment is initiated with terlipressin, midodrine, octreotide, and albumin infusion. Close monitoring of renal function, blood pressure, and fluid balance is essential. With appropriate management, the patient's renal function may improve, and the risk of complications is reduced.

By understanding the pathophysiology of HRS and the mechanisms of action of different treatment modalities, clinicians can effectively manage this life-threatening condition.

78. A. Cyclophosphamide

Explanation:

Cyclophosphamide is the most likely medication to improve respiratory status in a patient with systemic lupus erythematosus (SLE) and diffuse alveolar hemorrhage (DAH).

Why cyclophosphamide?

• Diffuse alveolar hemorrhage (DAH) is a severe and potentially life-threatening complication of SLE.

• It is an autoimmune-mediated condition where inflammation leads to bleeding into the lungs.

• Cyclophosphamide is a potent immunosuppressant that effectively suppresses the immune system, reducing inflammation and bleeding in the lungs.

Why other options are incorrect:

• **Azathioprine and mycophenolate mofetil:** While these are immunosuppressants, they are generally less potent than cyclophosphamide and have a slower onset of action. They are not the first-line treatment for DAH.

• **Rituximab:** This is a B-cell depleting agent primarily used in certain types of autoimmune diseases, but it is not the first-line treatment for DAH.

Case Study:

A 30-year-old woman with SLE presents to the ICU with acute onset of dyspnea, hemoptysis, and hypoxemia. Diagnosis of DAH is confirmed. The patient is initiated on high-dose intravenous methylprednisolone and cyclophosphamide. Supportive care, including oxygen therapy, blood transfusions, and mechanical ventilation, is provided as needed. With aggressive treatment, the patient's respiratory status gradually improves.

It's important to note that DAH is a medical emergency requiring prompt and aggressive treatment. Early recognition and initiation of appropriate therapy are crucial for improving patient outcomes.

79. A. Vancomycin and piperacillin/tazobactam

Explanation:

Vancomycin and piperacillin/tazobactam is the most appropriate empiric antibiotic regimen for a patient with CKD on hemodialysis who develops septic shock.

Why this combination?

• Patients with CKD, especially those on hemodialysis, are at increased risk for infections caused by resistant organisms, including methicillin-resistant Staphylococcus aureus (MRSA) and Pseudomonas aeruginosa.

• Vancomycin provides excellent coverage for MRSA, while piperacillin/tazobactam has broad-spectrum activity against gram-negative organisms, including Pseudomonas aeruginosa.

Why other options are incorrect:

• **Cefepime and metronidazole:** This combination lacks adequate coverage for MRSA, which is a common pathogen in this patient population.

• **Meropenem and vancomycin:** While both drugs have broad-spectrum activity, this combination may be overly broad and can increase the risk of adverse effects and development of resistance.

• **Levofloxacin and azithromycin:** This combination is not appropriate for severe infections like septic shock and lacks coverage for common resistant pathogens in this patient population.

Case Study:

A 60-year-old man with CKD on hemodialysis presents to the ICU with hypotension, tachycardia, and altered mental status. Blood cultures are obtained, and empiric therapy with vancomycin and piperacillin/tazobactam is initiated.

Once culture results are available, the antibiotic regimen can be adjusted accordingly.

By selecting a broad-spectrum antibiotic combination that covers common resistant pathogens, the risk of treatment failure and mortality in this critically ill patient is reduced.

80. D. Lung-protective ventilation with low tidal volumes and appropriate PEEP

Explanation:

Lung-protective ventilation is the cornerstone of managing patients with Acute Respiratory Distress Syndrome (ARDS), regardless of the underlying cause. It involves using low tidal volumes and appropriate positive end-expiratory pressure (PEEP).

Why lung-protective ventilation?

• ARDS is characterized by diffuse alveolar damage leading to decreased lung compliance and increased risk of ventilator-induced lung injury (VILI).

• High tidal volumes can increase lung injury by overdistending alveoli and causing shear stress.

• Low tidal volumes, typically 6-8 mL/kg of predicted body weight, minimize alveolar overdistension.

• PEEP helps to recruit collapsed alveoli and improve oxygenation without excessive pressure.

Why other options are incorrect:

• **High tidal volume ventilation:** This strategy is outdated and harmful, as it increases the risk of VILI.

• **Low PEEP:** Insufficient PEEP can lead to alveolar collapse and decreased oxygenation.

• **High respiratory rate:** Increasing respiratory rate can lead to increased dead space ventilation and worsening hypercapnia.

By implementing lung-protective ventilation strategies, the risk of VILI is reduced, and the patient's chances of recovery are improved.

81. A. Diltiazem

Explanation:

Diltiazem is the most appropriate medication for rate control in a patient with new-onset atrial fibrillation with rapid ventricular response (RVR), hypotension, and underlying coronary artery disease.

Why diltiazem?

- It is a calcium channel blocker that effectively slows down the heart rate without significantly decreasing blood pressure, which is crucial in this hypotensive patient.
- It has a relatively safe side effect profile and is suitable for patients with coronary artery disease.

Why other options are incorrect:

- **Amiodarone:** While effective for rate control, it has a long half-life and can cause hypotension, which would worsen the patient's condition.
- **Metoprolol:** A beta-blocker can lower heart rate but also has negative inotropic effects, which can further compromise cardiac output and blood pressure in a hypotensive patient.
- **Digoxin:** While effective for rate control, it has a narrow therapeutic index and requires careful monitoring, making it less ideal for rapid initiation in an acute setting.

Case Study:

A 72-year-old man with hypertension and coronary artery disease presents to the ICU with acute onset of atrial fibrillation with a rapid ventricular response of 150 beats per minute and hypotension (90/60 mmHg). Intravenous diltiazem is initiated, resulting in a gradual decrease in heart rate and improvement in blood pressure. The patient's condition stabilizes, and further management can be planned.

By choosing a medication that effectively controls heart rate without compromising blood pressure, the risk of hemodynamic instability is reduced.

82. D. All of the above

Explanation:

Acute lupus myocarditis is an inflammatory condition of the heart muscle caused by systemic lupus erythematosus (SLE). It can manifest with a variety of cardiac complications, including:

- **Elevated troponin levels:** Indicative of myocardial injury.
- **ST-segment elevations on ECG:** Suggestive of myocardial ischemia, although this is less common than non-ST elevation myocardial injury in lupus myocarditis.
- **Pericardial effusion on echocardiogram:** Often seen in patients with lupus myocarditis due to inflammation of the pericardium.

Therefore, all of these findings can be consistent with a diagnosis of acute lupus myocarditis. It's important to note that the specific combination of findings can vary depending on the severity and stage of the disease.

83. **B. Low-protein diet**
Explanation:
Low-protein diet is the most appropriate dietary modification for a patient with hepatic encephalopathy and elevated ammonia levels.
- **Hepatic encephalopathy** is a neuropsychiatric syndrome that occurs due to the accumulation of toxins in the blood, including ammonia.
- The liver normally converts ammonia into urea for excretion. However, in patients with cirrhosis, the liver's ability to process ammonia is impaired.
- **Protein breakdown** results in the production of ammonia. Therefore, reducing protein intake helps to lower ammonia levels and improve hepatic encephalopathy symptoms.

Why other options are incorrect:
- **High-protein diet:** Increasing protein intake would exacerbate ammonia levels and worsen hepatic encephalopathy.
- **High-carbohydrate diet:** While carbohydrates are important for energy, they do not directly impact ammonia levels.
- **Low-carbohydrate diet:** This is not indicated in hepatic encephalopathy and can lead to malnutrition.

It's important to note that dietary modifications should be done under the guidance of a healthcare professional, as complete protein restriction can lead to malnutrition. Other therapeutic measures, such as lactulose and rifaximin, are also essential in managing hepatic encephalopathy.

84. D. Dialysis

Explanation:

Uremic pericarditis is a complication of chronic kidney disease (CKD) that occurs due to the accumulation of uremic toxins. The most effective treatment for this condition is to remove these toxins from the body.

- **Dialysis** is the primary treatment for uremic pericarditis. It effectively removes uremic toxins from the blood, leading to improvement in pericardial inflammation and reducing the risk of complications like pericardial effusion and cardiac tamponade.

Why other options are incorrect:

- **Pericardiocentesis:** This procedure is indicated for refractory pericarditis with significant pericardial effusion causing hemodynamic compromise. It is not the first-line treatment.
- **Corticosteroids:** While sometimes used as adjunctive therapy in refractory cases, corticosteroids are not the primary treatment for uremic pericarditis.
- **NSAIDs:** These medications are contraindicated in patients with CKD due to the risk of acute kidney injury and worsening renal function.

By addressing the underlying cause of uremic pericarditis through dialysis, the risk of complications and mortality is significantly reduced.

85. D. Lung-protective ventilation with low tidal volumes and high PEEP

Explanation:

Lung-protective ventilation is the standard of care for patients with ARDS, regardless of the underlying cause. It involves:

- **Low tidal volumes:** This prevents overstretching of the injured lung tissue and reduces the risk of ventilator-induced lung injury (VILI).
- **High PEEP:** This helps to recruit collapsed alveoli and improve oxygenation without excessive pressure.

This strategy has been shown to improve oxygenation and reduce mortality in patients with ARDS.

Why other options are incorrect:

- **High tidal volume ventilation:** This is an outdated method that can worsen lung injury.
- **Low PEEP:** Insufficient PEEP can lead to alveolar collapse and decreased oxygenation.

- **High respiratory rate:** This can increase dead space ventilation and worsen hypercapnia without improving oxygenation.

86. Answer: D. Extracorporeal membrane oxygenation (ECMO)
Explanation:

Extracorporeal membrane oxygenation (ECMO) is the most appropriate mechanical circulatory support device for a 70-year-old woman with HFrEF in cardiogenic shock.

Cardiogenic shock is a severe condition where the heart cannot pump enough blood to meet the body's needs, leading to organ dysfunction. In this case, the patient's heart failure has deteriorated to the point where it can no longer sustain life.

ECMO provides both cardiac and respiratory support by removing blood from the body, oxygenating it, and returning it. It is a highly invasive procedure but is often life-saving in refractory cardiogenic shock.

Why other options are incorrect:

- **Intra-aortic balloon pump (IABP):** While IABP can improve coronary blood flow and reduce afterload, it is not sufficient for patients in cardiogenic shock. It provides limited circulatory support and is typically used as a bridge to more definitive therapy.

- **Impella:** This device provides left ventricular support by pumping blood from the left ventricle to the aorta. While it can be effective in some cases of cardiogenic shock, it may not be sufficient for a patient with severe heart failure and low cardiac output.

- **TandemHeart:** This device provides left ventricular unloading and circulatory support. However, it is generally indicated for patients with less severe heart failure compared to cardiogenic shock.

Case Study: A 70-year-old woman with a history of HFrEF is admitted to the ICU with hypotension, tachycardia, and altered mental status. Her echocardiogram shows severely reduced left ventricular ejection fraction and elevated pulmonary capillary wedge pressure. Despite maximal medical therapy, including vasopressors and inotropes, the patient remains in cardiogenic shock with persistent lactic acidosis. In this scenario, ECMO would be the most appropriate intervention to provide the necessary cardiac and respiratory support to stabilize the patient and allow for myocardial recovery or bridge to transplant.

In conclusion, for patients with refractory cardiogenic shock, ECMO is often the preferred mechanical circulatory support device due to its ability to provide both cardiac and respiratory support.

87. Answer: A. Continuous venovenous hemofiltration (CVVH)

Explanation:

Continuous venovenous hemofiltration (CVVH) is the most appropriate modality of renal replacement therapy (RRT) for a 45-year-old man with acute pancreatitis who has developed acute kidney injury (AKI).

Acute pancreatitis is an inflammatory condition of the pancreas that can lead to multi-organ dysfunction, including AKI. Patients with acute pancreatitis are often critically ill with hemodynamic instability and fluid shifts.

CVVH offers several advantages in this setting:

- **Continuous and gentle removal of fluids and solutes:** CVVH allows for gradual fluid removal, which helps maintain hemodynamic stability.
- **Reduced fluctuations in electrolytes and acid-base balance:** Unlike intermittent hemodialysis, CVVH provides a more stable internal environment.
- **Ability to remove larger molecules:** CVVH can effectively remove inflammatory mediators and other toxins associated with acute pancreatitis.

Why other options are incorrect:

- **Intermittent hemodialysis (IHD):** While effective for removing waste products, IHD can cause rapid fluid shifts and hemodynamic instability in critically ill patients, especially those with acute pancreatitis.
- **Peritoneal dialysis (PD):** This modality is generally not suitable for critically ill patients due to the risk of infection and the difficulty of managing fluid balance.
- **Sustained low-efficiency dialysis (SLED):** While this is a continuous modality, it is less efficient than CVVH in removing fluids and solutes, and may not be optimal for critically ill patients.

Case Study: A 45-year-old man with a history of alcoholism is admitted to the ICU with severe abdominal pain and elevated lipase levels, consistent with acute pancreatitis. Over the next few days, his creatinine level rises, and he develops oliguria. Despite aggressive fluid resuscitation, the patient remains hypotensive. In this case, initiating CVVH would help to stabilize the patient's fluid balance, remove inflammatory mediators, and support overall organ function.

In conclusion, CVVH is the preferred RRT modality for patients with acute pancreatitis and AKI due to its ability to provide continuous, gentle fluid removal and effective solute clearance while minimizing hemodynamic instability.

88. Answer: D. All of the above
Explanation:
All of the laboratory tests mentioned are crucial for monitoring potential complications of high-dose corticosteroids and cyclophosphamide therapy in a patient with lupus nephritis.
- **Complete blood count (CBC):** This test monitors for bone marrow suppression, which is a common side effect of both corticosteroids and cyclophosphamide. It can detect anemia, thrombocytopenia, and leukopenia.
- **Liver function tests (LFTs):** These tests assess liver function, as both medications can cause liver toxicity, leading to hepatitis or other liver complications.
- **Electrolytes:** Monitoring electrolytes is essential because corticosteroids can cause electrolyte imbalances, such as hypokalemia and hyponatremia, which can lead to serious complications.
Why other options are incorrect:
While each of the tests is important, focusing on only one would leave the patient at risk for undetected complications from the other areas.
Case Study: A 30-year-old woman with SLE is admitted to the ICU with lupus nephritis and started on high-dose corticosteroids and cyclophosphamide. Regular monitoring of CBC, LFTs, and electrolytes reveals:
- A decreasing white blood cell count, indicating bone marrow suppression.
- Elevated liver enzymes, suggesting potential liver toxicity.
- Decreasing potassium levels, indicating hypokalemia. This comprehensive monitoring allows for timely intervention to prevent severe complications.
In conclusion, a combination of CBC, LFTs, and electrolyte monitoring is essential for patients receiving high-dose corticosteroids and cyclophosphamide to detect and manage potential adverse effects effectively.

89. **Answer: A. Aspirin**

Explanation:

Aspirin is the most appropriate medication to prevent secondary stroke in a 60-year-old man with a history of hypertension and hyperlipidemia who has experienced an acute ischemic stroke and is not a candidate for reperfusion therapy.

- **Aspirin** is a platelet inhibitor that reduces the risk of clot formation, thereby decreasing the likelihood of another ischemic stroke.
- It is the cornerstone of stroke prevention and has been shown to be effective in reducing stroke recurrence.

Why other options are incorrect:

- **Clopidogrel:** While also a platelet inhibitor, it is generally used in combination with aspirin or as an alternative in patients who are aspirin-intolerant. It is not the first-line treatment for stroke prevention.
- **Warfarin:** This medication is an anticoagulant primarily used to prevent thromboembolic events in atrial fibrillation. It is not indicated for stroke prevention in patients without atrial fibrillation.
- **Apixaban:** Similar to warfarin, apixaban is an anticoagulant primarily used for atrial fibrillation and deep vein thrombosis prevention. It is not appropriate for stroke prevention in this patient.

Case Study: A 60-year-old man with a history of hypertension and hyperlipidemia presents to the ICU with right-sided weakness and slurred speech. A CT scan confirms a left middle cerebral artery stroke. Due to the time window for reperfusion therapy having elapsed, the patient is not a candidate for thrombolytic therapy. In this scenario, aspirin would be initiated promptly to reduce the risk of recurrent stroke.

In conclusion, aspirin is the standard of care for secondary stroke prevention in patients who have experienced an ischemic stroke and are not candidates for reperfusion therapy.

90. **Answer: A. Hypokalemia**

Explanation:

Hypokalemia is the most likely electrolyte abnormality to occur during the treatment of DKA.

Understanding the Pathophysiology:

• In DKA, insulin deficiency leads to increased gluconeogenesis and glycogenolysis, resulting in hyperglycemia.

• To compensate for the osmotic diuresis caused by hyperglycemia, the body loses significant amounts of potassium, sodium, and other electrolytes.

• Insulin administration promotes potassium shifting from the extracellular fluid into the intracellular space.

Treatment of DKA:

• Intravenous insulin therapy is crucial to correct hyperglycemia and ketoacidosis.

• Aggressive fluid resuscitation is necessary to correct dehydration.

The combination of insulin-induced intracellular potassium shift and fluid replacement can rapidly lead to hypokalemia.

Why other options are incorrect:

• **Hyperkalemia:** This is unlikely to occur during DKA treatment, as potassium is typically depleted. However, it can occur in severe cases before insulin therapy is initiated.

• **Hyponatremia:** While hyponatremia can occur in DKA due to fluid losses, it is usually corrected with fluid resuscitation.

• **Hypernatremia:** This is highly unlikely in DKA, as patients are typically dehydrated.

Case Study: A 50-year-old woman presents to the ICU with DKA, characterized by hyperglycemia, ketonuria, and metabolic acidosis. She is initiated on intravenous insulin and fluid resuscitation. Initial laboratory values reveal severe hypokalemia despite adequate potassium replacement. This is likely due to the rapid intracellular shift of potassium with insulin administration. Close monitoring and aggressive potassium replacement are essential to prevent life-threatening arrhythmias.

In conclusion, hypokalemia is a common complication of DKA treatment and requires vigilant monitoring and prompt intervention.

91. Answer: C. Congestive Heart Failure (CHF)

Explanation:

The most likely diagnosis for a 45-year-old woman with rheumatoid arthritis presenting with new-onset shortness of breath, tachycardia, hypotension, and bilateral pleural effusions is **Congestive Heart Failure (CHF)**.

Rationale:

- **Rheumatoid arthritis** is a systemic inflammatory disease that can affect multiple organs, including the heart.
- **CHF** is a common complication of rheumatoid arthritis due to inflammatory damage to the heart muscle.
- **Shortness of breath, tachycardia, and hypotension** are classic symptoms of CHF.
- **Bilateral pleural effusions** are a common finding in patients with CHF due to increased hydrostatic pressure in the pulmonary circulation.

Why other options are incorrect:

- **Acute Respiratory Distress Syndrome (ARDS):** While ARDS can present with similar symptoms, it typically involves more severe hypoxemia and bilateral infiltrates on chest x-ray, which are not described in this case.
- **Pulmonary Embolism (PE):** PE can cause shortness of breath and hypotension but is less likely to cause bilateral pleural effusions. Additionally, there is no specific risk factor for PE mentioned in the patient's history.
- **Pleural effusion secondary to rheumatoid arthritis:** While it's possible for rheumatoid arthritis to cause pleural effusions, the presence of other symptoms (shortness of breath, tachycardia, hypotension) strongly suggests an underlying cardiac cause.

Case Study: A 45-year-old woman with rheumatoid arthritis is admitted to the ICU with worsening shortness of breath, rapid heart rate, and low blood pressure. Chest x-ray reveals bilateral pleural effusions. An echocardiogram demonstrates decreased left ventricular ejection fraction, confirming the diagnosis of CHF.

In conclusion, the combination of rheumatoid arthritis, new-onset respiratory symptoms, hemodynamic instability, and bilateral pleural effusions strongly suggests CHF as the most likely diagnosis.

92. Answer: B. Prone positioning

Explanation:

Prone positioning is the most appropriate next intervention for a 75-year-old man with COPD experiencing deteriorating oxygenation despite increasing ventilator support.

Rationale:

• **Prone positioning** has been shown to improve oxygenation in patients with acute respiratory distress syndrome (ARDS) and can also be beneficial in patients with severe COPD exacerbations.

• By positioning the patient face down, the dependent lung regions (typically the lower lobes) are better ventilated and perfused, improving gas exchange.

• This intervention is relatively low-risk and can be implemented quickly.

Why other options are incorrect:

• **Inhaled nitric oxide:** While it can improve oxygenation in certain conditions, its efficacy in COPD-related respiratory failure is limited.

• **Extracorporeal membrane oxygenation (ECMO):** This is a highly invasive procedure reserved for patients with severe refractory hypoxemia who have exhausted other treatment options.

• **High-frequency oscillatory ventilation (HFOV):** This is another advanced ventilation mode that may be considered in certain cases, but prone positioning is generally a more appropriate first step.

Case Study: A 75-year-old man with COPD is intubated and placed on mechanical ventilation due to acute respiratory failure. Despite increasing ventilator support, his PaO2/FiO2 ratio continues to decline. The decision is made to initiate prone positioning. Within a few hours, his oxygenation improves significantly, and the need for additional ventilator support is reduced.

In conclusion, prone positioning is a valuable therapeutic option for patients with COPD experiencing refractory hypoxemia. It is important to note that this intervention should be performed under close monitoring in an ICU setting.

93. Answer: A. Vancomycin and gentamicin

Explanation:

Vancomycin and gentamicin is the most appropriate antibiotic regimen for a 30-year-old woman with a history of intravenous drug use presenting with infective endocarditis caused by methicillin-resistant Staphylococcus aureus (MRSA).

Rationale:

- **Vancomycin** is the drug of choice for treating MRSA infections due to its excellent activity against this organism.
- **Gentamicin** is added to the regimen to provide synergistic coverage and to potentially decrease the risk of vancomycin resistance.

Why other options are incorrect:

- **Daptomycin:** While effective against MRSA, it has limitations in the treatment of endocarditis, particularly left-sided endocarditis.
- **Linezolid:** This is an alternative option for MRSA endocarditis but is often reserved for cases where vancomycin is not tolerated or has failed.
- **Ceftaroline:** This antibiotic does not have activity against MRSA.

Case Study: A 30-year-old woman with a history of intravenous drug use presents with fever, chills, and a new heart murmur. Blood cultures grow MRSA. Given the severity of the infection and the risk of complications, the patient is started on intravenous vancomycin and gentamicin. After several weeks of therapy, the patient shows clinical improvement, and blood cultures become negative.

In conclusion, combination therapy with vancomycin and gentamicin is the recommended treatment for MRSA endocarditis due to its efficacy and potential to reduce the risk of complications.

94. Answer: A. Aspirin

Explanation:

Aspirin is the most appropriate medication to initiate within 48 hours of symptom onset to reduce the risk of recurrent stroke in a 65-year-old man with a history of hypertension and diabetes mellitus who has experienced an acute ischemic stroke and is not a candidate for reperfusion therapy.

- **Aspirin** is a platelet inhibitor that reduces the risk of clot formation, thereby decreasing the likelihood of another ischemic stroke.
- It is the cornerstone of stroke prevention and has been shown to be effective in reducing stroke recurrence.

Why other options are incorrect:

- **Clopidogrel:** While also a platelet inhibitor, it is generally used in combination with aspirin or as an alternative in patients who are aspirin-intolerant. It is not the first-line treatment for stroke prevention.
- **Warfarin:** This medication is an anticoagulant primarily used to prevent thromboembolic events in atrial fibrillation. It is not indicated for stroke prevention in patients without atrial fibrillation.
- **Statin:** Statins are used to lower cholesterol levels and reduce the risk of heart disease and stroke in the long term. While important for this patient, they do not have an immediate impact on stroke prevention like aspirin.

In conclusion, aspirin is the standard of care for secondary stroke prevention in patients who have experienced an ischemic stroke and are not candidates for reperfusion therapy.

95. Answer: A. Nonselective beta-blocker (e.g., propranolol)
Explanation:

Nonselective beta-blockers are the cornerstone of long-term management for patients with cirrhosis and varices.
- **Reduces portal pressure:** By decreasing heart rate and cardiac output, beta-blockers lower portal pressure, reducing the risk of variceal bleeding.
- **Proven efficacy:** Numerous studies have demonstrated the effectiveness of beta-blockers in preventing recurrent variceal bleeding.

Why other options are incorrect:
- **Endoscopic variceal band ligation (EVL):** While effective in acute variceal bleeding, EVL is a therapeutic intervention rather than a long-term management strategy.
- **Transjugular intrahepatic portosystemic shunt (TIPS):** TIPS is considered for patients with recurrent variceal bleeding despite optimal medical therapy or in those with refractory ascites. It is not typically the first-line treatment.
- **Liver transplantation:** Liver transplantation is the definitive treatment for end-stage liver disease but is reserved for patients with severe liver failure and limited life expectancy.

Case Study: A 50-year-old woman with cirrhosis is admitted to the ICU with acute variceal bleeding. She undergoes successful EVL and octreotide infusion. After stabilization, propranolol is initiated to reduce portal pressure and prevent recurrent bleeding. Regular follow-up with endoscopy and liver function tests is essential to monitor the patient's condition and adjust treatment as needed.

In conclusion, nonselective beta-blockers are the mainstay of long-term management for patients with cirrhosis and varices to prevent recurrent bleeding and improve overall prognosis.

96. Answer: A. Continuous venovenous hemofiltration (CVVH)

Explanation:

Continuous venovenous hemofiltration (CVVH) is the most appropriate modality of renal replacement therapy (RRT) for a 40-year-old man with acute pancreatitis who has developed acute kidney injury (AKI).

Rationale:

- **Continuous and gentle fluid removal:** CVVH allows for gradual fluid removal, which helps maintain hemodynamic stability.
- **Reduced fluctuations in electrolytes and acid-base balance:** Unlike intermittent hemodialysis, CVVH provides a more stable internal environment.
- **Ability to remove larger molecules:** CVVH can effectively remove inflammatory mediators and other toxins associated with acute pancreatitis.

Why other options are incorrect:

- **Intermittent hemodialysis (IHD):** While effective for removing waste products, IHD can cause rapid fluid shifts and hemodynamic instability in critically ill patients, especially those with acute pancreatitis.
- **Peritoneal dialysis (PD):** This modality is generally not suitable for critically ill patients due to the risk of infection and the difficulty of managing fluid balance.
- **Sustained low-efficiency dialysis (SLED):** While this is a continuous modality, it is less efficient than CVVH in removing fluids and solutes, and may not be optimal for critically ill patients.

In conclusion, CVVH is the preferred RRT modality for patients with acute pancreatitis and AKI due to its ability to provide continuous, gentle fluid removal and effective solute clearance while minimizing hemodynamic instability.

97. Answer: D. All of the above

Explanation:

All of the mentioned strategies are crucial in reducing the risk of ventilator-associated pneumonia (VAP) in a patient like this.

- **Oral chlorhexidine gluconate rinse:** This helps to reduce the bacterial load in the oral cavity, which is a common source of aspiration.
- **Elevation of the head of the bed to 30 degrees:** This reduces the risk of aspiration by preventing pooling of secretions in the back of the throat.
- **Daily "sedation vacations" and assessment of readiness to extubate:** Minimizing sedation and promoting early extubation can decrease the duration of intubation, thereby reducing the risk of VAP.

Implementing these evidence-based interventions together can significantly lower the incidence of VAP in critically ill patients.

98. Answer: B. Plasma exchange

Explanation:

Plasma exchange is the most likely intervention to improve oxygenation in a 35-year-old woman with systemic lupus erythematosus (SLE) and diffuse alveolar hemorrhage (DAH).

- **Diffuse alveolar hemorrhage** is a life-threatening condition characterized by bleeding into the lungs, leading to severe hypoxemia.
- **Plasma exchange** rapidly removes circulating autoantibodies and inflammatory mediators that contribute to the ongoing alveolar damage and hemorrhage.

Why other options are incorrect:

- **Intravenous corticosteroids:** While corticosteroids are often used in the management of SLE, they are not the primary treatment for DAH. They may have a role in reducing inflammation but do not directly address the underlying cause of bleeding.
- **Intravenous cyclophosphamide:** This immunosuppressive agent is used for severe lupus flares but is not a first-line treatment for DAH. It may be considered as adjunctive therapy after plasma exchange.

In conclusion, plasma exchange is the cornerstone of treatment for DAH in patients with SLE due to its ability to rapidly remove harmful antibodies and improve oxygenation.

99. **Answer: A. Dobutamine**
Explanation:
Dobutamine is the most appropriate inotropic agent for a 60-year-old man with acute decompensated heart failure (ADHF) who remains hypotensive and oliguric despite diuretic and vasodilator therapy.
- **Dobutamine** is a beta-1 agonist that primarily increases cardiac contractility without significantly increasing heart rate or peripheral vasoconstriction.
- This selective action makes it ideal for patients with ADHF as it improves cardiac output without exacerbating hypotension or renal dysfunction.

Why other options are incorrect:
- **Milrinone:** While it also increases cardiac output, it has more pronounced vasodilatory effects compared to dobutamine, which can worsen hypotension in this patient.
- **Dopamine:** At low doses, dopamine primarily increases renal blood flow, but at higher doses, it has vasoconstrictive properties that can worsen hypotension.
- **Norepinephrine:** Primarily a vasoconstrictor, norepinephrine would likely exacerbate hypotension and worsen renal perfusion in this patient.

In conclusion, dobutamine is the preferred inotropic agent for patients with ADHF and refractory hypotension due to its selective action on increasing cardiac contractility without causing significant vasoconstriction.

100. **Answer: D. All of the above**
Explanation:
A 50-year-old woman with rheumatoid arthritis presenting to the ICU with septic shock secondary to pneumonia is a critically ill patient requiring comprehensive and coordinated care. All of the mentioned bundles of care are essential for improving her outcomes.
- **Early Goal-Directed Therapy (EGDT):** This bundle focuses on rapid fluid resuscitation, vasopressor support, and blood transfusion to optimize hemodynamics and tissue perfusion in septic shock.
- **Surviving Sepsis Campaign bundle:** This encompasses a broader range of interventions, including early identification of sepsis, blood cultures, antibiotic administration, and lactate measurement, to improve overall survival.

- **ARDSNet protocol:** Since this patient is developing respiratory failure secondary to pneumonia, implementing ARDSNet protocols, which focus on lung protective ventilation strategies, can help prevent further lung injury.

By combining these evidence-based bundles, the ICU team can provide optimal care for this patient and increase her chances of survival and recovery.

101. Answer: C. Right coronary artery (RCA)

Explanation:

ST-segment elevations in leads II, III, and aVF are classic electrocardiographic findings indicative of an **inferior wall myocardial infarction**.

- The **right coronary artery (RCA)** is the primary blood supply to the inferior wall of the heart. Therefore, an occlusion of the RCA is the most likely cause of an inferior STEMI.

Why other options are incorrect:

- **Left anterior descending (LAD) artery:** This artery primarily supplies the anterior wall of the heart and is associated with ST-segment elevations in the anterior leads (V1-V4).
- **Left circumflex (LCx) artery:** This artery supplies the lateral wall of the heart and is associated with ST-segment elevations in the lateral leads (I, aVL, V5, V6).
- **Left main coronary artery (LMCA):** Occlusion of the LMCA typically results in a large anterior wall myocardial infarction with ST-segment elevations in multiple leads, including anterior, lateral, and inferior leads.

Understanding the coronary artery distribution to different regions of the heart is crucial for accurate diagnosis and management of myocardial infarction.

102. Answer: B. Serum lipase

Explanation:

Serum lipase is generally considered the more specific and sensitive marker for diagnosing acute pancreatitis.

- **Lipase** is an enzyme primarily produced by the pancreas. It is more specific to pancreatic injury than amylase, which can also be elevated in other conditions like salivary gland inflammation or renal failure.
- While **amylase** was traditionally used for diagnosing acute pancreatitis, its lower specificity has led to a shift towards lipase as the preferred marker.

Why other options are incorrect:

- **Serum alanine aminotransferase (ALT)** and **serum aspartate aminotransferase (AST)** are primarily liver enzymes and are not specific to pancreatic injury. They may be elevated in pancreatitis if there is associated liver involvement or biliary obstruction, but they are not diagnostic for the condition.

In conclusion, while both amylase and lipase can be elevated in acute pancreatitis, lipase is generally considered the more reliable marker for diagnosis.

103. Answer: B. Transesophageal echocardiogram (TEE)

Explanation:

Transesophageal echocardiogram (TEE) is the most appropriate diagnostic test to evaluate for the presence of vegetations on heart valves in a patient with infective endocarditis and septic embolic stroke.

- **TEE** provides a more detailed and accurate image of the heart and its valves compared to transthoracic echocardiography.
- It allows for better visualization of the left heart chambers, valves, and the aorta, which are often involved in infective endocarditis.
- In a patient with septic embolic stroke, TEE can help identify the source of the emboli, such as a vegetation on the mitral or aortic valve.

Why other options are incorrect:

- **Transthoracic echocardiogram (TTE):** While useful for initial evaluation, TTE may not provide sufficient detail, especially in patients with complex cardiac anatomy or when looking for smaller vegetations.
- **Cardiac magnetic resonance imaging (MRI):** Although excellent for assessing cardiac structure and function, MRI is not as good as echocardiography for visualizing heart valves and vegetations in real-time.
- **Cardiac computed tomography (CT) scan:** While CT can provide good anatomical information, it is not as effective as echocardiography in visualizing heart valves and cardiac structures in motion.

In conclusion, TEE is the gold standard for diagnosing infective endocarditis and assessing the severity of valvular involvement, especially in patients with complications such as septic embolic stroke.

104. Answer: A. Pseudomonas aeruginosa
Explanation:

Pseudomonas aeruginosa is the most likely cause of ventilator-associated pneumonia (VAP) in a 70-year-old woman with COPD who has been on mechanical ventilation for 48 hours.

• **Pseudomonas aeruginosa** is a common gram-negative bacterium often implicated in hospital-acquired infections, including VAP.

• It is particularly problematic in patients with chronic lung diseases, such as COPD, as it can colonize the respiratory tract and become opportunistic.

• The use of antibiotics and prolonged mechanical ventilation can contribute to the development of resistant strains of Pseudomonas aeruginosa.

Why other options are incorrect:

• **Staphylococcus aureus:** While a common cause of pneumonia, it is more typically associated with community-acquired pneumonia or healthcare-associated pneumonia.

• **Klebsiella pneumoniae:** This organism is also a common cause of pneumonia, but it is more often associated with urinary tract infections and bloodstream infections.

• **Escherichia coli:** Primarily a gastrointestinal pathogen, it is less likely to cause pneumonia compared to the other options.

In conclusion, Pseudomonas aeruginosa is a highly likely pathogen in patients with VAP, especially those with underlying chronic lung disease and prolonged mechanical ventilation.

105. Answer: C. Synchronized intermittent mandatory ventilation (SIMV)
Explanation:

Synchronized intermittent mandatory ventilation (SIMV) is the most appropriate ventilator mode for a 35-year-old man with severe community-acquired pneumonia (CAP) who requires intubation.

• **SIMV** allows for a combination of spontaneous and controlled breaths.

• It permits patient-initiated breaths, which helps maintain lung volume and prevent atelectasis.

• The ventilator delivers a preset number of mandatory breaths at a set tidal volume and respiratory rate.

- This mode provides a balance of patient-ventilator interaction and control, which is often beneficial in patients with acute respiratory failure.

Why other options are incorrect:

- **Assist control (AC):** This mode fully controls ventilation, and the patient has limited control over breathing. It may lead to overventilation and barotrauma.
- **Pressure control (PC):** While useful in certain conditions, PC mode may not be optimal for initial management of acute respiratory failure due to its potential for hyperventilation.
- **Pressure support ventilation (PSV):** This mode is typically used for weaning patients from mechanical ventilation, not for initial management of acute respiratory failure.

In conclusion, SIMV offers a flexible and adaptable approach to managing patients with severe CAP, allowing for patient-ventilator synchrony and minimizing the risk of ventilator-induced lung injury.

106. **Answer: A. Dobutamine**

Explanation:

Dobutamine is the most appropriate inotropic agent for a 65-year-old woman with HFrEF who is unresponsive to diuretics and vasodilators.

- **Dobutamine** primarily increases cardiac contractility with minimal effects on heart rate and peripheral vasoconstriction.
- This selective action improves cardiac output without exacerbating hypotension or renal dysfunction, which is crucial in patients with heart failure.

Why other options are incorrect:

- **Milrinone:** While it increases cardiac output, it has a more pronounced vasodilatory effect, which could worsen hypotension in a patient with decompensated heart failure.
- **Dopamine:** At low doses, dopamine primarily increases renal blood flow, but at higher doses, it has vasoconstrictive properties that can worsen hypotension.
- **Norepinephrine:** Primarily a vasoconstrictor, norepinephrine would likely exacerbate hypotension and worsen renal perfusion in a patient with decompensated heart failure.

In conclusion, dobutamine is the preferred inotropic agent for patients with HFrEF and refractory symptoms due to its selective action on increasing cardiac contractility without causing significant vasoconstriction.

107. **Answer: C. Model for End-Stage Liver Disease (MELD) score**
Explanation:

The **Model for End-Stage Liver Disease (MELD) score** is the most important prognostic factor for survival in patients with hepatorenal syndrome (HRS).

• The MELD score is a validated prognostic model that incorporates key factors of liver disease severity, including bilirubin, creatinine, and INR.

• A higher MELD score indicates more severe liver disease and a higher risk of complications, including HRS and mortality.

• It is widely used to prioritize patients for liver transplantation and to assess the prognosis of patients with advanced liver disease.

Why other options are incorrect:

• **Serum creatinine level:** While elevated creatinine is a hallmark of HRS, it reflects the renal dysfunction rather than the underlying liver disease severity.

• **Serum bilirubin level:** Bilirubin is a component of the MELD score but does not fully capture the overall severity of liver disease.

• **Response to treatment with terlipressin:** While terlipressin can improve renal function in some patients with HRS, it does not predict long-term survival as accurately as the MELD score.

In conclusion, the MELD score is the most comprehensive and reliable prognostic indicator for patients with HRS.

108. **Answer: C. Noninvasive positive pressure ventilation (NIPPV)**
Explanation:

Noninvasive positive pressure ventilation (NIPPV) is the most appropriate next intervention for a 25-year-old woman with status asthmaticus who is deteriorating despite maximal medical therapy.

• **NIPPV** can improve oxygenation and reduce the work of breathing by providing continuous positive airway pressure.

• It can delay or prevent the need for invasive mechanical ventilation.

Why other options are incorrect:

• **Intravenous ketamine:** While ketamine has been studied for refractory asthma, it is not a first-line treatment and requires further research.

• **Inhaled heliox:** While it can improve gas exchange in some cases, it is not typically considered a first-line intervention for severe asthma.

- **Endotracheal intubation and mechanical ventilation:** These should be considered as a last resort when NIPPV fails to improve the patient's condition.

In conclusion, NIPPV is a valuable tool in the management of severe asthma exacerbations and can help prevent the need for invasive ventilation.

109. **Answer: C. Medical therapy with beta-blockers and blood pressure control**

Explanation:

Medical therapy with beta-blockers and blood pressure control is the most appropriate initial management strategy for a hemodynamically stable patient with an acute aortic dissection.

- **Immediate goal:** Reduce aortic shear stress by lowering blood pressure and heart rate.
- **Beta-blockers:** Decrease heart rate and myocardial contractility, reducing aortic wall stress.
- **Blood pressure control:** Lowering blood pressure helps to reduce the force exerted on the aortic wall.

Why other options are incorrect:

- **Surgical repair:** Indicated for hemodynamically unstable patients, patients with rapidly expanding aortic dissection, or those with complications such as organ malperfusion or impending rupture.
- **Endovascular repair:** Considered for specific types of aortic dissection (Type B) and in selected patients. Not the initial management for hemodynamically stable patients.
- **Percutaneous transluminal angioplasty (PTA):** Not applicable in the management of aortic dissection.

In conclusion, initial management of a hemodynamically stable patient with acute aortic dissection focuses on medical therapy to stabilize the patient and prevent dissection progression. Surgical or endovascular intervention may be considered later based on the patient's clinical course.

110. **Answer: A. Pericardiocentesis**
Explanation:
Pericardiocentesis is the most appropriate treatment for a 70-year-old woman with CKD who has developed uremic pericarditis and subsequent cardiac tamponade.

• **Cardiac tamponade** is a life-threatening condition where fluid accumulates in the pericardial sac, compressing the heart and impairing its ability to pump blood effectively.

• **Pericardiocentesis** involves draining the excess fluid from the pericardial space, relieving the pressure on the heart and restoring cardiac output.

Why other options are incorrect:

• **Corticosteroids:** While they can be used in the management of uremic pericarditis, they are not a primary treatment for cardiac tamponade.

• **Nonsteroidal anti-inflammatory drugs (NSAIDs):** These medications are generally avoided in patients with CKD due to the risk of renal impairment and are not effective in treating cardiac tamponade.

• **Dialysis:** While essential for managing CKD, dialysis alone is not sufficient to treat the immediate life-threatening consequences of cardiac tamponade.

In conclusion, pericardiocentesis is a life-saving procedure for patients with cardiac tamponade, regardless of the underlying cause.

111. **Answer: A. Nitroglycerin**
Explanation:
Nitroglycerin is the most appropriate medication to reduce afterload in a patient with acute decompensated heart failure (ADHF).

• **Afterload** is the resistance the heart must overcome to eject blood. By reducing afterload, the heart can work more efficiently.

• **Nitroglycerin** is a potent vasodilator that primarily decreases preload but also has a significant effect on reducing afterload.

• This reduction in afterload can improve cardiac output and alleviate symptoms of ADHF.

Why other options are incorrect:

• **Furosemide:** A diuretic, primarily used to reduce preload by promoting fluid loss.

- **Dobutamine:** An inotropic agent that increases cardiac contractility, primarily used to improve cardiac output.
- **Nesiritide:** A synthetic form of BNP, primarily used to reduce preload and afterload, but its role in routine ADHF management is still being evaluated.

In conclusion, nitroglycerin is a cornerstone in the management of ADHF to reduce afterload and improve cardiac function.

112. Answer: B. Proteinuria and hematuria

Explanation:

Proteinuria and hematuria are the most consistent laboratory findings with lupus nephritis.

- **Lupus nephritis** is a kidney inflammation that occurs as a complication of systemic lupus erythematosus (SLE).
- Damage to the kidney's filtering units results in the leakage of protein and red blood cells into the urine, leading to proteinuria and hematuria.

Why other options are incorrect:

- **Decreased serum creatinine:** This would indicate improved kidney function, which is opposite to what occurs in lupus nephritis.
- **Normal complement levels:** Complement levels are often decreased in patients with lupus nephritis due to immune complex deposition in the kidneys.
- **Negative antinuclear antibody (ANA) titer:** ANA is a common autoantibody found in patients with SLE. A negative ANA titer would be inconsistent with a diagnosis of SLE.

In conclusion, proteinuria and hematuria are key diagnostic indicators of lupus nephritis.

113. Answer: D. Lung-protective ventilation with low tidal volumes and high PEEP

Explanation:

Lung-protective ventilation with low tidal volumes and high PEEP is the most appropriate ventilator setting to improve ventilation-perfusion (V/Q) mismatch in a patient with COPD experiencing an acute exacerbation.

- **Ventilation-perfusion mismatch** occurs when there is an imbalance between the amount of air reaching the alveoli (ventilation) and the amount of blood flowing through the pulmonary capillaries (perfusion).

- **Low tidal volumes** help to prevent overdistension of the lungs and reduce the risk of ventilator-induced lung injury (VILI).
- **High PEEP** helps to recruit and open collapsed alveoli, improving oxygenation and reducing dead space.

Why other options are incorrect:

- **High tidal volume ventilation:** Can lead to overdistension of the lungs, barotrauma, and worsening V/Q mismatch.
- **Low PEEP:** Insufficient PEEP may not adequately open collapsed alveoli, leading to hypoxemia.
- **High respiratory rate:** Can increase dead space and worsen V/Q mismatch.

In conclusion, lung-protective ventilation with low tidal volumes and high PEEP is the cornerstone of mechanical ventilation in patients with COPD to optimize oxygenation and minimize lung injury.

114. Answer: D. All of the above

Explanation:

All of the mentioned interventions are crucial in reducing the risk of ventilator-associated pneumonia (VAP) in a patient on mechanical ventilation.

- **Oral chlorhexidine gluconate rinse:** Reduces bacterial load in the oral cavity, a common source of aspiration.
- **Elevation of the head of the bed to 30 degrees:** Prevents aspiration by reducing pooling of secretions in the back of the throat.
- **Daily "sedation vacations" and assessment of readiness to extubate:** Minimizes sedation, promotes spontaneous breathing, and facilitates early extubation, all of which reduce the risk of VAP.

Implementing these evidence-based interventions together significantly lowers the incidence of VAP in critically ill patients.

115. Answer: D. Extracorporeal membrane oxygenation (ECMO)

Explanation:

Extracorporeal membrane oxygenation (ECMO) is the most appropriate mechanical circulatory support device for a 65-year-old man with HFrEF in cardiogenic shock who remains hypotensive and oliguric despite inotropic and vasopressor support.

- **Cardiogenic shock** is a severe condition where the heart cannot pump enough blood to meet the body's needs, leading to organ dysfunction.
- **ECMO** provides both cardiac and respiratory support by oxygenating the blood outside the body, allowing the heart and lungs to rest and recover.

Why other options are incorrect:
- **Intra-aortic balloon pump (IABP):** While IABP can improve coronary blood flow and reduce afterload, it is not sufficient for patients in cardiogenic shock.
- **Impella:** This device provides left ventricular support but may not be enough for patients with severe heart failure and low cardiac output.
- **TandemHeart:** This device provides left ventricular unloading and circulatory support but is generally indicated for patients with less severe heart failure compared to cardiogenic shock.

In conclusion, ECMO is the most advanced and comprehensive form of mechanical circulatory support and is often the life-saving intervention for patients with refractory cardiogenic shock.

116. **Answer: A. Nonselective beta-blocker (e.g., propranolol)**
Explanation:
Nonselective beta-blockers are the cornerstone of long-term management for patients with cirrhosis and varices.
- **Reduces portal pressure:** By decreasing heart rate and cardiac output, beta-blockers lower portal pressure, reducing the risk of variceal bleeding.
- **Proven efficacy:** Numerous studies have demonstrated the effectiveness of beta-blockers in preventing recurrent variceal bleeding.

Why other options are incorrect:
- **Endoscopic variceal band ligation (EVL):** While effective in acute variceal bleeding, EVL is a therapeutic intervention rather than a long-term management strategy.
- **Transjugular intrahepatic portosystemic shunt (TIPS):** TIPS is considered for patients with recurrent variceal bleeding despite optimal medical therapy or in those with refractory ascites. It is not typically the first-line treatment.
- **Liver transplantation:** Liver transplantation is the definitive treatment for end-stage liver disease but is reserved for patients with severe liver failure and limited life expectancy.

In conclusion, nonselective beta-blockers are the mainstay of long-term management for patients with cirrhosis and varices to prevent recurrent bleeding and improve overall prognosis.

117. Answer: A. Heliox

Explanation:

Heliox, a mixture of helium and oxygen, is the most likely adjunctive therapy to improve the patient's respiratory status in this case.

- **Heliox** reduces airway resistance by decreasing the density of the gas mixture. This is particularly beneficial in patients with severe airway obstruction, like those with status asthmaticus. The lower density gas mixture flows more easily through narrowed airways, improving oxygen delivery.

Why other options are incorrect:

- **Ketamine:** While ketamine has bronchodilator properties and can be used in refractory status asthmaticus, it is not the first-line adjunctive therapy. It is typically reserved for severe cases when other measures have failed.

- **Noninvasive positive pressure ventilation (NIPPV):** NIPPV can be beneficial in managing severe asthma exacerbations, but in this case, the patient is already in the ICU and has failed to respond to initial therapies. NIPPV might not be sufficient to address the severity of the respiratory distress.

- **Extracorporeal membrane oxygenation (ECMO):** ECMO is a life-saving intervention for patients with severe respiratory failure who are unresponsive to other treatments. It is reserved for critically ill patients as a last resort and would not be the initial choice in this scenario.

In summary, heliox is the most appropriate adjunctive therapy to improve the patient's respiratory status due to its ability to reduce airway resistance and improve oxygen delivery in severe airway obstruction.

118. Answer: B. Computed tomography angiography (CTA) of the chest

Explanation:

Computed tomography angiography (CTA) of the chest is the most appropriate diagnostic test to evaluate the extent of an aortic dissection in a hemodynamically stable patient.

- **CTA** provides a rapid and accurate assessment of the aorta, including its size, location, and extent of the dissection. It can also identify complications such as aortic rupture or involvement of branch vessels.

Why other options are incorrect:

- **Chest X-ray:** While a chest X-ray can show mediastinal widening, which is suggestive of aortic dissection, it is not specific enough to diagnose the condition or determine the extent of the dissection.
- **Transesophageal echocardiogram (TEE):** TEE is an excellent tool for evaluating the aortic arch and proximal descending aorta. However, it may not visualize the entire thoracic and abdominal aorta. Moreover, it is an invasive procedure with potential complications.
- **Magnetic resonance imaging (MRI) of the chest:** MRI is highly sensitive for diagnosing aortic dissection but is time-consuming and requires the patient to lie still for an extended period. In a hemodynamically unstable patient, MRI may not be feasible.

In summary, CTA is the preferred imaging modality for diagnosing and evaluating the extent of an acute aortic dissection in a hemodynamically stable patient due to its speed, accuracy, and ability to provide comprehensive information about the aorta.

119. Answer: C. Pulsus paradoxus

Explanation:

Pulsus paradoxus is the most consistent hemodynamic finding in cardiac tamponade.

- **Pulsus paradoxus** is a decrease in systolic blood pressure by more than 10 mmHg during inspiration. This occurs because the increased intrathoracic pressure during inspiration impairs venous return to the right ventricle, which is already compromised by the pericardial effusion. This leads to a decrease in cardiac output and systolic blood pressure.

Why other options are incorrect:

- **Increased cardiac output:** Cardiac tamponade actually leads to decreased cardiac output due to impaired ventricular filling caused by the pericardial effusion.

- **Decreased central venous pressure (CVP):** In cardiac tamponade, CVP is typically elevated due to increased right atrial pressure caused by the restricted ventricular filling.
- **Widened pulse pressure:** Pulse pressure is the difference between systolic and diastolic blood pressure. In cardiac tamponade, pulse pressure tends to be narrowed due to decreased cardiac output and increased systemic vascular resistance.

In summary, pulsus paradoxus is a classic sign of cardiac tamponade and is caused by the impaired venous return during inspiration in the presence of a pericardial effusion.

120. Answer: D. All of the above
Explanation:

All of the listed interventions - early goal-directed therapy (EGDT), low-dose corticosteroids, and tight glycemic control - have been shown to improve mortality in patients with septic shock.

- **Early goal-directed therapy (EGDT):** This involves rapid assessment and aggressive management of hemodynamic parameters, including mean arterial pressure, central venous pressure, and lactate levels. EGDT has been shown to improve outcomes in patients with septic shock.
- **Low-dose corticosteroids:** While controversial in the past, recent studies have demonstrated that low-dose corticosteroids can improve survival in patients with septic shock, especially those with refractory hypotension.
- **Tight glycemic control:** Maintaining blood glucose levels within a target range (e.g., 80-110 mg/dL) has been associated with reduced mortality in critically ill patients, including those with septic shock.

In summary, implementing all three interventions - EGDT, low-dose corticosteroids, and tight glycemic control - can contribute to improved outcomes in patients with septic shock. It is important to note that these interventions should be part of a comprehensive management plan for septic shock and should be tailored to the individual patient's clinical condition.

121. Answer: A. Ventricular septal rupture

Explanation:

A new-onset holosystolic murmur at the apex radiating to the axilla in a patient with STEMI is highly suggestive of **ventricular septal rupture (VSR)**.

• **VSR** occurs when a portion of the septum between the left and right ventricles tears, allowing blood to flow from the high-pressure left ventricle to the lower-pressure right ventricle during systole. This creates a turbulent blood flow, resulting in a holosystolic murmur.

Why other options are incorrect:

• **Papillary muscle rupture:** While this can also cause a murmur, it is typically a mitral regurgitation murmur, which is often heard at the apex and radiates to the axilla. However, it would not be a holosystolic murmur.

• **Free wall rupture:** This is a catastrophic complication of STEMI that usually results in rapid hemodynamic collapse and death. It does not typically present with a new murmur.

• **Acute pericarditis:** Pericarditis can cause a pericardial friction rub, which is a scratching sound, not a holosystolic murmur.

In summary, the combination of a new-onset holosystolic murmur and recent STEMI is highly indicative of ventricular septal rupture, a serious and life-threatening complication.

Note: This is a critical condition requiring immediate intervention.

122. Answer: C. Magnetic resonance imaging (MRI) of the brain

Explanation:

Magnetic resonance imaging (MRI) of the brain is the most helpful diagnostic test to confirm the suspected diagnosis of posterior reversible encephalopathy syndrome (PRES) in this patient.

• **MRI** is the gold standard for diagnosing PRES. It typically shows characteristic findings of vasogenic edema in the posterior regions of the brain, such as the occipital and parietal lobes.

Why other options are incorrect:

• **Electroencephalogram (EEG):** While EEG can be helpful in evaluating seizure activity, it is not specific for diagnosing PRES.

- **Lumbar puncture:** Lumbar puncture is generally avoided in patients with suspected increased intracranial pressure, such as those with PRES. It may also be misleading, as cerebrospinal fluid (CSF) findings are often normal in PRES.
- **Computed tomography (CT) scan of the head:** CT scan may not be sensitive enough to detect the early changes of PRES. Additionally, it involves exposure to ionizing radiation.

In summary, MRI is the imaging modality of choice for confirming the diagnosis of PRES due to its ability to visualize the characteristic brain lesions associated with this condition.

123. Answer: B. Hypokalemia
Explanation:

Hypokalemia is the most commonly associated electrolyte abnormality in Diabetic Ketoacidosis (DKA).

- **Hypokalemia** occurs due to several factors:
  - Insulin deficiency leads to increased renal potassium excretion.
  - Cellular shift of potassium into the intracellular space as insulin promotes glucose uptake.
  - Severe osmotic diuresis caused by hyperglycemia leads to potassium loss.

Why other options are incorrect:

- **Hyperkalemia:** This is actually uncommon in DKA due to the abovementioned factors. However, it's important to monitor potassium levels closely, as it can occur if the patient is severely dehydrated or has concomitant renal failure.
- **Hypernatremia:** While hyperglycemia can contribute to osmotic diuresis and fluid loss, hypernatremia is less common in DKA compared to hypokalemia.
- **Hyponatremia:** This is usually not a primary electrolyte abnormality in DKA and can occur due to dilutional effects from aggressive fluid resuscitation.

In summary, hypokalemia is a critical electrolyte imbalance to monitor and correct in patients with DKA. It is essential to closely monitor potassium levels and replace it as needed to prevent potentially fatal arrhythmias.

124. Answer: B. Endoscopic variceal band ligation (EVL)
Explanation:

Endoscopic variceal band ligation (EVL) is the most effective initial endoscopic therapy for controlling acute variceal bleeding.

- **EVL** involves placing rubber bands around the base of varices to occlude blood flow and promote necrosis of the varices. This is generally more effective than sclerotherapy in achieving immediate hemostasis and preventing rebleeding.

Why other options are incorrect:

- **Endoscopic variceal sclerotherapy (EVS):** While EVS can be effective, it is generally less effective than EVL in achieving immediate hemostasis. Additionally, it carries a higher risk of complications such as esophageal perforation and severe esophagitis.

- **Balloon tamponade:** Balloon tamponade can be used as a temporary measure to control bleeding while other therapies are being prepared. However, it has a high rate of complications, including aspiration, vomiting, and arrhythmias. It is not a definitive treatment for variceal bleeding.

- **Transjugular intrahepatic portosystemic shunt (TIPS):** TIPS is a radiologic procedure that creates a shunt between the portal vein and the hepatic vein to reduce portal pressure. It is an effective treatment for preventing recurrent variceal bleeding but is not the initial treatment of choice for acute bleeding.

In summary, EVL is the preferred endoscopic therapy for the initial management of acute variceal bleeding due to its effectiveness in achieving hemostasis and preventing rebleeding.

Note: Adjunctive therapies such as octreotide, vasopressin, and blood products are also crucial in the management of acute variceal bleeding.

125. Answer: B. Low tidal volume ventilation with high PEEP

Explanation:

Low tidal volume ventilation with high PEEP is the most effective ventilator strategy for improving oxygenation while minimizing lung injury in patients with acute respiratory distress syndrome (ARDS).

- **Low tidal volume:** This strategy helps to prevent overdistension of injured lung alveoli, reducing the risk of further lung damage.

- **High PEEP (Positive End-Expiratory Pressure):** This keeps alveoli open, preventing collapse and improving oxygenation.

Why other options are incorrect:

- **High tidal volume ventilation:** This can lead to overdistension of injured lung alveoli, causing further damage and worsening the ARDS.

- **Low or high tidal volume with low PEEP:** Low PEEP allows alveoli to collapse, reducing oxygenation. High PEEP with high tidal volume increases the risk of overdistension and barotrauma.

The ARDSNet study demonstrated that low tidal volume ventilation (6 mL/kg predicted body weight) and PEEP titration to optimize oxygenation without excessive alveolar pressures significantly improved survival rates in patients with ARDS.

In summary, the combination of low tidal volume and high PEEP is crucial in managing ARDS and optimizing patient outcomes.

126. Answer: A. Low respiratory rate and short inspiratory time

Explanation:

Low respiratory rate and short inspiratory time is the most appropriate ventilator setting to manage airflow obstruction and air trapping in a patient with status asthmaticus.

- **Low respiratory rate:** This allows for longer expiratory time, which is crucial for patients with air trapping to exhale trapped air effectively.
- **Short inspiratory time:** This prevents excessive lung inflation, which can exacerbate air trapping and worsen the patient's condition.

Why other options are incorrect:

- **High respiratory rate:** This would increase air trapping and worsen hyperinflation.
- **Long inspiratory time:** This would also contribute to air trapping and overdistension of the lungs.

Additional considerations for ventilator management in status asthmaticus:

- **Permissive hypercapnia:** Allowing a slightly higher than normal PaCO2 can be tolerated to avoid excessive ventilator pressures and further lung injury.
- **Low tidal volumes:** To prevent volutrauma.
- **Sedation:** To reduce oxygen consumption and improve patient-ventilator synchrony.
- **Neuromuscular blockade:** In severe cases, to improve ventilation and oxygenation.

In summary, the goal of ventilator management in status asthmaticus is to allow adequate time for expiration, prevent overdistension of the lungs, and minimize the risk of complications.

Note: Close monitoring of the patient's clinical condition and blood gases is essential to adjust ventilator settings as needed.

127. Answer: A. Beta-blockers

Explanation:

Beta-blockers are the most appropriate medication for long-term blood pressure control in a patient with a history of aortic dissection.

• **Beta-blockers** reduce myocardial contractility and heart rate, leading to decreased shear stress on the aorta. This is crucial in preventing the propagation of an aortic dissection or the development of a new dissection.

Why other options are incorrect:

• **Calcium channel blockers:** While they can lower blood pressure, they do not have the specific protective effect on the aorta that beta-blockers provide.

• **ACE inhibitors and ARBs:** These medications are effective for blood pressure control but can increase shear stress on the aorta, potentially increasing the risk of aortic dissection. They are generally avoided in patients with a history of aortic dissection.

In summary, beta-blockers are the cornerstone of long-term blood pressure management in patients with aortic dissection due to their ability to reduce myocardial contractility and shear stress on the aorta.

Note: Other medications, such as statins for lipid management and antiplatelet agents, may also be indicated depending on the individual patient's risk factors.

128. Answer: A. Tachycardia

Explanation:

Tachycardia is a potential adverse effect of norepinephrine.

• **Norepinephrine** is a potent vasoconstrictor with both alpha and beta-adrenergic effects. While its primary action is to increase blood pressure through vasoconstriction (alpha-adrenergic effect), it can also stimulate beta-1 receptors, leading to increased heart rate and contractility.

Why other options are incorrect:

- **Hypotension:** Norepinephrine is primarily used to treat hypotension, so this is unlikely.
- **Bradycardia:** While norepinephrine can cause reflex bradycardia due to increased blood pressure, this is less common than tachycardia.
- **Hyperglycemia:** Norepinephrine does not directly cause hyperglycemia.

In summary, while norepinephrine is a valuable tool for managing septic shock, it is essential to monitor for potential adverse effects, including tachycardia. Close hemodynamic monitoring and titration of the dose are crucial to optimize the benefits while minimizing risks.

129. Answer: A. Sodium bicarbonate infusion

Explanation:

The patient presents with a severe metabolic acidosis (pH 7.20, HCO3- 12 mEq/L) with compensatory respiratory alkalosis (PaCO2 30 mmHg). The most appropriate initial intervention is to correct the metabolic acidosis directly.

- **Sodium bicarbonate infusion** is used to rapidly correct severe metabolic acidosis. It directly increases the bicarbonate level in the blood, helping to restore normal pH.

Why other options are incorrect:

- **Intravenous insulin and glucose:** This is the treatment for diabetic ketoacidosis, a different metabolic acidosis.
- **Hemodialysis:** While hemodialysis can correct metabolic acidosis, it is a slower process and not indicated as the initial intervention in this acutely ill patient with severe acidosis.
- **Thiamine supplementation:** Thiamine deficiency can cause metabolic acidosis, but it is not the primary problem in this case.

In summary, sodium bicarbonate infusion is the most rapid and effective way to correct severe metabolic acidosis in this patient. However, it's important to monitor closely for potential complications like overcorrection and worsening hypernatremia.

Note: The underlying cause of the metabolic acidosis should also be investigated and treated concurrently.

130. Answer: A. Fresh frozen plasma (FFP)

Explanation:

Fresh frozen plasma (FFP) is the most appropriate blood product to correct coagulopathy in a patient with acute alcoholic hepatitis.

• **FFP** contains all clotting factors, including those deficient in liver disease. It is effective in reversing coagulopathy caused by a lack of clotting factor synthesis.

Why other options are incorrect:

• **Cryoprecipitate:** Primarily contains fibrinogen and factor VIII. While it can be useful in specific clotting factor deficiencies, it is not as comprehensive as FFP in addressing the multiple clotting factor deficiencies seen in liver disease.

• **Platelets:** While important for primary hemostasis, they are not the primary issue in coagulopathy due to liver disease. Platelets are indicated for thrombocytopenia, not factor deficiencies.

• **Prothrombin complex concentrate (PCC):** While PCC can rapidly correct specific clotting factor deficiencies, it is often reserved for specific bleeding conditions, such as vitamin K deficiency or warfarin overdose, rather than the global coagulopathy seen in liver disease.

In summary, FFP is the broadest and most effective blood product for correcting the coagulopathy associated with acute alcoholic hepatitis.

Note: It is essential to monitor the patient closely for response to the FFP and potential complications such as fluid overload.

131. Answer: A. Spironolactone

Explanation:

Spironolactone is the most appropriate medication to add to this patient's regimen to improve symptoms and reduce hospital readmission.

• **Spironolactone** is a mineralocorticoid receptor antagonist (MRA) that effectively reduces fluid retention, improves symptoms, and decreases the risk of hospitalization in patients with heart failure. It works by blocking the action of aldosterone, a hormone that promotes sodium and water retention.

Why other options are incorrect:

• **Sacubitril/valsartan:** While this combination is an excellent choice for chronic heart failure with reduced ejection fraction, it is not the best initial choice for acute decompensated heart failure. It takes time to exert its beneficial effects.

- **Ivabradine:** This medication is used to reduce heart rate in patients with heart failure with reduced ejection fraction and sinus rhythm. It is not indicated in acute decompensated heart failure.
- **Digoxin:** While digoxin can be used in heart failure, it has a narrow therapeutic index and is associated with increased risk of toxicity. It is not the first-line treatment for acute decompensated heart failure.

In summary, spironolactone is a valuable addition to the treatment of acute decompensated heart failure due to its ability to reduce fluid overload, improve symptoms, and decrease the risk of hospitalization.

Note: Other treatments, such as intravenous diuretics, inotropes, and oxygen therapy, may be required to manage acute decompensated heart failure.

132. Answer: C. Prone positioning
Explanation:

Prone positioning is the most effective intervention to improve oxygenation and reduce mortality in patients with ARDS.

- **How it works:** Placing the patient face-down improves oxygenation by:
  o Redistributing lung fluids and improving ventilation-perfusion matching
  o Reducing alveolar collapse
  o Increasing lung compliance
- **Evidence:** Numerous studies have demonstrated that prone positioning significantly improves oxygenation, reduces the need for higher levels of PEEP, and decreases mortality in ARDS patients.

Why other options are incorrect:

- **A. High tidal volume ventilation:** This was once a common practice but has been shown to increase ventilator-induced lung injury (VILI) and mortality. Lower tidal volumes are now recommended.
- **B. Low positive end-expiratory pressure (PEEP):** While PEEP is important in ARDS management, low levels are generally insufficient to prevent alveolar collapse. Adequate PEEP is crucial but should be titrated carefully to balance oxygenation and lung injury.
- **D. Inhaled nitric oxide:** While it can improve oxygenation in some cases, its effect is often modest and inconsistent. It is not considered a first-line treatment for ARDS.

Case Study:

A 55-year-old woman develops ARDS following sepsis. Her PaO2/FiO2 ratio is 100, and she requires high levels of PEEP to maintain adequate oxygenation. The decision is made to initiate prone positioning. Within a few hours, her PaO2 improves significantly, allowing for a reduction in PEEP and ventilator settings.

By understanding the pathophysiology of ARDS and the evidence-based interventions, nurses can play a crucial role in optimizing care for these critically ill patients.

133. Answer: B. Cyclophosphamide

Explanation:

Cyclophosphamide is the standard of care for induction therapy in patients with diffuse proliferative lupus nephritis (Class IV). It is a highly effective immunosuppressant that has been shown to induce remission and prevent progression of kidney disease in this patient population.

- **How it works:** Cyclophosphamide is an alkylating agent that suppresses the immune system by inhibiting cell proliferation.

Why other options are incorrect:

- **A. Mycophenolate mofetil (MMF):** While MMF is an effective immunosuppressant, it is typically used as maintenance therapy after induction with cyclophosphamide. It is not as potent as cyclophosphamide and may not be sufficient for rapidly controlling severe lupus nephritis.
- **C. Rituximab:** Rituximab is a B-cell depleting agent that is used in the treatment of lupus nephritis, but it is not the first-line therapy for induction. It is often used as an alternative for patients who are intolerant or resistant to cyclophosphamide.
- **D. Belimumab:** Belimumab is a monoclonal antibody that targets B-lymphocyte stimulator (BLyS). It is approved for the treatment of lupus but is not considered a first-line therapy for lupus nephritis.

Case Study:

A 35-year-old woman with a history of SLE presents with rapidly progressive renal failure. A renal biopsy confirms diffuse proliferative lupus nephritis. The patient is initiated on intravenous cyclophosphamide for induction therapy. After achieving remission, she is transitioned to mycophenolate mofetil for maintenance therapy.

It is essential to monitor patients closely for adverse effects of cyclophosphamide, such as infection and bone marrow suppression.

134. Answer: A. Aspirin
Explanation:
Aspirin is the recommended medication to initiate within 24 hours of symptom onset in a patient with acute ischemic stroke who is not a candidate for intravenous thrombolysis or mechanical thrombectomy.
- **How it works:** Aspirin is an antiplatelet agent that inhibits platelet aggregation, reducing the risk of clot formation and subsequent stroke.

Why other options are incorrect:
- **B. Clopidogrel:** While clopidogrel is also an antiplatelet agent, aspirin is preferred for initial treatment of acute ischemic stroke due to its rapid onset of action.
- **C. Warfarin:** Warfarin is an anticoagulant, not an antiplatelet agent. It takes several days to achieve therapeutic effect and is not recommended for acute stroke treatment.
- **D. Apixaban:** Apixaban is a newer anticoagulant that is not indicated for acute stroke treatment. It is primarily used for stroke prevention in patients with atrial fibrillation.

Case Study:
A 70-year-old man presents to the emergency department with symptoms of acute ischemic stroke. Due to the time window for thrombolysis having elapsed, he is not a candidate for this treatment. Aspirin is administered immediately to reduce the risk of recurrent stroke.

Early initiation of aspirin has been shown to reduce the risk of recurrent stroke and improve outcomes in patients with acute ischemic stroke.

135. Answer: D. Any of the above
Explanation:
All of the listed beta-blockers (propranolol, nadolol, and carvedilol) are effective in preventing rebleeding in patients with cirrhosis and acute variceal bleeding.

- **How they work:** Beta-blockers reduce portal pressure by decreasing cardiac output and reducing blood flow to the liver. This helps to lower the risk of variceal bleeding.

Why other options are incorrect:
- **A, B, and C:** While each of these beta-blockers is effective, there is no specific preference for one over the other. The choice of beta-blocker often depends on factors such as patient tolerance, comorbidities, and availability.

Case Study:

A 50-year-old man with cirrhosis and a history of variceal bleeding is admitted to the ICU with acute variceal bleeding. After successful EVL, propranolol is initiated to prevent rebleeding. The patient tolerates the medication well and remains free of rebleeding during hospitalization.

The decision of which beta-blocker to use should be made in consultation with the patient's hepatologist and based on individual patient factors.

136. **Answer: A. Lactulose**

Explanation:

Lactulose is the first-line treatment for hepatic encephalopathy. It is a synthetic disaccharide that acts as a laxative and is effective in reducing ammonia levels.

- **How it works:** Lactulose acidifies the colon, leading to the conversion of ammonia into ammonium ions. Ammonium ions are less readily absorbed from the gut into the bloodstream, thereby reducing ammonia levels.

Why other options are incorrect:
- **B. Rifaximin:** Rifaximin is a non-absorbable antibiotic that reduces intestinal bacteria, which produce ammonia. While effective, it is often used as an adjunct to lactulose, not as first-line therapy.
- **C. Neomycin:** Neomycin is another antibiotic used to reduce intestinal bacteria, but it carries a higher risk of side effects, including nephrotoxicity and ototoxicity. It is generally reserved for cases refractory to other treatments.
- **D. L-ornithine L-aspartate (LOLA):** While LOLA can improve mental status in hepatic encephalopathy, it does not directly reduce ammonia levels. It is often used as adjunctive therapy.

Case Study:

A 45-year-old man with cirrhosis develops hepatic encephalopathy with increasing confusion. Lactulose is initiated, and within 24 hours, his mental status improves significantly. Ammonia levels also decrease.

Lactulose is generally well-tolerated, but it can cause diarrhea. Monitoring fluid and electrolyte balance is essential during treatment.

137. Answer: B. Low respiratory rate

Explanation:

Low respiratory rate is the most appropriate ventilator setting to reduce the risk of barotrauma and dynamic hyperinflation in a patient with status asthmaticus.

- **How it works:** A lower respiratory rate allows for longer expiratory time, which helps to prevent air trapping and reduce the risk of dynamic hyperinflation. This, in turn, decreases the risk of barotrauma.

Why other options are incorrect:

- **A. High tidal volume ventilation:** This would increase the risk of barotrauma and lung injury, which is detrimental in patients with status asthmaticus.
- **C. High inspiratory flow rate:** While a high inspiratory flow rate can improve gas exchange, it can also contribute to air trapping and dynamic hyperinflation.
- **D. Low inspiratory:expiratory (I:E) ratio:** A low I:E ratio means a shorter expiratory time, which can lead to air trapping and dynamic hyperinflation.

Case Study:

A 30-year-old woman with severe asthma is intubated for status asthmaticus. Initial ventilator settings include a low respiratory rate (8-10 breaths/min), low tidal volume, and prolonged expiratory time. These settings help to prevent air trapping and reduce the risk of barotrauma.

It is important to monitor the patient closely for signs of dynamic hyperinflation, such as increasing peak inspiratory pressures and decreased oxygenation. Adjusting ventilator settings as needed is crucial.

138. Answer: B. Clopidogrel

Explanation:

Clopidogrel is the recommended medication to be added to aspirin to reduce the risk of stent thrombosis in patients who undergo percutaneous coronary intervention (PCI) with drug-eluting stent placement.

- **How it works:** Clopidogrel, like aspirin, is an antiplatelet agent that prevents platelet aggregation, reducing the risk of clot formation on the stent. This combination therapy provides dual antiplatelet protection.

Why other options are incorrect:

- **A. Aspirin:** Aspirin is already a standard component of antiplatelet therapy after PCI. While essential, it is not sufficient on its own to prevent stent thrombosis.
- **C. Ticagrelor and D. Prasugrel:** These are newer antiplatelet agents that are equally effective as clopidogrel in preventing stent thrombosis. However, they have a higher risk of bleeding compared to clopidogrel. In this case, clopidogrel is a reasonable choice due to the patient's history of hypertension and coronary artery disease, which increases the bleeding risk.

Case Study:

A 65-year-old man with a history of hypertension and diabetes mellitus presents with acute ST-elevation myocardial infarction. He undergoes successful PCI with placement of a drug-eluting stent in the left anterior descending artery. Aspirin and clopidogrel are initiated to prevent stent thrombosis.

Dual antiplatelet therapy with aspirin and clopidogrel is typically continued for at least 12 months after PCI with drug-eluting stents. Regular follow-up is essential to monitor for complications and adjust medication as needed.

139. **Answer: D. All of the above**

Explanation:

All of the listed electrolyte abnormalities (hypokalemia, hyperkalemia, and hypophosphatemia) can occur during the treatment of HHS. Close monitoring of these electrolytes is crucial to prevent life-threatening complications.

- **Hypokalemia:** Insulin promotes potassium shift from the extracellular to the intracellular space. This, combined with urinary potassium losses due to osmotic diuresis, can lead to hypokalemia.
- **Hyperkalemia:** Although less common, hyperkalemia can occur in severe cases of HHS, especially if the patient has renal insufficiency.
- **Hypophosphatemia:** Insulin promotes phosphate uptake into cells, and severe hypophosphatemia can occur during HHS treatment, particularly in patients with malnutrition or severe illness.

Case Study:

A 55-year-old woman with type 2 diabetes is admitted to the ICU with HHS. Despite aggressive fluid resuscitation, her serum potassium level drops rapidly. She is supplemented with potassium chloride infusion to prevent hypokalemia. Additionally, serum phosphate levels are monitored closely, and phosphate replacement is initiated as needed.

Regular electrolyte monitoring and prompt replacement are essential for preventing complications associated with HHS treatment.

140. **Answer: C. Torsemide**

Explanation:

Torsemide is the most appropriate diuretic for a patient with chronic kidney disease (CKD) and acute pulmonary edema.

- **Why Torsemide:**
  - **Potency:** Torsemide is a loop diuretic with a longer duration of action and greater potency than furosemide. This makes it more effective in removing excess fluid in patients with reduced kidney function.
  - **Kidney-sparing effects:** Compared to other loop diuretics, torsemide has shown some kidney-protective effects in certain studies, making it a potentially better choice for patients with CKD.

Why other options are incorrect:

- **A. Furosemide:** While furosemide is a potent loop diuretic, it has a shorter duration of action compared to torsemide and may not be as effective in patients with reduced kidney function.
- **B. Bumetanide:** Similar to furosemide, bumetanide is a loop diuretic but with less potency. It may not be as effective in rapidly removing excess fluid in severe pulmonary edema.
- **D. Ethacrynic acid:** This is another loop diuretic but is less commonly used due to its potential for ototoxicity and other side effects. It is generally reserved for patients who are allergic to sulfonamide-based diuretics (like furosemide and torsemide).

Additional Considerations:

- **Careful monitoring:** Regardless of the diuretic chosen, close monitoring of renal function, electrolytes, and hemodynamic status is essential.

- **Adjunctive therapies:** Diuretics should be used in conjunction with other treatments for pulmonary edema, such as oxygen therapy, positive pressure ventilation, and vasodilators.

By carefully selecting the appropriate diuretic and monitoring the patient closely, it is possible to improve outcomes in patients with CKD and acute pulmonary edema.

141. Answer: D. Fibrinolytic therapy

Explanation:

Fibrinolytic therapy is not routinely recommended for the initial management of NSTEMI. It is primarily reserved for patients with ST-segment elevation myocardial infarction (STEMI) to rapidly dissolve the clot blocking the coronary artery.

Why other options are correct:

- **A. Aspirin:** This is a cornerstone of treatment for NSTEMI, helping to prevent platelet aggregation and reduce the risk of further clot formation.
- **B. Ticagrelor:** This is a potent antiplatelet agent that, along with aspirin, helps to prevent stent thrombosis and reduce the risk of ischemic events.
- **C. Enoxaparin:** This is an anticoagulant that helps to prevent clot formation and reduce the risk of ischemic complications.

In NSTEMI, the focus is on stabilizing the patient, preventing further myocardial damage, and determining the best revascularization strategy (either through percutaneous coronary intervention or coronary artery bypass graft). Fibrinolytic therapy carries a higher risk of bleeding complications compared to the benefits in NSTEMI patients.

142. Answer: D. All of the above

Explanation:

All of the listed options are absolute indications for surgical intervention in a patient with infective endocarditis complicated by a large vegetation on the mitral valve.

- **New-onset heart failure:** This indicates severe valve dysfunction, which is a life-threatening complication of infective endocarditis. Surgical intervention is necessary to repair or replace the damaged valve.

- **Persistent bacteremia despite appropriate antibiotic therapy:** This suggests that medical management alone is insufficient to eradicate the infection. Surgery is often required to remove the infected vegetation and prevent further complications.

- **Embolic events despite appropriate antibiotic therapy:** Embolic events, such as stroke or septic emboli, are serious complications of infective endocarditis. Surgical intervention is often necessary to prevent further embolic events and reduce the risk of mortality.

In summary, these three conditions represent critical situations where medical management alone is unlikely to be successful, and surgical intervention is essential to improve patient outcomes.

143. **Answer: A. Piperacillin/tazobactam and vancomycin**

Explanation:

Piperacillin/tazobactam and vancomycin is the most appropriate empiric antibiotic regimen for a patient with COPD who develops ventilator-associated pneumonia (VAP) after 72 hours on mechanical ventilation.

- **Rationale:**
  - **Piperacillin/tazobactam:** This combination covers a broad spectrum of gram-negative bacteria, including Pseudomonas aeruginosa, which is a common pathogen in VAP.
  - **Vancomycin:** This antibiotic is used to cover for potential methicillin-resistant Staphylococcus aureus (MRSA), a common cause of hospital-acquired infections, including VAP.

Why other options are incorrect:

- **B. Cefepime and metronidazole:** Cefepime has good coverage for gram-negative organisms but lacks adequate coverage for gram-positive organisms like MRSA. Metronidazole primarily covers anaerobic bacteria, which may not be the primary pathogen in VAP.

- **C. Meropenem and vancomycin:** While meropenem provides excellent coverage for gram-negative organisms, including Pseudomonas aeruginosa, the combination with vancomycin might be considered overkill in some cases and could increase the risk of adverse effects.

- **D. Levofloxacin and azithromycin:** This combination is not recommended as empiric therapy for VAP due to increasing resistance patterns of these antibiotics to common VAP pathogens.

Additional considerations:

- **De-escalation:** Once culture and sensitivity results are available, the antibiotic regimen can be de-escalated to a narrower-spectrum agent if appropriate.
- **Duration of therapy:** The duration of antibiotic therapy for VAP typically ranges from 7 to 14 days, depending on the severity of illness and clinical response.

144. Answer: D. All of the above

Explanation:

All of the listed interventions have been shown to improve mortality in patients with septic shock.

- **A. Early goal-directed therapy (EGDT):** This involves rapid identification and treatment of sepsis, with a focus on achieving specific physiological targets such as mean arterial pressure, central venous pressure, and urine output. EGDT has been shown to improve outcomes in septic shock.
- **B. Low-dose corticosteroids:** Studies have demonstrated that low-dose corticosteroids can improve survival in patients with septic shock, especially those with persistent hypotension despite fluid resuscitation and vasopressors.
- **C. Tight glycemic control:** While initially thought to improve outcomes, more recent studies have shown that tight glycemic control does not reduce mortality and may increase the risk of hypoglycemia. However, hyperglycemia should still be managed to prevent complications.

It's important to note that while these interventions have been shown to be beneficial, they should be implemented as part of a comprehensive approach to the management of septic shock, which includes early recognition, source control, and appropriate antimicrobial therapy.

145. Answer: C. Ultrafiltration

Explanation:

Ultrafiltration is the most appropriate intervention for a patient with HFpEF who remains refractory to diuretics and vasodilators.

- **How it works:** Ultrafiltration is a process that removes excess fluid from the body using a semipermeable membrane. It is particularly effective in removing fluid overload in patients with heart failure.

Why other options are incorrect:

- **A. Impella:** This is a mechanical circulatory support device primarily used in patients with cardiogenic shock or severe heart failure with reduced ejection fraction. It is not typically indicated in HFpEF.
- **B. Intra-aortic balloon pump (IABP):** This is another mechanical circulatory support device that is primarily used in patients with acute coronary syndromes or cardiogenic shock. It is not indicated in HFpEF.
- **D. Inhaled nitric oxide:** This is a vasodilator that can be used in pulmonary arterial hypertension, but it is not effective in treating fluid overload in HFpEF.

Ultrafiltration can rapidly reduce pulmonary and peripheral congestion, improve symptoms, and decrease the need for invasive interventions in patients with refractory HFpEF.

146. Answer: D. Hepatorenal syndrome

Explanation:

Hepatorenal syndrome (HRS) is the most likely type of AKI in a patient with alcoholic hepatitis.

- **Hepatorenal syndrome:** This is a renal dysfunction caused by severe liver disease. It occurs due to a complex interplay of factors, including splanchnic vasoconstriction, circulatory dysfunction, and renal hypoperfusion.

Why other options are incorrect:

- **A. Prerenal AKI:** This is caused by decreased blood flow to the kidneys. While hypovolemia can contribute to AKI in patients with liver disease, hepatorenal syndrome is a more specific diagnosis.
- **B. Intrinsic AKI:** This involves direct damage to the kidney tissue. While alcoholic hepatitis can cause systemic inflammation, it is less likely to directly damage the kidneys.
- **C. Postrenal AKI:** This is caused by obstruction of the urinary tract. While this can occur in patients with liver disease due to complications such as hepatocellular carcinoma, it is less common than hepatorenal syndrome in this setting.

Hepatorenal syndrome is a severe complication of liver disease with a high mortality rate. Early recognition and appropriate management are crucial for improving patient outcomes.

147. Answer: C. pH 7.25, PaCO2 60 mmHg
Explanation:
The ABG findings that are most concerning for impending respiratory arrest in a patient with status asthmaticus are:
- **pH 7.25:** This indicates severe acidosis, which is a sign of worsening respiratory failure.
- **PaCO2 60 mmHg:** This elevated PaCO2 level signifies significant hypercapnia, a hallmark of respiratory failure due to inadequate alveolar ventilation.

Why other options are incorrect:
- **A. pH 7.35, PaCO2 45 mmHg:** These values are within normal ranges and do not indicate impending respiratory arrest.
- **B. pH 7.45, PaCO2 35 mmHg:** These values represent a normal acid-base balance and do not indicate respiratory failure.
- **D. pH 7.55, PaCO2 25 mmHg:** This indicates respiratory alkalosis, which can occur in acute asthma exacerbations but is not as critical as the acidosis and hypercapnia seen in option C.

A pH of 7.25 and PaCO2 of 60 mmHg suggest that the patient is experiencing severe respiratory failure with impending respiratory arrest. Immediate intervention is required to improve ventilation and oxygenation.

148. Answer: C. Surgical repair
Explanation:
Stanford Type A aortic dissection is a life-threatening condition that requires immediate surgical intervention. This type of dissection involves the ascending aorta and aortic arch, placing the patient at high risk for complications such as aortic rupture, cardiac tamponade, or stroke.

Why other options are incorrect:
- **A. Medical therapy with beta-blockers and blood pressure control:** While medical management is crucial to stabilize the patient before surgery, it is not sufficient on its own to address the underlying problem of the aortic dissection.

- **B. Endovascular repair:** This is an option for Stanford Type B dissections, but it is not suitable for Type A dissections due to the involvement of the ascending aorta.
- **D. Percutaneous transluminal angioplasty (PTA):** This is a procedure used for coronary artery disease, not for aortic dissection.

Immediate surgical repair is the gold standard treatment for Stanford Type A aortic dissection to prevent catastrophic complications and improve patient survival.

149. Answer: A. Right atrial collapse

Explanation:

Right atrial collapse is the most consistent echocardiographic finding in cardiac tamponade.

- **Cardiac tamponade:** This occurs when excess fluid accumulates in the pericardial sac, compressing the heart and impairing its ability to fill.
- **Right atrial collapse:** Due to increased pressure in the pericardial sac, the right atrium is compressed during inspiration, causing it to collapse. This is a hallmark sign of cardiac tamponade on echocardiogram.

Why other options are incorrect:

- **B. Left ventricular hypertrophy:** This is a chronic condition and not specifically associated with cardiac tamponade.
- **C. Mitral valve prolapse:** This is a valvular heart disease and not directly related to pericardial effusion.
- **D. Aortic stenosis:** This is another valvular heart disease unrelated to cardiac tamponade.

Right atrial collapse is a specific and reliable echocardiographic finding that helps to diagnose cardiac tamponade in patients with uremic pericarditis.

150. Answer: A. Hypernatremia

Explanation:

Vasopressin is an antidiuretic hormone that reduces water loss by the kidneys. One of the potential adverse effects of vasopressin is the retention of water, which can lead to an increase in sodium concentration in the blood, resulting in **hypernatremia**.

Why other options are incorrect:

- **B. Hyponatremia:** This is the opposite of hypernatremia and is not associated with vasopressin use.
- **C. Hyperglycemia and D. Hypoglycemia:** Vasopressin does not directly affect glucose metabolism, so these options are incorrect.

Therefore, close monitoring of sodium levels is essential in patients receiving vasopressin.

151. A. Octreotide

Explanation:

- **Octreotide** is a synthetic analogue of somatostatin, a hormone that inhibits the release of various substances, including vasoactive peptides. In the context of esophageal varices, octreotide is highly effective in reducing portal hypertension by decreasing splanchnic blood flow. This reduction in portal pressure helps to prevent further bleeding from the varices.
- Additionally, octreotide has a direct vasoconstrictive effect on the varices themselves, further contributing to its efficacy in controlling acute variceal bleeding.

Why other options are wrong:

- **Propranolol** and **Nadolol** are beta-blockers. While they are effective in preventing the initial development of varices and reducing the risk of rebleeding in patients with cirrhosis, they are not the first-line treatment for acute variceal bleeding. They work by reducing portal pressure over time, but their effect is slower compared to octreotide.
- **Spironolactone** is a potassium-sparing diuretic primarily used for managing ascites in patients with cirrhosis. It has a minor role in reducing portal pressure but is not as effective as octreotide in acute variceal bleeding.

Case Study:

A 55-year-old male with a history of alcohol abuse is admitted to the ICU with severe hematemesis and melena. Endoscopy confirms large esophageal varices with active bleeding. The patient is immediately started on IV octreotide infusion. Within hours, the bleeding is controlled, and the patient's hemodynamic status stabilizes. Propranolol is initiated after the acute bleeding episode to prevent rebleeding.

In conclusion, octreotide is the most effective medication for the acute management of variceal bleeding due to its rapid onset of action and ability to reduce portal pressure. hypertension and prevent variceal rebleeding.

152. D. Diffuse proliferative lupus nephritis

Explanation:

• **Diffuse proliferative lupus nephritis (DPLN)** is the most likely histological finding in a patient with SLE presenting with acute kidney injury (AKI) and nephrotic syndrome. It is a severe form of lupus nephritis characterized by widespread inflammation and proliferation of cells within the glomeruli.

• DPLN is associated with rapid progression to kidney failure, heavy proteinuria, and hematuria.

Why other options are wrong:

• **Minimal change disease** is characterized by effacement of the podocyte foot processes on electron microscopy. While it can cause nephrotic syndrome, it is typically associated with a less severe clinical course and is not typically seen in patients with SLE.

• **Focal segmental glomerulosclerosis (FSGS)** involves scarring in only some parts of the glomeruli. It is more commonly associated with HIV infection, heroin use, and obesity.

• **Membranous nephropathy** is characterized by thickening of the glomerular basement membrane due to immune complex deposition. While it can occur in patients with SLE, it is less likely to cause AKI and nephrotic syndrome as rapidly as DPLN.

Case Study:

A 38-year-old woman with a known history of SLE is admitted to the ICU with rapidly worsening renal function and significant proteinuria. A renal biopsy is performed, which reveals diffuse glomerular hypercellularity, glomerular necrosis, and crescent formation consistent with DPLN. The patient is initiated on high-dose corticosteroids and immunosuppressive therapy.

In conclusion, DPLN is the most likely diagnosis in a patient with SLE presenting with AKI and nephrotic syndrome. Early recognition and aggressive treatment are crucial to prevent progression to end-stage kidney disease.

153. B. Bilevel positive airway pressure (BiPAP)

Explanation:

• **BiPAP** is the most appropriate noninvasive ventilation (NIV) mode for a patient with COPD exacerbation and hypercapnic respiratory failure.

• It delivers two levels of positive pressure: a higher inspiratory positive airway pressure (IPAP) to improve oxygenation and a lower expiratory positive airway pressure (EPAP) to prevent alveolar collapse.

• This combination effectively addresses the underlying pathophysiology of COPD, which includes air trapping, hyperinflation, and hypoventilation.

Why other options are wrong:

• **CPAP** delivers a single, constant level of positive pressure. While it can improve oxygenation, it is less effective than BiPAP in addressing the hypercapnia associated with COPD exacerbation.

• **ASV** is an automated mode that adjusts ventilator settings based on patient-generated waveforms. While it can be effective in some patients, it may be more complex to set up and monitor compared to BiPAP in the acute setting.

• **HFNC** can improve oxygenation but does not provide the positive pressure support needed to address hypercapnia and improve ventilation in patients with acute COPD exacerbation.

Case Study:

A 75-year-old man with COPD presents to the ICU with worsening dyspnea, increased sputum production, and worsening hypoxemia. ABG analysis reveals hypercapnia. BiPAP is initiated, and the patient's respiratory rate and oxygen saturation improve within hours. The patient's condition stabilizes, and he avoids intubation.

In conclusion, BiPAP is the preferred NIV mode for patients with COPD exacerbation and hypercapnic respiratory failure due to its ability to improve both oxygenation and ventilation.

154. A. 30 mL/kg crystalloid bolus over 30 minutes

Explanation:

• **Early goal-directed therapy (EGDT)** for septic shock emphasizes rapid fluid resuscitation to improve hemodynamics and tissue perfusion.

- A **30 mL/kg crystalloid bolus** is the recommended initial fluid resuscitation strategy. Crystalloids are the first-line choice due to their rapid distribution and effectiveness in expanding intravascular volume.
- Administering the bolus over **30 minutes** allows for gradual volume expansion and monitoring of hemodynamic response.

Why other options are wrong:

- **B, C, and D** are incorrect because they either involve smaller fluid volumes, faster infusion rates, or the use of colloids. While colloids can be considered in refractory cases, crystalloids are the initial fluid of choice.

Case Study:

A 30-year-old woman presents to the ICU with hypotension, tachycardia, and altered mental status. She is diagnosed with septic shock secondary to a pelvic abscess. A 30 mL/kg bolus of normal saline is administered over 30 minutes. Her blood pressure improves, and her mental status clears.

In conclusion, a 30 mL/kg crystalloid bolus over 30 minutes is the most appropriate initial fluid resuscitation strategy for a patient with septic shock.

155. A. Intra-aortic balloon pump (IABP)

Explanation:

- **IABP** is the most appropriate mechanical circulatory support device for a patient with cardiogenic shock secondary to heart failure with reduced ejection fraction (HFrEF) and severe aortic insufficiency.
- The IABP improves coronary perfusion, reduces afterload, and augments cardiac output. This is particularly beneficial in patients with aortic insufficiency, as it helps to reduce the regurgitant volume returning to the left ventricle.

Why other options are wrong:

- **Impella** is a left ventricular assist device that can significantly augment cardiac output. However, in patients with severe aortic insufficiency, the increased left ventricular outflow can worsen aortic regurgitation.
- **TandemHeart** is a right ventricular assist device primarily used for patients with right ventricular failure. It is not indicated in this case.
- **ECMO** is a more invasive form of mechanical circulatory support that provides both respiratory and cardiac support. It is generally reserved for patients with refractory cardiogenic shock or those requiring respiratory support. In this case, the patient's primary issue is hemodynamic instability, not respiratory failure.

Case Study:

A 65-year-old man with HFrEF presents to the ICU with cardiogenic shock. Despite inotropes and vasopressors, he remains hypotensive and oliguric. An echocardiogram reveals severe aortic insufficiency. An IABP is inserted, leading to improved blood pressure, increased urine output, and decreased pulmonary congestion.

In conclusion, IABP is the most appropriate initial mechanical circulatory support device for a patient with cardiogenic shock secondary to HFrEF and severe aortic insufficiency due to its ability to improve coronary perfusion, reduce afterload, and augment cardiac output without exacerbating aortic regurgitation.

156. B. Prolonged prothrombin time (PT)

Explanation:

• **Prolonged prothrombin time (PT)** is the most indicative of poor prognosis and increased mortality in a patient with severe alcoholic hepatitis and acute liver failure.

• PT reflects the liver's ability to synthesize clotting factors, which are essential for hemostasis. In severe liver disease, the liver's synthetic function is impaired, leading to decreased production of clotting factors and prolonged PT.

• A prolonged PT is a strong predictor of developing hepatic encephalopathy, bleeding complications, and overall mortality in patients with acute liver failure.

Why other options are wrong:

• **Elevated serum bilirubin** is a common finding in liver disease but is less predictive of mortality compared to prolonged PT.

• **Elevated serum ammonia** is associated with hepatic encephalopathy, a complication of liver failure. While it indicates liver dysfunction, it is not as directly linked to mortality as prolonged PT.

• **Decreased serum albumin** reflects chronic liver disease and malnutrition but is less specific to the severity of acute liver failure and its associated mortality risk.

Case Study:

A 40-year-old man with a history of alcoholism is admitted to the ICU with jaundice, ascites, and encephalopathy. Laboratory tests reveal elevated bilirubin, ammonia, and a prolonged PT. Despite treatment, the patient's PT continues to worsen, and he develops severe bleeding from the gastrointestinal tract.

In conclusion, a prolonged PT is a critical laboratory marker of severity and prognosis in patients with alcoholic hepatitis and acute liver failure. It is essential to monitor PT closely and initiate appropriate management strategies to prevent complications.

157. **D. All of the above**

Explanation:

All of the listed medications are essential components in the management of status asthmaticus, a severe, life-threatening exacerbation of asthma.

- **Albuterol:** A beta-2 agonist, it directly relaxes airway smooth muscle, leading to bronchodilation. It's a cornerstone in the treatment of acute asthma exacerbations.

- **Ipratropium bromide:** An anticholinergic, it also relaxes airway smooth muscle by blocking acetylcholine receptors. It has an additive effect to beta-agonists in improving lung function.

- **Magnesium sulfate:** While not a bronchodilator in the traditional sense, it has bronchodilatory effects by interfering with calcium-mediated smooth muscle contraction. It's often used as an adjunct therapy in severe asthma, especially when beta-agonists and anticholinergics are not providing adequate relief.

In a patient with status asthmaticus requiring intubation and mechanical ventilation, a combination of these medications is often necessary to achieve optimal bronchodilation and improve lung function.

Case Study:

A 25-year-old woman with a history of asthma presents to the ICU with severe respiratory distress, wheezing, and hypoxemia. Despite aggressive treatment with nebulized albuterol and ipratropium, her condition deteriorates, requiring intubation. Magnesium sulfate is added to the treatment regimen, and in combination with the other bronchodilators, her respiratory status gradually improves.

In conclusion, a multi-modal approach using albuterol, ipratropium bromide, and magnesium sulfate is essential in the management of status asthmaticus.

158. A. Medical therapy with beta-blockers and blood pressure control

Explanation:

• **Stanford Type B aortic dissection** involves the descending aorta and its branches. In patients who are hemodynamically stable, the initial management focuses on aggressive medical management to reduce aortic wall stress.

• **Beta-blockers** are the cornerstone of treatment as they decrease heart rate and blood pressure, reducing the shearing forces on the aortic wall.

• **Blood pressure control** is essential to lower aortic pressure and prevent dissection propagation.

Why other options are wrong:

• **Surgical repair** and **Endovascular repair** are generally reserved for complicated Type B dissections with complications such as aortic rupture, persistent pain despite medical management, or rapidly expanding aortic diameter.

• **Percutaneous transluminal angioplasty (PTA)** is not indicated in the management of aortic dissection.

Case Study:

A 55-year-old man presents to the ICU with acute onset of severe chest pain radiating to the back. Imaging confirms a Stanford Type B aortic dissection. He is hemodynamically stable. Immediate initiation of beta-blockers and blood pressure control is started. The patient is monitored closely for complications, and surgical or endovascular intervention is considered if his condition deteriorates.

In conclusion, medical management with beta-blockers and blood pressure control is the initial treatment of choice for hemodynamically stable patients with Stanford Type B aortic dissection.

159. B. Pulsus paradoxus

Explanation:

• **Pulsus paradoxus** is a characteristic finding in cardiac tamponade. It refers to an exaggerated decrease in systolic blood pressure during inspiration. This occurs because the increased intrathoracic pressure during inspiration impairs venous return to the heart, leading to a drop in cardiac output and blood pressure.

Why other options are wrong:

- **Hypertension** is typically not associated with cardiac tamponade. In fact, hypotension is more common due to decreased cardiac output.
- **Widened pulse pressure** is the opposite of what is seen in cardiac tamponade. A narrow pulse pressure (difference between systolic and diastolic blood pressure) is more characteristic.
- **Kussmaul's sign** is an increase in jugular venous pressure during inspiration, which is seen in conditions like constrictive pericarditis, not cardiac tamponade.

Case Study:

A 70-year-old woman with CKD presents to the ICU with uremic pericarditis. She develops worsening dyspnea, tachycardia, and hypotension. Physical examination reveals muffled heart sounds and pulsus paradoxus. An echocardiogram confirms cardiac tamponade, requiring urgent pericardiocentesis.

In conclusion, pulsus paradoxus is a hallmark sign of cardiac tamponade and should prompt immediate evaluation and intervention.

160. D. All of the above

Explanation:

All of the listed laboratory tests are crucial to monitor for potential complications of norepinephrine therapy:

- **Serum lactate:** This is a marker of tissue perfusion and oxygenation. Elevated lactate levels can indicate inadequate tissue perfusion, a potential complication of vasopressor therapy.
- **Troponin:** This is a cardiac marker. Norepinephrine can increase myocardial oxygen demand, potentially leading to myocardial ischemia or injury. Monitoring troponin levels can help detect cardiac complications.
- **Creatinine kinase (CK):** This is a muscle enzyme. Norepinephrine can cause decreased blood flow to peripheral tissues, leading to tissue hypoxia and potential muscle damage. Monitoring CK levels can help detect rhabdomyolysis.

Case Study:

A 50-year-old woman with rheumatoid arthritis develops septic shock secondary to pneumonia. Norepinephrine is initiated to maintain adequate blood pressure. Close monitoring of serum lactate, troponin, and CK levels is essential to detect early signs of tissue hypoperfusion, myocardial injury, or rhabdomyolysis.

In conclusion, all three laboratory tests are important for monitoring patients receiving norepinephrine therapy to identify and manage potential complications effectively.

161. C. Serum lactate

Explanation:

- **Serum lactate** is the most reliable and direct indicator of tissue perfusion in a patient with septic shock. It reflects the balance between oxygen supply and demand at the cellular level.
- An elevated lactate level indicates inadequate tissue oxygenation and perfusion, despite adequate fluid resuscitation and vasopressor support.
- Serial lactate measurements can be used to assess the response to treatment and guide further interventions.

Why other options are wrong:

- **Central venous pressure (CVP)** and **Pulmonary capillary wedge pressure (PCWP)** are indirect measures of fluid volume status. They can be helpful in guiding fluid resuscitation but do not directly reflect tissue perfusion.
- **Mixed venous oxygen saturation (SvO2)** is a valuable parameter in assessing global oxygen delivery and consumption. However, it is less sensitive to changes in tissue perfusion compared to lactate and is more influenced by factors such as hemoglobin concentration and oxygen delivery.

Case Study:

A 72-year-old woman with hypertension and type 2 diabetes mellitus develops septic shock secondary to a urinary tract infection. Despite adequate fluid resuscitation and initiation of norepinephrine, the patient's blood pressure remains low, and there are signs of organ dysfunction. Serial lactate measurements are elevated, indicating persistent tissue hypoperfusion. Further interventions, such as increasing vasopressor dose or considering additional hemodynamic support, are guided by the lactate trends.

In conclusion, serum lactate is the most reliable and direct marker of tissue perfusion in septic shock and should be monitored closely to guide treatment decisions.

162. A. Prolonged QT interval

Explanation:

Hypocalcemia can significantly affect the heart's electrical activity. A low calcium level disrupts the normal function of cardiac muscle cells, leading to prolonged repolarization. This prolonged repolarization manifests as a **prolonged QT interval** on the ECG.

Why other options are wrong:

- **Shortened QT interval:** This is typically associated with hypercalcemia, not hypocalcemia.
- **Peaked T waves:** While often seen in hyperkalemia, they are not characteristic of hypocalcemia.
- **U waves:** These are small, positive deflections following the T wave, often seen in hypokalemia, not hypocalcemia.

Case Study:

A 48-year-old man with acute pancreatitis develops severe hypocalcemia. An ECG is obtained, which reveals a prolonged QT interval. This finding, in conjunction with the low calcium level, confirms the diagnosis of hypocalcemia and highlights the risk of cardiac arrhythmias.

In conclusion, a prolonged QT interval is the most likely ECG finding in a patient with severe hypocalcemia. It's essential to monitor these patients closely for arrhythmias and treat the underlying cause of hypocalcemia.

163. D. Either A or B

Explanation:

- **Intravenous immunoglobulin (IVIG)** and **plasma exchange (PLEX)** are both effective treatments for Guillain-Barré syndrome (GBS). They work by different mechanisms but have similar outcomes in terms of accelerating recovery and reducing the severity of the illness.
- IVIG provides antibodies that block damaging immune responses, while PLEX removes harmful antibodies from the blood.
- The choice between IVIG and PLEX often depends on factors such as the severity of the illness, the patient's overall condition, and available resources.

Why other options are wrong:

- **Corticosteroids** are not effective in treating GBS and may even worsen the condition.

In conclusion, both IVIG and PLEX are considered first-line treatments for GBS, and the decision of which to use is typically made on a case-by-case basis.

Would you like to know more about the specific indications for IVIG and PLEX in GBS?

164. A. Low respiratory rate

Explanation:

Reducing cardiac workload in a patient with cardiogenic shock following an acute myocardial infarction is crucial. The ventilator settings should aim to minimize the negative impact on cardiac function.

• **Low respiratory rate:** This reduces the work of breathing, decreases intrathoracic pressure fluctuations, and improves venous return to the heart. It allows for better cardiac filling and increases cardiac output.

Why other options are wrong:

• **High tidal volume ventilation:** This can increase intrathoracic pressure, reduce venous return, and increase afterload on the heart, worsening cardiac function.

• **High inspiratory flow rate:** While important for oxygen delivery, a high flow rate can increase peak inspiratory pressure and negatively impact cardiac function.

• **Low inspiratory:expiratory (I:E) ratio:** While important in certain respiratory conditions, it does not directly impact cardiac workload.

Case Study:

A 65-year-old man with a history of coronary artery disease is admitted to the ICU with cardiogenic shock post-MI. He is intubated and placed on mechanical ventilation. The ventilator settings are adjusted to a low respiratory rate to minimize the negative impact on cardiac function. This, combined with other supportive measures, helps to improve cardiac output and hemodynamic stability.

In conclusion, a low respiratory rate is the most appropriate ventilator setting to reduce cardiac workload in a patient with cardiogenic shock.

165. A. High-dose corticosteroids

Explanation:

• **High-dose corticosteroids** are the initial treatment of choice for diffuse alveolar hemorrhage (DAH) associated with systemic lupus erythematosus (SLE). They have a rapid onset of action and are effective in reducing inflammation and controlling bleeding.

Why other options are wrong:

• **Cyclophosphamide** and **rituximab** are immunosuppressive agents used for the management of lupus nephritis and other severe manifestations of SLE, but they have a slower onset of action and are not the first-line treatment for DAH.

• **Plasma exchange** can be considered as a rescue therapy for severe, refractory DAH, but it is not the initial treatment of choice.

Case Study:

A 50-year-old woman with SLE presents to the ICU with acute respiratory failure and hemoptysis. DAH is suspected, and high-dose corticosteroids are initiated immediately. Within a few days, the patient's respiratory status improves, and the bleeding subsides.

In conclusion, high-dose corticosteroids are the cornerstone of treatment for DAH associated with SLE due to their rapid onset of action and effectiveness in controlling inflammation and bleeding.

166. A. Trimethoprim-sulfamethoxazole (TMP-SMX)

Explanation:

• **Trimethoprim-sulfamethoxazole (TMP-SMX)** is the first-line treatment for Pneumocystis pneumonia (PCP) in patients with HIV infection. It is highly effective, well-tolerated, and has a good safety profile.

Why other options are wrong:

• **Pentamidine:** This is a second-line treatment for PCP, typically used in patients who are intolerant or allergic to TMP-SMX.

• **Clindamycin and primaquine:** This combination is not used for the treatment of PCP. Clindamycin is an antibiotic primarily used for bacterial infections, while primaquine is an antimalarial drug.

• **Atovaquone:** This is an alternative treatment for PCP but is not the first-line choice.

Case Study:

A 40-year-old man with HIV infection presents to the ICU with shortness of breath, fever, and dry cough. Chest X-ray shows bilateral diffuse infiltrates consistent with PCP. The patient is initiated on TMP-SMX therapy, and his condition improves significantly within a few days.

In conclusion, TMP-SMX is the preferred treatment for PCP in patients with HIV infection due to its efficacy, safety, and cost-effectiveness.

167. A. Serum sodium

Explanation:

- **Serum sodium** is the most important laboratory test to monitor for potential complications of vasopressin therapy.

- Vasopressin, also known as anti-diuretic hormone (ADH), promotes water reabsorption by the kidneys, which can lead to **hyponatremia** (low sodium levels).

- Close monitoring of serum sodium is crucial to prevent the development of severe hyponatremia, which can have serious neurological consequences.

Why other options are wrong:

- **Serum potassium**, **serum glucose**, and **serum creatinine** are important to monitor in critically ill patients, but they are not specifically related to vasopressin therapy complications.

Case Study:

A 75-year-old man with septic shock is treated with norepinephrine and vasopressin. Regular monitoring of serum sodium levels reveals a gradual decline. The vasopressin dose is adjusted, and fluid management is optimized to prevent further hyponatremia.

In conclusion, close monitoring of serum sodium levels is essential in patients receiving vasopressin therapy to prevent the development of hyponatremia and its associated complications.

168. A. Angiotensin-converting enzyme (ACE) inhibitor

Explanation:

- **Angiotensin-converting enzyme (ACE) inhibitors** are the cornerstone of treatment for scleroderma renal crisis (SRC). They effectively lower blood pressure and improve renal perfusion by blocking the renin-angiotensin-aldosterone system (RAAS).

- ACE inhibitors have been shown to halt the progression of renal disease and even improve renal function in some cases.

Why other options are wrong:

- **Angiotensin II receptor blockers (ARBs)** can be considered as an alternative to ACE inhibitors if the patient cannot tolerate ACE inhibitors, but they are generally less effective.

- **Calcium channel blockers** and **beta-blockers** are not first-line treatments for SRC and may not be as effective in controlling blood pressure and protecting renal function.

Case Study:

A 30-year-old woman with systemic sclerosis presents to the ICU with rapidly worsening renal function and hypertension. Scleroderma renal crisis is suspected. Immediate initiation of an ACE inhibitor, such as captopril, is started. Close monitoring of blood pressure and renal function is essential.

In conclusion, ACE inhibitors are the most effective and recommended treatment for scleroderma renal crisis due to their ability to lower blood pressure, improve renal perfusion, and potentially halt the progression of renal disease.

169. A. Ciprofloxacin

Explanation:

- **Ciprofloxacin** is the most commonly used prophylactic antibiotic to prevent spontaneous bacterial peritonitis (SBP) in patients with cirrhosis and ascites.

- It has excellent coverage against the most common bacteria causing SBP, such as *Escherichia coli* and *Klebsiella pneumoniae*.

Why other options are wrong:

- **Norfloxacin:** While also a fluoroquinolone, ciprofloxacin is generally preferred for SBP prophylaxis due to its broader spectrum of coverage.

- **Trimethoprim-sulfamethoxazole (TMP-SMX):** This antibiotic is primarily used for prophylaxis against Pneumocystis jirovecii pneumonia (PCP) in immunocompromised patients, not for SBP prevention.

- **Cefotaxime:** This is a third-generation cephalosporin with good coverage against gram-negative bacteria. However, it is not the first-line choice for SBP prophylaxis due to the potential for increased antibiotic resistance.

Case Study:

A 60-year-old man with cirrhosis develops acute variceal bleeding and undergoes EVL and octreotide therapy. To prevent SBP, he is started on ciprofloxacin prophylaxis. Regular monitoring of ascites and liver function is essential.

In conclusion, ciprofloxacin is the recommended prophylactic antibiotic for patients with cirrhosis and ascites to prevent SBP.

170. A. Joint aspiration and antibiotics

Explanation:

• **Septic arthritis** is a serious infection of the joint that requires prompt diagnosis and treatment to prevent joint damage and systemic complications.

• The initial management involves **joint aspiration** to obtain synovial fluid for culture and sensitivity testing. This fluid analysis helps identify the causative organism and guide antibiotic therapy.

• Simultaneously, **antibiotics** should be initiated based on the suspected pathogen (often Staphylococcus aureus).

Why other options are wrong:

• **Surgical drainage and debridement** may be necessary in cases of severe infection, joint instability, or persistent infection despite medical management. However, it is not the initial treatment.

• **Intra-articular corticosteroid injection** is used for inflammatory conditions, not infections. It would be contraindicated in septic arthritis.

• **Immobilization and physical therapy** are part of the rehabilitation process after the infection is controlled, but they are not initial management strategies.

Case Study:

A 55-year-old woman with rheumatoid arthritis presents with severe knee pain, swelling, and redness. Joint aspiration is performed, and the synovial fluid is cloudy with a white blood cell count of 50,000 cells/mm^3. Gram stain reveals gram-positive cocci in clusters. The patient is immediately started on intravenous vancomycin pending culture results.

In conclusion, joint aspiration and initiation of appropriate antibiotics are crucial for the management of septic arthritis.

171. Answer: A. Bacterial meningitis

Explanation:

The patient's presentation, including fever, confusion, nuchal rigidity, and the cerebrospinal fluid (CSF) findings of elevated white blood cell count with a predominance of neutrophils, low glucose, and elevated protein, strongly point to a diagnosis of **bacterial meningitis**.

- **Elevated white blood cell count with a predominance of neutrophils** is a classic hallmark of bacterial meningitis, indicating an acute inflammatory response to the bacterial infection.
- **Low glucose level** in the CSF is another crucial finding, as bacteria consume glucose for their metabolism.
- **Elevated protein** is a nonspecific finding but supports the diagnosis of meningitis.

Why other options are incorrect:

- **Viral meningitis** typically presents with a lower white blood cell count, a higher glucose level, and a lymphocytic predominance in the CSF.
- **Fungal meningitis** is less common and usually affects immunocompromised individuals. The CSF findings in fungal meningitis are typically different, with a lower white blood cell count and a higher opening pressure.
- **Tuberculous meningitis** is a chronic infection with a gradual onset. The CSF findings in tuberculous meningitis include a low glucose level, elevated protein, and a lymphocytic predominance.

Case Study:

A 65-year-old woman with rheumatoid arthritis, a condition that can suppress the immune system, is at increased risk for infections. The rapid onset of symptoms, including fever, confusion, and stiff neck, coupled with the critical CSF findings, made bacterial meningitis the most likely diagnosis. Immediate initiation of appropriate antibiotic therapy was crucial to improve the patient's outcome.

Note: Bacterial meningitis is a medical emergency requiring prompt diagnosis and treatment.

172. Answer: A. Staphylococcus aureus

Explanation:

The patient's history of IV drug use is a significant risk factor for infective endocarditis (IE). In this population, **Staphylococcus aureus** is the most common causative organism.

- **Staphylococcus aureus** is a virulent bacterium that can easily spread via contaminated needles used for IV drug injection. It has a propensity for causing right-sided endocarditis, which is often associated with tricuspid valve involvement.

- The patient's presentation of fever, chills, and a new murmur is consistent with IE, and the echocardiographic finding of a large vegetation on the tricuspid valve further supports this diagnosis.

Why other options are incorrect:

- **Streptococcus viridans** is more commonly associated with endocarditis on native, previously damaged heart valves.

- **Enterococcus faecalis** is often found in patients with urinary tract infections or those who have undergone recent genitourinary procedures.

- **Pseudomonas aeruginosa** is a gram-negative organism that is typically associated with hospital-acquired infections and is less likely to cause community-acquired IE.

Case Study:

A 45-year-old man with a long history of IV heroin use presented to the emergency department with fever, chills, and a new heart murmur. Blood cultures were positive for Staphylococcus aureus, and echocardiography revealed a large vegetation on the tricuspid valve. The patient was immediately started on intravenous vancomycin and underwent surgical intervention to remove the vegetation.

Note: Early diagnosis and treatment of infective endocarditis are crucial to prevent severe complications such as embolization, heart failure, and death.

173. Answer: A. Noninvasive ventilation (NIV)

Explanation:

In a patient with COPD experiencing acute exacerbation and hypercapnic respiratory failure, **noninvasive ventilation (NIV)** is the preferred initial intervention. NIV has been shown to improve oxygenation, reduce the risk of intubation, and improve patient outcomes in this population.

- **NIV** delivers positive pressure support through a mask, which helps to improve ventilation and oxygenation without the need for invasive procedures.
- It can reverse acidosis, reduce the work of breathing, and improve gas exchange.

Why other options are incorrect:

- **Invasive mechanical ventilation** should be considered if NIV fails to improve the patient's condition or if the patient develops severe respiratory acidosis or hemodynamic instability.
- **High-flow nasal cannula (HFNC)** can provide supplemental oxygen but does not offer the same level of respiratory support as NIV in patients with hypercapnic respiratory failure.
- **Tracheostomy** is a definitive airway management option but is generally reserved for patients with prolonged need for mechanical ventilation or complex airway management issues.

Case Study:

A 70-year-old man with COPD presented to the ICU with worsening dyspnea, increased sputum production, and hypoxemia. Despite aggressive medical management, his $PaCO_2$ continued to rise. NIV was initiated, and within a few hours, his respiratory status improved significantly, avoiding the need for intubation.

Note: Early initiation of NIV in patients with acute exacerbation of COPD and hypercapnic respiratory failure is crucial to prevent further deterioration and improve patient outcomes.

174. D. Arterial blood gas (ABG)

Explanation:

Arterial blood gas (ABG) is the most critical parameter for assessing the effectiveness of mechanical ventilation in a patient with severe CAP. ABG analysis provides direct information about the patient's oxygenation (PaO_2), ventilation ($PaCO_2$), and acid-base balance. These values are essential for determining the adequacy of oxygen delivery, the efficiency of CO_2 removal, and the overall respiratory status.

- **PaO2** reflects the oxygenation status and helps to adjust the FiO2 (fraction of inspired oxygen) accordingly.
- **PaCO2** reflects the ventilation status and helps to adjust the ventilator settings to maintain optimal CO2 elimination.
- **pH** provides information about acid-base balance, which can be affected by respiratory dysfunction.

Why other options are incorrect:
- **Tidal volume** is important, but it is just one component of ventilation. It does not provide information about gas exchange or acid-base balance.
- **Respiratory rate** is influenced by various factors, including sedation, pain, and the patient's underlying condition. It is not a reliable indicator of the effectiveness of ventilation.
- **Peak inspiratory pressure** reflects the pressure required to deliver a tidal volume, but it does not provide information about gas exchange or ventilation.

Case Study:
A 30-year-old woman was admitted to the ICU with severe CAP and required intubation and mechanical ventilation. Initial ABG analysis showed severe hypoxemia (low PaO2) and hypercapnia (high PaCO2), indicating inadequate gas exchange. By carefully monitoring ABG values, the ventilator settings were adjusted, and the patient's respiratory status gradually improved.

Note: ABG analysis is essential for optimizing ventilator management and preventing complications associated with mechanical ventilation.

175. D. Nesiritide

Explanation:
In a patient with acute decompensated heart failure (ADHF) and refractory fluid overload, despite optimal diuretic therapy, **nesiritide** is a suitable option to enhance diuresis.
- **Nesiritide** is a recombinant form of B-type natriuretic peptide (BNP), a hormone with potent vasodilatory and natriuretic effects.
- It reduces preload and afterload, leading to increased cardiac output and diuresis.
- It is particularly useful in patients with HFpEF, as it can improve hemodynamics and reduce pulmonary congestion.

Why other options are incorrect:

- **Spironolactone** is a potassium-sparing diuretic primarily used for long-term management of heart failure to reduce morbidity and mortality. It has a slower onset of action and is not the best choice for acute diuresis.
- **Sacubitril/valsartan** is an angiotensin receptor-neprilysin inhibitor (ARNI) used for chronic heart failure management. It is not indicated for acute diuresis.
- **Dopamine** is a vasopressor with inotropic effects. While it can increase renal blood flow and diuresis at low doses, it is generally reserved for patients with hypotension and is associated with increased mortality in patients with heart failure.

Case Study:

A 65-year-old woman with HFpEF was admitted to the ICU with acute pulmonary edema. Despite high-dose loop diuretics, her urine output remained low, and she remained hypoxic. Nesiritide was initiated, leading to a rapid increase in urine output, improvement in oxygenation, and reduction in pulmonary congestion.

Note: Nesiritide should be used cautiously due to the risk of hypotension. Hemodynamic monitoring is essential during treatment.

176. B. Terlipressin

Explanation:

Hepatorenal syndrome (HRS) is a severe complication of liver disease characterized by rapid deterioration of kidney function without intrinsic kidney damage. The underlying pathophysiology involves splanchnic vasodilation and renal vasoconstriction.

- **Terlipressin**, a synthetic analogue of vasopressin, is the recommended first-line treatment for HRS. It causes vasoconstriction, improving renal perfusion and increasing urine output.

Why other options are incorrect:

- **Albumin infusion:** While albumin can increase intravascular volume, it does not specifically address the underlying pathophysiology of HRS and is not as effective as vasoconstrictors in improving renal function.
- **Midodrine and octreotide:** This combination has been used in the past, but its efficacy is less established than terlipressin, and it is often associated with more adverse effects.

- **Hemodialysis:** While hemodialysis can manage the complications of renal failure, it does not address the underlying cause of HRS and is considered a supportive measure rather than a curative treatment.

Case Study:

A 40-year-old man with alcoholic hepatitis developed HRS with rapidly declining renal function. Terlipressin was initiated, and within a few days, there was a significant improvement in urine output and stabilization of renal function. The patient was eventually bridged to liver transplantation.

Note: Early recognition and treatment of HRS are crucial for improving patient outcomes. Liver transplantation is the definitive treatment for HRS.

177. D. Endotracheal intubation and mechanical ventilation

Explanation:

The patient is experiencing severe, refractory status asthmaticus despite maximal medical therapy, including inhaled bronchodilators, systemic corticosteroids, and intravenous magnesium sulfate. In such cases, **endotracheal intubation and mechanical ventilation** are indicated to protect the airway, improve gas exchange, and prevent respiratory failure.

Why other options are incorrect:

- **Inhaled heliox:** While heliox can improve gas flow in some cases of severe asthma, it is not a first-line treatment for refractory status asthmaticus.
- **Intravenous ketamine:** Ketamine has been studied in the management of status asthmaticus, but its role is not well-established, and it is not a standard of care.
- **Subcutaneous terbutaline:** Subcutaneous terbutaline is no longer recommended for the management of status asthmaticus due to its limited efficacy and potential adverse effects.

Case Study:

A 25-year-old woman presented to the ICU with severe wheezing, dyspnea, and hypoxemia despite aggressive medical management for status asthmaticus. Her PEFR remained critically low, and she developed increasing respiratory distress. To prevent respiratory failure and protect the airway, endotracheal intubation and mechanical ventilation were initiated.

Note: Early recognition of impending respiratory failure in status asthmaticus is crucial to prevent irreversible damage.

178. C. Surgical repair

Explanation:

Stanford type A aortic dissection is a life-threatening condition that involves the ascending aorta. It carries a high risk of rupture and mortality. Therefore, **surgical repair** is the definitive treatment.

- Surgery involves replacing the damaged portion of the aorta with a synthetic graft. This procedure stabilizes the dissection, reduces the risk of rupture, and improves patient outcomes.

Why other options are incorrect:

- **Medical therapy with beta-blockers and blood pressure control:** While these medications are crucial for initial stabilization and reducing aortic shear stress, they are not definitive treatments and cannot prevent dissection progression or rupture.
- **Endovascular repair:** This is an option for Stanford type B dissections, but it is not suitable for type A dissections due to the involvement of the proximal aorta.
- **Percutaneous transluminal angioplasty (PTA):** This is a procedure used for peripheral arterial disease, not for aortic dissection.

Case Study:

A 55-year-old man presented to the ICU with severe chest pain, hypotension, and signs of cardiac tamponade. A CT scan confirmed a Stanford type A aortic dissection. The patient underwent emergency surgical repair, which successfully stabilized the dissection and prevented further complications.

Note: Early diagnosis and prompt surgical intervention are crucial for improving survival rates in patients with Stanford type A aortic dissection.

179. A. Chest pain

Explanation:

The most common presenting symptom of uremic pericarditis is **chest pain**. This pain is often described as sharp, pleuritic, and worsens with deep inspiration or lying flat.

- **Dyspnea**, while a potential symptom, is more commonly associated with advanced uremic pericarditis leading to cardiac tamponade.
- **Pericardial friction rub** is a physical exam finding, not a presenting symptom.

- **Fever** is not a typical symptom of uremic pericarditis.

Case Study:

A 70-year-old woman with CKD presented to the ICU with complaints of acute onset chest pain. An echocardiogram revealed pericardial effusion, and the diagnosis of uremic pericarditis was confirmed.

Note: Early recognition of uremic pericarditis is crucial to prevent complications such as cardiac tamponade.

180. C. Peripheral ischemia

Explanation:

Norepinephrine is a potent vasoconstrictor used to treat hypotension in septic shock. However, excessive vasoconstriction can lead to **peripheral ischemia.**

- **Peripheral ischemia** occurs when blood flow to the extremities is reduced, resulting in tissue damage. Symptoms include cold, pale extremities, pain, and numbness.

Why other options are incorrect:

- **Hypotension** is the indication for norepinephrine, so it is unlikely to occur.
- **Bradycardia** is not a common side effect of norepinephrine. In fact, it can cause tachycardia.
- **Hypoglycemia** is not associated with norepinephrine use.

Case Study:

A 50-year-old woman with septic shock required increasing doses of norepinephrine to maintain adequate blood pressure. The nursing staff closely monitored her peripheral pulses and capillary refill to detect early signs of peripheral ischemia.

Note: Close monitoring of peripheral perfusion is essential when using norepinephrine.

181. B. Vasopressin

Explanation:

In a patient with septic shock who remains hypotensive despite adequate fluid resuscitation and norepinephrine, **vasopressin** is a suitable second-line agent.

- **Vasopressin** is a potent vasoconstrictor that can improve mean arterial pressure (MAP) by increasing systemic vascular resistance. It is particularly useful in patients with refractory hypotension and distributive shock.

- The patient's underlying conditions of hypertension, diabetes, and chronic kidney disease do not contraindicate the use of vasopressin.

Why other options are incorrect:

- **Epinephrine:** While epinephrine can be used as a second-line vasopressor, it has a broader effect on both alpha and beta receptors, which can lead to increased heart rate and myocardial oxygen demand. It should be reserved for patients with refractory shock and evidence of myocardial depression.

- **Phenylephrine:** Primarily an alpha-1 agonist, phenylephrine can increase blood pressure but may cause reflex bradycardia and reduced cardiac output. It is not typically the first choice for septic shock.

- **Dobutamine:** Primarily an inotropic agent, dobutamine increases cardiac output but has minimal vasoconstrictive effects. It is not indicated for hypotension in septic shock.

Case Study:

A 68-year-old woman with septic shock remained hypotensive despite adequate fluid resuscitation and increasing doses of norepinephrine. Vasopressin was added to the regimen, resulting in a significant improvement in MAP and hemodynamic stability.

Note: Vasopressin should be used cautiously due to the risk of myocardial ischemia and should be titrated carefully. Close monitoring of blood pressure, heart rate, and urine output is essential.

182. A. Emergency colectomy

Explanation:

Toxic megacolon is a life-threatening complication of inflammatory bowel disease characterized by colonic dilation, systemic toxicity, and the risk of perforation. Given the patient's severe presentation with fever, tachycardia, and hypotension, **emergency colectomy** is the most appropriate initial management.

Why other options are incorrect:

- **Intravenous corticosteroids:** While corticosteroids are often used in the management of ulcerative colitis, they are not effective in the setting of toxic megacolon and can delay definitive treatment.

- **Intravenous antibiotics and fluids:** While supportive care with antibiotics and fluids is important, it is not sufficient on its own to address the underlying problem of colonic dilation and the risk of perforation.

- **Nasogastric decompression and bowel rest:** These measures can be helpful in reducing colonic distension, but they are not definitive treatments for toxic megacolon and should be considered adjuncts to surgical management.

Case Study:

A 35-year-old man with ulcerative colitis presented to the ICU with severe abdominal pain, fever, tachycardia, and hypotension. A CT scan confirmed toxic megacolon with colonic dilation. The patient underwent emergency colectomy and recovered successfully.

Note: Toxic megacolon is a surgical emergency requiring prompt intervention to prevent catastrophic complications.

183. A. Increased alveolar-capillary permeability

Explanation:

The most likely pathophysiologic mechanism underlying ARDS in a patient with SLE is **increased alveolar-capillary permeability**.

- **SLE** is an autoimmune disease characterized by inflammation and damage to various organs, including the lungs.
- The inflammatory process in SLE can lead to increased permeability of the alveolar-capillary membrane, allowing fluid and proteins to leak into the alveoli.
- This results in pulmonary edema, impaired gas exchange, and the development of ARDS.

Why other options are incorrect:

- **Decreased surfactant production** is a common cause of ARDS in preterm infants but is less likely in adults with SLE.
- **Pulmonary embolism** can cause acute respiratory distress, but it is not the most likely cause in a patient with SLE and ARDS.
- **Aspiration pneumonitis** is another potential cause of ARDS, but it is less likely in a patient with SLE without a history of aspiration.

Case Study:

A 50-year-old woman with a history of SLE developed acute respiratory distress, hypoxemia, and bilateral pulmonary infiltrates. The diagnosis of ARDS was made. The underlying pathophysiology was attributed to increased alveolar-capillary permeability due to the inflammatory process associated with SLE.

Note: ARDS is a severe condition with high mortality, and early recognition and aggressive management are crucial.

184. D. All of the above

Explanation:

All of the listed hemodynamic parameters are crucial in managing cardiogenic shock:

- **Mean arterial pressure (MAP) > 65 mmHg:** Adequate blood pressure is essential to maintain perfusion to vital organs.
- **Cardiac index (CI) > 2.2 L/min/m2:** Cardiac index reflects cardiac output relative to body size and is a key indicator of tissue perfusion.
- **Central venous pressure (CVP) 8-12 mmHg:** While not as precise as other parameters, CVP can provide initial guidance on fluid responsiveness.

Achieving and maintaining these targets requires a balanced approach involving fluid resuscitation, vasopressors, and inotropes as needed.

Note: It's important to remember that these are general guidelines and individual patient needs may vary. Continuous monitoring and adjustment of therapy are essential.

185. A. Bleeding

Explanation:

While the primary goal of endoscopic variceal ligation (EVL) is to control acute variceal bleeding, it's important to understand that **re-bleeding** is the most common complication. Despite successful initial hemostasis, new varices can form or previously ligated varices can re-bleed.

Why other options are incorrect:

- **Infection:** While infection is a potential complication of any invasive procedure, it's less common than re-bleeding in the context of EVL.
- **Stricture formation:** Stricture formation can occur as a late complication of EVL but is not as frequent as re-bleeding.
- **Esophageal perforation:** This is a serious but rare complication of EVL.

Note: To prevent re-bleeding, patients often require multiple sessions of EVL, and prophylactic medications like beta-blockers are commonly used.

186. D. Decompressive craniectomy

Explanation:

A GCS score of 6 indicates severe traumatic brain injury (TBI). In patients with severe TBI and intracranial hypertension refractory to medical management,

decompressive craniectomy can be considered to reduce intracranial pressure (ICP) and potentially improve neurological outcome.

• **Hyperventilation** was once used to lower ICP but is now generally avoided due to potential negative effects on cerebral blood flow and oxygenation.

• **Mannitol** is an osmotic diuretic that can temporarily reduce ICP but has limitations and potential side effects.

• **Hypothermia** has been studied in TBI management but its role is still evolving and not considered a first-line intervention.

Note: Decompressive craniectomy is a complex procedure with potential risks and benefits. It should be considered in carefully selected patients based on specific criteria and in consultation with neurosurgical experts.

187. Answer: B. Initiation of hydrocortisone

Explanation:

Elevated lactate in the setting of septic shock despite adequate fluid resuscitation and vasopressor therapy suggests persistent tissue hypoperfusion. One of the key strategies to improve tissue oxygenation and perfusion in this scenario is the use of corticosteroids.

Hydrocortisone has been shown to improve hemodynamics and reduce mortality in patients with septic shock who require vasopressors. It works by modulating the inflammatory response and improving microvascular circulation.

Why other options are incorrect:

• **A. Transfusion of packed red blood cells (PRBCs):** While anemia can contribute to tissue hypoxia, the primary issue in this patient is likely microcirculatory dysfunction rather than oxygen-carrying capacity. There is no evidence to suggest that anemia is significantly contributing to the elevated lactate.

• **C. Addition of dobutamine:** Dobutamine is an inotropic agent that increases cardiac output. While it may improve hemodynamics, it is not specifically targeted at addressing the underlying issue of microcirculatory dysfunction, which is the primary cause of elevated lactate in this case.

• **D. Increase in norepinephrine dose:** Increasing the dose of norepinephrine may further increase blood pressure but may not necessarily improve tissue perfusion. In fact, excessive vasoconstriction can worsen microcirculatory dysfunction.

Case Study:

A 65-year-old male presents to the ICU with septic shock secondary to pneumonia. Despite adequate fluid resuscitation and initiation of norepinephrine, his lactate level remains elevated at 4.5 mmol/L. He is started on hydrocortisone, and within 6 hours, his lactate level decreases to 2.8 mmol/L, and his mean arterial pressure improves.

By understanding the pathophysiology of septic shock and the role of corticosteroids in improving microcirculation, the nurse practitioner can effectively manage this critical condition and improve patient outcomes.

188. Answer: D. All of the above

Explanation:

All of the options presented can be considered to reduce airway resistance and improve ventilation in a patient with status asthmaticus who is refractory to standard bronchodilator therapy.

• **Inhaled helium-oxygen mixture (heliox):** This gas mixture has lower density than air, which reduces airway resistance and improves airflow. It can be beneficial in patients with severe airway obstruction.

• **Intravenous magnesium sulfate:** Magnesium has bronchodilator properties and can also stabilize mast cells, reducing inflammatory mediator release. It has been shown to be effective in some cases of severe asthma.

• **Inhaled corticosteroids:** While primarily anti-inflammatory, corticosteroids can also have a bronchodilator effect by reducing airway edema and mucus production.

In a patient with severe status asthmaticus, a combination of these therapies may be necessary to optimize airway management and improve ventilation.

Why other options are incorrect:

There is no single best answer in this case, as all options can be considered based on the patient's specific clinical condition and response to treatment.

Case Study: A 32-year-old male presents to the ICU with severe status asthmaticus. Despite aggressive bronchodilator therapy, his peak airway pressures remain high. He is started on inhaled heliox, intravenous magnesium sulfate, and high-dose inhaled corticosteroids. After several hours, there is a gradual improvement in his respiratory status, with a decrease in peak airway pressures and improved oxygenation.

It is important to note that the choice of therapy should be individualized based on the patient's clinical presentation, severity of illness, and response to treatment.

189. Answer: A. High-dose corticosteroids

Explanation:

High-dose corticosteroids are the cornerstone of treatment for lupus myocarditis. They rapidly suppress the inflammatory process, which is the underlying cause of the myocardial damage. By reducing inflammation, corticosteroids improve cardiac function and prevent further myocardial injury.

Why other options are incorrect:

• **B. Cyclophosphamide:** While cyclophosphamide is a potent immunosuppressant used in the treatment of lupus nephritis and severe lupus flares, it is not the first-line treatment for lupus myocarditis. It takes longer to work compared to corticosteroids and carries a higher risk of side effects.

• **C. Mycophenolate mofetil:** This immunosuppressant is generally used for maintenance therapy in lupus nephritis and is not as effective as corticosteroids in rapidly controlling acute inflammation in lupus myocarditis.

• **D. Rituximab:** Rituximab is a B-cell depleting agent primarily used in the treatment of lupus nephritis and refractory lupus. It has a slower onset of action and is not the initial treatment choice for acute lupus myocarditis.

Case Study:

A 45-year-old woman with a history of SLE presents to the ICU with acute onset of dyspnea, chest pain, and tachycardia. Echocardiogram reveals decreased left ventricular ejection fraction and evidence of myocardial inflammation. The patient is diagnosed with lupus myocarditis and initiated on high-dose intravenous methylprednisolone. Within a few days, her symptoms improve, and echocardiogram shows improvement in cardiac function.

It is important to note that while corticosteroids are the initial treatment, other immunosuppressive agents may be added depending on the severity of the myocarditis and the patient's response to therapy.

190. Answer: A. Continuous venovenous hemofiltration (CVVH)
Explanation:
Continuous venovenous hemofiltration (CVVH) is the most appropriate modality of renal replacement therapy (RRT) for a critically ill patient with acute pulmonary edema secondary to chronic kidney disease (CKD).
- **Continuous:** CVVH provides continuous and gentle fluid removal, which is crucial in managing fluid overload associated with acute pulmonary edema.
- **Venovenous:** This access method is less invasive than arteriovenous access required for hemodialysis and is suitable for critically ill patients.
- **Hemofiltration:** This process removes fluid and small solutes without the need for a dialysate bath, which is beneficial in patients with hemodynamic instability.

Why other options are incorrect:
- **B. Intermittent hemodialysis (IHD):** IHD involves rapid fluid removal and can lead to hemodynamic instability in critically ill patients. It is less suitable for patients with acute pulmonary edema.
- **C. Peritoneal dialysis (PD):** PD is not suitable for critically ill patients due to the risk of infection and the inability to achieve rapid fluid removal required in acute pulmonary edema.
- **D. Sustained low-efficiency dialysis (SLED):** While SLED offers continuous removal of fluids and solutes, it is less efficient than CVVH in removing fluid rapidly, which is crucial in managing acute pulmonary edema.

Case Study:
A 72-year-old man with a history of CKD presents to the ICU with acute pulmonary edema. He is intubated and mechanically ventilated. CVVH is initiated, and within 24 hours, there is a significant improvement in his respiratory status with decreased pulmonary congestion.

CVVH offers several advantages in managing critically ill patients with acute kidney injury, including hemodynamic stability, electrolyte balance, and removal of inflammatory mediators.

191. Answer: D. Esmolol
Explanation:
Esmolol is the most appropriate initial choice for rate control in this patient due to its rapid onset and short half-life, allowing for precise titration.

- **Rapid onset:** Esmolol acts within minutes, which is crucial in a hemodynamically unstable patient with atrial fibrillation with rapid ventricular response (RVR) and hypotension.
- **Short half-life:** The short half-life allows for quick titration of the dose based on the patient's response, minimizing the risk of hypotension.
- **Hemodynamic stability:** Esmolol has a relatively neutral effect on blood pressure, making it suitable for patients with hypotension, such as this patient with heart failure.

Why other options are incorrect:
- **A. Amiodarone:** While amiodarone is effective for rate control and rhythm conversion in atrial fibrillation, it has a long onset of action and can cause hypotension, making it less suitable for initial management in this hemodynamically unstable patient.
- **B. Diltiazem:** Diltiazem can cause hypotension, especially in patients with heart failure, and its onset of action is slower than esmolol.
- **C. Digoxin:** Digoxin has a slower onset of action and a narrow therapeutic index, making it less suitable for rapid rate control in a critically ill patient.

Case Study:

A 60-year-old male with a history of COPD and heart failure presents to the ICU with new-onset atrial fibrillation with a rapid ventricular rate of 170 beats per minute and hypotension. Esmolol is initiated as a continuous infusion. Within minutes, the heart rate decreases to 120 beats per minute, and blood pressure improves. The esmolol infusion is titrated to maintain a target heart rate while monitoring for hypotension.

By using esmolol as the initial rate control agent, the healthcare provider can rapidly improve hemodynamics and stabilize the patient while planning for further management of atrial fibrillation.

192. Answer: A. Aggressive blood pressure control
Explanation:

Aggressive blood pressure control is the cornerstone of management for PRES. The condition is often triggered by rapid increases in blood pressure, leading to endothelial dysfunction and vasogenic edema in the brain. By rapidly lowering blood pressure, the underlying cause of the condition can be addressed, and the risk of further neurological damage is reduced.

Why other options are incorrect:

• **B. Intravenous immunoglobulin (IVIG):** While IVIG may be considered in severe cases of PRES or when there is evidence of autoimmune involvement, it is not the first-line treatment.

• **C. Plasma exchange:** Plasma exchange is indicated in severe cases of lupus nephritis or thrombotic thrombocytopenic purpura (TTP) but not typically for PRES.

• **D. Corticosteroid therapy:** Corticosteroids are the mainstay of treatment for lupus flares but are not specifically indicated for PRES. They may have a role in refractory cases but are not the initial management strategy.

Case Study:

A 40-year-old woman with SLE presents to the ICU with new-onset seizures, headache, and visual disturbances. Blood pressure is 180/110 mmHg. Brain MRI confirms PRES. The patient is immediately treated with antihypertensive medications to rapidly lower blood pressure. Over the next 24 hours, her neurological symptoms improve, and blood pressure stabilizes.

It is important to note that while aggressive blood pressure control is crucial, it should be done cautiously to avoid precipitating hypotension and further brain injury. Close monitoring of blood pressure and neurological status is essential.

193. Answer: D. Airway pressure release ventilation (APRV)

Explanation:

Airway pressure release ventilation (APRV) is the most appropriate ventilator setting for a patient with COPD and hypercapnic respiratory failure. This mode allows for prolonged inspiratory times with higher mean airway pressures, which can improve gas exchange and reduce work of breathing in patients with air trapping and hyperinflation, as seen in COPD.

• APRV provides continuous positive airway pressure (CPAP) during most of the respiratory cycle, which helps to recruit and stabilize alveoli.

• It allows for spontaneous breaths, which can help to maintain respiratory muscle tone and reduce ventilator-induced lung injury.

Why other options are incorrect:

• **A. Pressure-controlled ventilation (PCV):** While PCV can be used in certain situations, it may not be optimal for patients with COPD due to the potential for overdistension of the lungs.

- **B. Volume-controlled ventilation (VCV):** VCV can lead to high peak inspiratory pressures, which can be detrimental to the lungs of patients with COPD.
- **C. Pressure support ventilation (PSV):** PSV is typically used for weaning patients from mechanical ventilation and may not provide adequate support for patients with severe hypercapnia.

Case Study:

A 72-year-old man with severe COPD is admitted to the ICU with an acute exacerbation and hypercapnic respiratory failure. He is intubated and placed on APRV. Within 24 hours, his PaCO2 decreases, and his oxygenation improves. The APRV settings are adjusted as needed to optimize gas exchange and minimize ventilator-induced lung injury.

APRV is a complex mode of ventilation and requires careful monitoring and titration. However, it can be a valuable tool in managing patients with COPD and hypercapnic respiratory failure.

194. Answer: D. All of the above

Explanation:

All of the options listed can be considered as adjunctive therapies to improve hemodynamic status in a patient with septic shock secondary to severe community-acquired pneumonia (CAP).

- **Low-dose hydrocortisone:** As discussed earlier, low-dose hydrocortisone has been shown to improve hemodynamics and reduce mortality in patients with septic shock who require vasopressors.
- **Vitamin C:** Vitamin C is an antioxidant that has been shown to improve hemodynamics and reduce organ dysfunction in patients with sepsis. It acts by reducing oxidative stress and modulating the inflammatory response.
- **Thiamine:** Thiamine deficiency is common in critically ill patients, including those with sepsis. Thiamine plays a crucial role in glucose metabolism and cellular energy production. Correcting thiamine deficiency can improve hemodynamic stability.

Why other options are incorrect:

There is no single best answer in this case, as all options can be considered based on the patient's specific clinical condition and response to treatment.

Case Study:

A 32-year-old woman presents to the ICU with severe CAP and rapidly progresses to septic shock despite appropriate antibiotic therapy. She is initiated on low-dose hydrocortisone, vitamin C, and thiamine. Within 24 hours, there is an improvement in her hemodynamic parameters, including increased mean arterial pressure and reduced lactate levels.

It is important to note that these therapies are adjunctive to standard care for septic shock, including fluid resuscitation, vasopressors, and appropriate antibiotic therapy.

195. Answer: C. Extracorporeal membrane oxygenation (ECMO)
Explanation:

Extracorporeal membrane oxygenation (ECMO) is the most appropriate intervention for a patient with refractory cardiogenic shock despite maximal medical therapy, including inotropes and vasopressors. ECMO provides both respiratory and circulatory support by oxygenating blood and pumping it back to the body, effectively taking over the functions of the heart and lungs.

Why other options are incorrect:

• **A. Impella:** While Impella can augment cardiac output, it is primarily a cardiac support device and may not be sufficient for patients with severe cardiogenic shock and refractory hypotension.

• **B. Intra-aortic balloon pump (IABP):** IABP is a less invasive support device that can improve coronary blood flow and reduce afterload, but it is generally not as effective as ECMO in severe cardiogenic shock.

• **D. Ventricular assist device (VAD):** VADs are durable, long-term support devices, but they require complex surgical implantation and are not typically considered as the initial therapy for acute cardiogenic shock.

Case Study:

A 68-year-old man with a history of HFrEF presents to the ICU with cardiogenic shock refractory to inotropes and vasopressors. Despite maximal medical therapy, he remains hypotensive and oliguric. ECMO is initiated, and within hours, there is an improvement in hemodynamics, and the patient's condition stabilizes.

ECMO is a complex and high-risk therapy, but it can be lifesaving for patients with refractory cardiogenic shock. Careful patient selection and management are essential for optimal outcomes.

196. Answer: D. Urine neutrophil gelatinase-associated lipocalin (NGAL)
Explanation:
Urine neutrophil gelatinase-associated lipocalin (NGAL) is the most specific biomarker for the diagnosis of acute tubular necrosis (ATN). It is released early in the course of ATN and its levels correlate with the severity of kidney injury.
Why other options are incorrect:
- **A. Blood urea nitrogen (BUN):** While BUN is elevated in AKI, it is not specific to ATN and can be increased due to other factors such as dehydration, protein catabolism, and decreased renal blood flow.
- **B. Serum creatinine:** Similar to BUN, serum creatinine is a marker of kidney function but lacks specificity for ATN. It can be elevated in various types of AKI.
- **C. Fractional excretion of sodium (FeNA):** FeNA is a useful tool to differentiate between prerenal and intrinsic renal AKI. However, it is not specific for ATN and can be affected by other factors such as diuretic use.
Case Study:
A 45-year-old man with a history of alcohol abuse is admitted to the ICU with acute pancreatitis. His serum creatinine starts to rise, and urine NGAL levels are significantly elevated, supporting the diagnosis of ATN as the cause of his AKI.
By using NGAL as a biomarker, clinicians can earlier identify patients with ATN and initiate appropriate management strategies.

197. Answer: C. Rapid shallow breathing index (RSBI)
Explanation:
The **rapid shallow breathing index (RSBI)** is the most important predictor of successful extubation in a patient with status asthmaticus. It is calculated by dividing the respiratory rate by the tidal volume. A lower RSBI (typically <105 breaths/min/L) is associated with a higher likelihood of successful extubation.
Why other options are incorrect:
- **A. Peak expiratory flow rate (PEFR):** While PEFR is a useful measure of lung function in asthma, it is less reliable in predicting extubation success in critically ill patients.
- **B. Forced expiratory volume in 1 second (FEV1):** Similar to PEFR, FEV1 is a measure of lung function but is not as predictive of extubation success as RSBI.
- **D. Negative inspiratory force (NIF):** NIF is a measure of respiratory muscle strength, but it is not as consistently predictive of extubation success as RSBI.

Case Study:

A 28-year-old woman with severe asthma is intubated for status asthmaticus. After a few days of treatment, her RSBI is calculated to be 85 breaths/min/L. This value indicates a good likelihood of successful extubation, and the decision is made to proceed with a spontaneous breathing trial.

By using RSBI as a predictor of extubation success, clinicians can make more informed decisions about the timing of extubation and reduce the risk of extubation failure.

198. Answer: B. Computed tomography angiography (CTA) of the chest

Explanation:

Computed tomography angiography (CTA) of the chest is the most appropriate imaging modality for long-term surveillance of a Stanford Type B aortic dissection.

- **Excellent visualization:** CTA provides detailed images of the aorta and its branches, allowing for accurate assessment of the dissection's extent, progression, or complications.
- **Non-invasive:** CTA is a less invasive procedure compared to other options.
- **Rapid:** CTA can be performed quickly, making it suitable for follow-up imaging.

Why other options are incorrect:

- **A. Chest X-ray:** While a chest X-ray can show widening of the mediastinum, it is not specific for aortic dissection and cannot accurately assess the extent of the dissection.
- **C. Transesophageal echocardiogram (TEE):** TEE provides excellent images of the heart and proximal aorta but is limited in its ability to visualize the descending aorta.
- **D. Magnetic resonance imaging (MRI) of the chest:** MRI can provide excellent images of the aorta but is more time-consuming and expensive than CTA. Additionally, it requires patients to lie still for an extended period, which can be challenging for critically ill patients.

CTA is the preferred imaging modality for follow-up of Stanford Type B aortic dissections due to its combination of accuracy, speed, and non-invasive nature.

199. Answer: A. Hemodialysis

Explanation:

Hemodialysis is the most effective treatment for uremic pericarditis. This condition is caused by the buildup of uremic toxins in the blood due to kidney failure. By removing these toxins through hemodialysis, the underlying cause of the pericarditis is addressed.

Why other options are incorrect:

- **B. Pericardiocentesis:** While pericardiocentesis can relieve symptoms if there's a large pericardial effusion causing cardiac tamponade, it doesn't address the underlying cause of uremic pericarditis.
- **C. Corticosteroids:** Corticosteroids have a limited role in uremic pericarditis and are not considered first-line treatment. They may be used as adjunctive therapy in refractory cases.
- **D. Nonsteroidal anti-inflammatory drugs (NSAIDs):** NSAIDs are generally avoided in patients with kidney disease due to their potential to worsen renal function. They are not effective in treating uremic pericarditis.

By initiating or intensifying hemodialysis, the risk of pericardial effusion and cardiac tamponade can be significantly reduced, improving patient outcomes.

200. Answer: D. All of the above

Explanation:

To effectively assess the effectiveness of norepinephrine therapy in a patient with septic shock, it is crucial to monitor multiple hemodynamic parameters.

- **Mean arterial pressure (MAP):** This is a direct measure of perfusion pressure and is the primary target for vasopressor therapy. An increase in MAP indicates improved perfusion.
- **Central venous pressure (CVP):** While not as direct as MAP, CVP can provide information about fluid status. Adequate fluid resuscitation is essential for optimizing the response to vasopressors.
- **Cardiac index (CI):** This parameter assesses cardiac output relative to body size and is crucial for determining if the patient is adequately perfused. A low CI may indicate the need for additional inotropic support or addressing underlying cardiac issues.

By monitoring all three parameters, healthcare providers can gain a comprehensive understanding of the patient's hemodynamic status and make appropriate adjustments to therapy.

201. Answer: A. Cholesterol embolism
Explanation:

Given the patient's history of coronary artery disease and the development of acute limb ischemia following an NSTEMI, the most likely cause of the limb ischemia is a **cholesterol embolism**.

- **Cholesterol embolism** occurs when atherosclerotic plaques rupture and release cholesterol crystals into the bloodstream. These crystals can then embolize to various organs, including the kidneys, skin, and limbs, causing tissue damage. This condition is often associated with coronary artery disease and is more common in older patients.

Why other options are incorrect:

- **B. Deep vein thrombosis (DVT):** While DVT can lead to pulmonary embolism, it typically presents with leg swelling, pain, and redness. Acute limb ischemia would be a less common presentation.
- **C. Peripheral arterial disease (PAD):** PAD is a chronic condition that gradually progresses over time. Acute limb ischemia would be an abrupt onset and not typically associated with an NSTEMI.
- **D. Acute compartment syndrome:** This condition is characterized by increased pressure within a muscle compartment, leading to impaired blood flow. It typically presents with severe pain, swelling, and muscle tenderness, and is not directly related to coronary artery disease.

In conclusion, the sudden onset of acute limb ischemia in a patient with recent NSTEMI strongly suggests cholesterol embolism as the most likely cause.

202. Answer: A. Vancomycin and gentamicin for 4-6 weeks
Explanation:

Vancomycin and gentamicin are the most appropriate initial antibiotic regimen for a patient with infective endocarditis complicated by a perivalvular abscess, especially in the context of intravenous drug use.

- **Coverage:** This combination provides excellent coverage against the most common pathogens causing infective endocarditis in this population, including

Staphylococcus aureus (methicillin-sensitive and resistant) and other gram-positive organisms.

- **Duration:** A prolonged course of 4-6 weeks is typically required to eradicate the infection and prevent relapse.

Why other options are incorrect:

- **B. Daptomycin:** While effective against gram-positive organisms, daptomycin is not the preferred initial choice for complicated infective endocarditis due to potential limitations in efficacy against certain staphylococcal strains and its lack of activity against gram-negative organisms.
- **C. Ceftaroline:** This antibiotic primarily covers gram-positive and some gram-negative organisms but is not the optimal choice for severe infections like endocarditis with perivalvular abscess.
- **D. Penicillin G:** While effective against some streptococcal species, penicillin G lacks coverage against many common pathogens associated with infective endocarditis in intravenous drug users.

It's important to note that this is an initial empiric regimen, and the specific antibiotics may be adjusted based on the results of blood cultures and susceptibility testing. Additionally, surgical intervention is often required to address the perivalvular abscess.

203. Answer: A. Daily spontaneous awakening trial (SAT) and spontaneous breathing trial (SBT)

Explanation:

Daily spontaneous awakening trial (SAT) and spontaneous breathing trial (SBT) have been shown to be the most effective weaning strategy in reducing the duration of mechanical ventilation and the risk of complications in patients with COPD exacerbations.

- **SAT:** This involves waking the patient daily to assess their readiness for weaning and to prevent delirium.
- **SBT:** This involves disconnecting the patient from the ventilator for a predetermined period to assess their ability to breathe independently.

By combining SAT and SBT, healthcare providers can identify patients who are ready to be weaned earlier and reduce the overall duration of mechanical ventilation.

Why other options are incorrect:

- **B. Once-daily SBT only:** While SBT is important, daily assessment of the patient's readiness for weaning through SAT is also crucial.
- **C. Intermittent mandatory ventilation (IMV):** IMV is an older weaning method that has been largely replaced by spontaneous breathing trials due to its potential for increased ventilator-induced lung injury.
- **D. Pressure support ventilation (PSV) only:** PSV is a mode of ventilation, not a weaning strategy. It can be used as part of a weaning protocol but is not as effective as SAT and SBT.

By implementing a standardized weaning protocol that includes daily SAT and SBT, healthcare providers can improve patient outcomes and reduce the length of stay in the ICU.

204. Answer: B. MAP > 65 mmHg
Explanation:

The most appropriate target for mean arterial pressure (MAP) in a patient with septic shock, such as this 30-year-old woman, is **MAP > 65 mmHg**.

This guideline is based on the Surviving Sepsis Campaign recommendations. The goal is to restore adequate perfusion to vital organs.

- **MAP > 60 mmHg:** While this might be sufficient in some stable patients, it may not be adequate to ensure optimal tissue perfusion in severe septic shock.
- **MAP > 70 mmHg or > 75 mmHg:** There is insufficient evidence to support targeting a MAP higher than 65 mmHg routinely. Higher MAP targets might increase the risk of complications such as myocardial ischemia or intracranial hypertension without proven benefits.

It's important to note that the MAP goal is an initial target, and individual patient factors, such as comorbidities and response to therapy, should be considered when making treatment decisions. Continuous monitoring of MAP and other hemodynamic parameters is essential to optimize care.

205. Answer: B. Ultrafiltration
Explanation:

Ultrafiltration is the most appropriate next step in this patient with HFpEF and refractory diuresis. It is a rapid and effective method for removing excess fluid volume without the need for dialysis.

- **Ultrafiltration** works by applying a pressure gradient across a semipermeable membrane to remove fluid from the blood. This can rapidly improve congestion and diuresis.

Why other options are incorrect:

- **A. Continuous renal replacement therapy (CRRT):** While CRRT can remove fluid, it is typically reserved for patients with acute kidney injury or severe electrolyte imbalances. It is not the first-line treatment for refractory diuresis in HFpEF.

- **C. High-dose loop diuretics:** Increasing the dose of loop diuretics may lead to ototoxicity and electrolyte imbalances without significant improvement in diuresis, especially in patients with refractory fluid overload.

- **D. Vasodilator therapy:** While vasodilators can improve cardiac output in some patients with HFpEF, they are not primarily used to increase diuresis.

By using ultrafiltration, the patient's fluid overload can be rapidly addressed, leading to improved symptoms and hemodynamic stability.

206. Answer: C. AKI characterized by renal vasoconstriction in the setting of advanced liver disease

Explanation:

Hepatorenal syndrome (HRS) is a complex condition characterized by the development of acute kidney injury (AKI) in patients with advanced liver disease. It's primarily due to renal vasoconstriction caused by the body's response to the underlying liver dysfunction.

- **Renal vasoconstriction:** This is the key pathophysiological mechanism. As the liver fails, it leads to systemic vasodilation. The body compensates by activating the renin-angiotensin-aldosterone system (RAAS) and sympathetic nervous system, causing renal vasoconstriction. This decreased blood flow to the kidneys ultimately leads to AKI.

Why other options are incorrect:

- **A. AKI caused by direct nephrotoxicity of alcohol:** While alcohol can cause direct kidney damage, HRS is not directly related to this mechanism.

- **B. AKI caused by hypovolemia due to gastrointestinal bleeding:** While hypovolemia can lead to AKI, HRS is a specific type of AKI related to liver disease.

- **D. AKI caused by obstruction of the urinary tract:** This is a post-renal cause of AKI, unrelated to liver disease.

Understanding the pathophysiology of HRS is crucial for effective management, as it guides therapeutic interventions aimed at improving renal perfusion.

207. Answer: D. All of the above
Explanation:
All of the listed adjunctive therapies have shown some benefit in managing severe asthma exacerbations, including status asthmaticus:
- **Magnesium sulfate:** This has bronchodilator properties and can stabilize mast cells, reducing inflammation.
- **Ketamine:** This has been explored as a potential bronchodilator and sedative in refractory status asthmaticus, with some promising results.
- **Heliox:** A mixture of helium and oxygen, it reduces airway resistance and can improve gas exchange.

While evidence for the use of these agents is still evolving, they can be considered as additional options when standard treatments fail to achieve adequate control. It's important to note that these therapies should be used under close monitoring in a critical care setting.

208. Answer: C. SBP < 140 mmHg
Explanation:
The goal for blood pressure management in a patient with a stable Stanford Type B aortic dissection is to **maintain a systolic blood pressure (SBP) below 140 mmHg**.
- **Lowering blood pressure excessively** can reduce blood flow to the organs perfused by the distal aorta.
- **Maintaining a slightly elevated blood pressure** can help maintain perfusion to the distal organs while minimizing the shear stress on the aorta.

It's important to note that this is a general guideline, and individual patient factors should be considered when determining the optimal blood pressure goal. Close monitoring of blood pressure and clinical status is essential.

209. Answer: A. Pericardiocentesis
Explanation:
Pericardiocentesis is the most definitive treatment for cardiac tamponade, regardless of the underlying cause (in this case, uremic pericarditis). It involves

draining the excess fluid from the pericardial sac, relieving the pressure on the heart and restoring cardiac output.

Why other options are incorrect:
- **B. Pericardial window:** This is a more invasive procedure that involves creating a permanent opening in the pericardium to allow fluid to drain continuously. It is usually reserved for recurrent pericardial effusions.
- **C. Pericardiectomy:** This is a surgical procedure to remove the pericardium and is indicated only in rare cases of recurrent, refractory pericarditis or constrictive pericarditis.
- **D. Corticosteroids:** While corticosteroids can be helpful in reducing inflammation in some cases of pericarditis, they are not effective in treating cardiac tamponade.

In a patient with cardiac tamponade, rapid intervention with pericardiocentesis is crucial to prevent hemodynamic collapse.

210. Answer: D. All of the above
Explanation:

Given the patient's critical condition and persistent septic shock despite initial antibiotic therapy, a comprehensive approach is necessary.

- **Change empiric antibiotic therapy:** If the patient is not responding to the initial antibiotics, it's essential to consider changing the regimen based on clinical findings, potential pathogens, and local resistance patterns.
- **Add antifungal therapy:** Given the patient's immunocompromised state due to rheumatoid arthritis and the potential for invasive fungal infections in severe sepsis, adding antifungal therapy should be considered.
- **Search for an alternative source of infection:** It's crucial to re-evaluate the patient for other potential sources of infection, such as urinary tract infection, skin and soft tissue infections, or intra-abdominal infections.

A multidisciplinary approach involving infectious disease specialists can be helpful in optimizing the management of this complex case.

211. Answer: D. Esmolol

Explanation:

Esmolol is the most appropriate initial medication for rate control in this patient due to its rapid onset and offset of action, allowing for quick titration to achieve desired heart rate without causing significant hemodynamic instability.

Patient Profile:

- Elderly patient with multiple comorbidities (hypertension, coronary artery disease, COPD, heart failure)
- Acute onset of atrial fibrillation with rapid ventricular response (RVR)
- Hypotensive (BP 90/60 mmHg)

Medication Breakdown:

- **Amiodarone (A):** While effective for rate control in atrial fibrillation, it has a long half-life and can cause hypotension, bradycardia, and thyroid dysfunction. It is not ideal for rapid onset rate control, especially in a hypotensive patient.

- **Diltiazem (B):** A calcium channel blocker with some rate-control properties, it can cause hypotension and is less effective in rapid rate control compared to esmolol. It is also associated with increased risk of heart failure exacerbation in patients with HFrEF.

- **Digoxin (C):** While effective for rate control, digoxin has a narrow therapeutic index and requires careful monitoring. It is not the first-line choice for rapid rate control and can exacerbate heart failure.

- **Esmolol (D):** A short-acting beta-blocker with a rapid onset and offset of action. It is ideal for rapid rate control in hemodynamically unstable patients like this one. It can be titrated quickly to achieve the desired heart rate and has minimal negative inotropic effects.

Rationale for Esmolol:

- **Rapid onset and offset:** Allows for quick titration to achieve desired heart rate without causing significant hemodynamic instability.

- **Minimal negative inotropic effects:** Important in a patient with HFrEF.

- **Safe in hypotension:** Can be used cautiously while monitoring blood pressure closely.

Case Study: A 78-year-old man with a history of hypertension, coronary artery disease, COPD, and HFrEF presents to the ICU with new-onset atrial fibrillation with RVR and hypotension. Esmolol is initiated as a bolus followed by continuous infusion. The patient's heart rate gradually decreases, and blood pressure stabilizes. Esmolol infusion is titrated to maintain a heart rate of 100-110 bpm.

Conclusion: Esmolol is the most appropriate initial medication for rate control in this patient due to its rapid onset and offset of action, allowing for quick titration to achieve desired heart rate without causing significant hemodynamic instability. It is also safe to use in a hypotensive patient with HFrEF, and it has minimal negative inotropic effects.

212. Answer: D. All of the above
Explanation:

Posterior Reversible Encephalopathy Syndrome (PRES) is a condition characterized by headache, seizures, altered mental status, and visual disturbances. It is often associated with rapidly increasing blood pressure, but other factors can contribute to its development.

In this case, the patient has multiple risk factors for PRES:

• **Hypertension:** A common cause of PRES, leading to increased intracranial pressure and endothelial dysfunction.

• **Immunosuppressive therapy:** Used to treat SLE, can contribute to PRES by affecting vascular endothelial cells and causing fluid shifts.

• **Active lupus flare:** Inflammation associated with lupus can also induce endothelial dysfunction and contribute to PRES.

Therefore, all of the listed options can contribute to the development of PRES in this patient.

It's important to note that while hypertension is often the primary trigger for PRES, the presence of underlying conditions like SLE can increase the risk and severity of the condition.

Case Study: A 42-year-old woman with SLE on immunosuppressive therapy presents with severe headache, seizures, and altered mental status. Blood pressure is found to be significantly elevated.Brain MRI confirms PRES. The patient is treated with blood pressure control, supportive care, and management of her lupus flare.

Conclusion: In this case, hypertension, immunosuppressive therapy, and active lupus flare all contributed to the development of PRES. Addressing all these factors is crucial for effective management and prevention of complications.

213. Answer: D. Lung-protective ventilation with low tidal volumes and appropriate PEEP

Explanation:

Ventilator-induced lung injury (VILI) is a serious complication of mechanical ventilation that can lead to acute respiratory distress syndrome (ARDS). It is primarily caused by excessive lung distension and shear stress.

- **High tidal volume ventilation (A):** This can lead to overdistension of the lungs, causing VILI.
- **High plateau pressure (B):** Similarly, high plateau pressure indicates overdistension and is associated with VILI.
- **Low positive end-expiratory pressure (PEEP) (C):** Insufficient PEEP can lead to alveolar collapse and atelectasis, worsening oxygenation and potentially increasing the risk of VILI.

Lung-protective ventilation with **low tidal volumes** and **appropriate PEEP** is the cornerstone of preventing VILI. This strategy aims to maintain adequate oxygenation while minimizing lung injury. By using lower tidal volumes, the risk of overdistension is reduced. Applying appropriate PEEP helps to prevent alveolar collapse and improve oxygenation without excessive pressure.

Case Study: A 75-year-old man with COPD is intubated for acute respiratory failure. The ventilator is set to a low tidal volume (6-8 ml/kg predicted body weight) and PEEP is titrated to optimize oxygenation while minimizing plateau pressure. This approach helps to protect the lungs from injury and improve patient outcomes.

Conclusion: Lung-protective ventilation with low tidal volumes and appropriate PEEP is the most effective strategy to reduce the risk of VILI in patients with COPD requiring mechanical ventilation.

214. Answer: D. All of the above

Explanation:

This patient is presenting with severe sepsis secondary to community-acquired pneumonia. Improving oxygen delivery is a critical component of management.

- **Transfusion of packed red blood cells (PRBCs):** If the patient is anemic, transfusion can increase oxygen-carrying capacity, thus improving oxygen delivery.

- **Inotropic support with dobutamine:** This can increase cardiac output, leading to improved tissue perfusion and oxygen delivery.
- **Increase in the fraction of inspired oxygen (FiO2):** Increasing the oxygen concentration delivered to the patient can improve oxygenation, though it's important to balance this with the risk of oxygen toxicity.

All three of these interventions can be considered, and the optimal approach will depend on the specific clinical circumstances of the patient. For example, if the patient is hypovolemic, fluid resuscitation might be prioritized before blood transfusion.

Case Study: A 30-year-old woman with severe CAP develops septic shock. Her blood pressure is low, and lactate is elevated.Initial management includes fluid resuscitation and appropriate antibiotics. Despite these measures, her oxygenation continues to deteriorate. A hemoglobin level is checked and found to be low. The patient receives a transfusion of PRBCs. Additionally, dobutamine is initiated to improve cardiac output. The FiO2 is increased to maintain adequate oxygenation.

Conclusion: In a patient with severe sepsis secondary to pneumonia, improving oxygen delivery is crucial. Transfusion of PRBCs, inotropic support, and increasing FiO2 are all potential interventions that can be considered to achieve this goal.

215. Answer: A. Intra-aortic balloon pump (IABP)
Explanation:

This patient is experiencing refractory cardiogenic shock, meaning he is not responding to standard medical treatments. Given the contraindications to Impella and ECMO, the most appropriate next step would be an **intra-aortic balloon pump (IABP)**.

- **IABP (A):** This device provides temporary circulatory support by improving coronary blood flow and reducing afterload. It is less invasive than Impella or ECMO and can be a bridge to recovery or more definitive therapy.
- **TandemHeart (B):** This is a partial ventricular assist device that requires surgical implantation, which is not suitable in this scenario due to the patient's critical condition and the need for a rapidly deployable therapy.
- **Ventricular assist device (VAD) (C):** VADs are complex devices requiring surgical implantation and are generally considered for long-term support or

bridge to transplant. They are not suitable for immediate management of refractory cardiogenic shock.

- **Percutaneous left ventricular assist device (pLVAD) (D):** While less invasive than traditional VADs, pLVADs still require surgical implantation and are not the most appropriate choice for immediate management of this patient's acute condition.

In summary, the IABP is the most suitable option for this patient due to its rapid deployment, less invasive nature, and ability to improve hemodynamics.

216. Answer: A. Hyperkalemia

Explanation:

Hyperkalemia is the most common electrolyte abnormality associated with Acute Tubular Necrosis (ATN).

- **Hyperkalemia (A):** The kidneys play a crucial role in potassium excretion. When kidney function declines, as in ATN, potassium accumulates in the body, leading to hyperkalemia.
- **Hypokalemia (B):** This is less common in ATN. It can occur in specific conditions like severe vomiting or diarrhea but is not the typical electrolyte imbalance.
- **Hypernatremia (C):** This is associated with water loss rather than kidney dysfunction. It's more common in conditions like dehydration.
- **Hyponatremia (D):** This is also related to water imbalance, not primarily kidney dysfunction. It can occur in conditions like excessive water intake or syndrome of inappropriate antidiuretic hormone (SIADH).

In summary, hyperkalemia is the most frequent electrolyte disturbance in patients with ATN due to the kidneys' impaired ability to excrete potassium.

217. Answer: A. Administration of neuromuscular blocking agents

Explanation:

Status asthmaticus is a severe, life-threatening exacerbation of asthma that is unresponsive to standard therapy. In this situation, the patient is already intubated and on mechanical ventilation, indicating the severity of the condition.

- **Administration of neuromuscular blocking agents (A):** This is often necessary in severe status asthmaticus to improve gas exchange and reduce peak airway pressures. By paralyzing the muscles, it allows the ventilator to take over completely, reducing the patient's work of breathing and decreasing airway resistance.

- **Use of inhaled anesthetics (B):** While inhaled anesthetics can relax bronchial smooth muscle, they are generally not the first-line treatment for severe status asthmaticus and may have other adverse effects.
- **Increasing the respiratory rate (C):** Increasing the respiratory rate can actually worsen air trapping and increase peak airway pressures in patients with status asthmaticus.
- **Increasing the tidal volume (D):** Increasing tidal volume can also lead to increased peak airway pressures and barotrauma in this setting.

Therefore, in a patient with severe status asthmaticus who is already intubated and on mechanical ventilation, the administration of neuromuscular blocking agents is the most likely strategy to reduce peak airway pressures and improve ventilation.

218. Answer: A. Morphine
Explanation:
Morphine is the most appropriate choice for pain control in a patient with a Stanford Type B aortic dissection who is hemodynamically stable.

- **Morphine (A):** It is a potent opioid with a proven efficacy in managing severe pain. It also has vasodilatory properties, which can be beneficial in reducing afterload in patients with aortic dissection.
- **Fentanyl (B):** While a potent analgesic, fentanyl has a shorter duration of action compared to morphine. It may require more frequent dosing, which could be less practical in this setting.
- **Hydromorphone (C):** This is another opioid option, but morphine is generally preferred for its vasodilatory effects in this specific patient population.

It's crucial to monitor blood pressure closely when using morphine due to its potential hypotensive effects. However, in a hemodynamically stable patient with a Stanford Type B aortic dissection, the benefits of pain control often outweigh the risks.

Note: The choice of analgesic should always be individualized based on the patient's specific condition and response to treatment.

219. Answer: A. Diastolic collapse of the right ventricle
Explanation:
- **Diastolic collapse of the right ventricle (A):** This is the most specific echocardiographic finding for pericardial effusion. As the pericardial effusion increases, it exerts pressure on the heart, causing the right ventricle to collapse during diastole due to its thinner wall compared to the left ventricle.
- **Left ventricular hypertrophy (B):** This is a common finding in patients with chronic kidney disease but is not specific for pericardial effusion.
- **Mitral valve prolapse (C):** This is an unrelated valvular heart disease and not associated with pericardial effusion.
- **Aortic stenosis (D):** This is another unrelated valvular heart disease and not associated with pericardial effusion.

Therefore, the diastolic collapse of the right ventricle is the most specific echocardiographic finding for pericardial effusion in this patient with uremic pericarditis.

220. Answer: A. Lung
Explanation:
The most common site of infection in patients with rheumatoid arthritis who develop septic shock is the lung.
Patients with rheumatoid arthritis are at increased risk for developing respiratory complications, including pneumonia, due to several factors:
- **Immunosuppression:** The use of immunosuppressive medications to manage rheumatoid arthritis can weaken the immune system, making them more susceptible to infections.
- **Chronic inflammation:** The chronic inflammatory process associated with rheumatoid arthritis can affect lung tissue, increasing the risk of pneumonia.
- **Aspiration risk:** Some patients with rheumatoid arthritis may have difficulty swallowing, increasing the risk of aspiration pneumonia.

While other sites of infection, such as the urinary tract, skin, and gastrointestinal tract, can occur in patients with rheumatoid arthritis, pneumonia is the most common cause of septic shock in this population.

221. Answer: C. Intravenous tissue plasminogen activator (tPA)
Explanation:

Intravenous tissue plasminogen activator (tPA) is the most appropriate treatment for a patient presenting within the thrombolysis window with a confirmed ischemic stroke like a right MCA infarction.

- **tPA (C):** This is a thrombolytic agent that dissolves blood clots, restoring blood flow to the ischemic brain tissue. It is crucial to administer tPA within a specific time window (usually 3-4.5 hours) from symptom onset to maximize its effectiveness in reducing stroke-related disability.

- **Aspirin (A):** Aspirin is a platelet inhibitor used for stroke prevention but is not effective in acutely treating an ongoing ischemic stroke.

- **Clopidogrel (B):** Similar to aspirin, clopidogrel is an antiplatelet agent used for secondary prevention but not for acute stroke treatment.

- **Warfarin (D):** Warfarin is an anticoagulant used for long-term prevention of stroke in atrial fibrillation but carries a risk of bleeding and is not indicated for acute stroke treatment.

It's important to note that tPA administration has strict inclusion and exclusion criteria, and it should only be administered by experienced healthcare providers in a setting equipped for managing potential complications.

222. Answer: D. All of the above
Explanation:

Patients who undergo surgery for infective endocarditis with perivalvular abscess are at high risk for several complications. Close monitoring of the following is crucial:

- **Arrhythmias (A):** Given the cardiac surgery and potential for inflammation and damage to the heart, arrhythmias are a common complication.

- **Heart failure (B):** The surgical procedure itself, along with the underlying infection, can weaken the heart muscle, leading to heart failure.

- **Stroke (C):** Embolization of infected material or thrombus formation on the prosthetic valve can lead to stroke.

Therefore, all of the listed options should be closely monitored in the postoperative period.

223. Answer: A. Piperacillin/tazobactam

Explanation:

Pseudomonas aeruginosa is a gram-negative bacterium that is often resistant to many antibiotics. Therefore, choosing an appropriate antibiotic is crucial for successful treatment.

- **Piperacillin/tazobactam (A):** This is a combination antibiotic that covers a wide range of gram-negative bacteria, including Pseudomonas aeruginosa. It is often considered a good first-line choice for treating Pseudomonas pneumonia in hospitalized patients.
- **Cefepime (B):** While effective against some Pseudomonas strains, resistance is increasing. It's generally not the preferred first-line choice.
- **Meropenem (C):** A carbapenem with good activity against Pseudomonas, but it's often reserved for more severe infections or when other options have failed due to the increasing risk of carbapenem resistance.
- **Levofloxacin (D):** A fluoroquinolone, it has activity against Pseudomonas, but resistance is also increasing. It's generally not the first-line choice for severe infections like pneumonia.

In conclusion, piperacillin/tazobactam is the most appropriate initial antibiotic choice for treating Pseudomonas aeruginosa pneumonia in a hospitalized patient with COPD. However, antibiotic selection should be based on local susceptibility patterns and the severity of the infection.

224. Answer: C. CVP 8-12 mmHg

Explanation:

The goal for central venous pressure (CVP) in a patient with septic shock is to maintain adequate preload and tissue perfusion. While there is no universally agreed-upon "perfect" CVP value, a target range of **8-12 mmHg** is often used as a starting point.

- **CVP 0-5 mmHg (A):** This indicates hypovolemia and inadequate preload. Aggressive fluid resuscitation is needed to optimize tissue perfusion.
- **CVP 5-10 mmHg (B):** This is on the lower end of the acceptable range and may indicate inadequate fluid resuscitation.
- **CVP 8-12 mmHg (C):** This is generally considered a reasonable target for CVP in septic shock patients, suggesting adequate preload and fluid resuscitation.

- **CVP > 12 mmHg (D):** This may indicate fluid overload and increased risk of pulmonary edema. Careful fluid management is necessary to avoid this complication.

It's important to note that CVP is just one parameter and should be interpreted in conjunction with other hemodynamic parameters, such as mean arterial pressure, cardiac output, and lactate levels.

225. Answer: C. Vasodilator therapy
Explanation:

In a patient with HFpEF and refractory diuresis despite intravenous diuretics, **vasodilator therapy** is often the next logical step.

- **Vasodilator therapy (C):** By reducing preload and afterload, vasodilators can improve cardiac filling and output, leading to increased diuresis. Medications like nitroprusside or nitroglycerin can be used for this purpose.
- **Continuous renal replacement therapy (CRRT) (A):** While CRRT can help manage fluid overload and electrolyte imbalances, it's typically reserved for patients with acute kidney injury or severe electrolyte disturbances.
- **High-dose loop diuretics (B):** Increasing the dose of loop diuretics may provide some additional diuresis, but in patients with refractory diuresis, the benefit may be limited.
- **Inotropic therapy (D):** While inotropes can improve cardiac output, they can also increase myocardial oxygen demand and worsen congestion. They are generally not the first-line treatment for HFpEF with refractory diuresis.

By improving cardiac function and reducing congestion, vasodilator therapy can enhance diuresis and improve overall hemodynamics in patients with HFpEF.

226. Answer: D. All of the above
Explanation:

Hepatorenal syndrome (HRS) is a renal dysfunction that occurs as a complication of severe liver disease. It is characterized by:

- **Increased serum creatinine (A):** This indicates impaired kidney function, a hallmark of HRS.
- **Decreased urine sodium (B):** The kidneys fail to adequately concentrate urine in HRS, leading to low urine sodium levels.

- **Dilute urine (C):** As a result of the kidney's inability to concentrate urine, the urine becomes dilute.

Therefore, all of the listed laboratory findings are characteristic of HRS.

227. Answer: A. Low respiratory rate and short inspiratory time
Explanation:

In a patient with status asthmaticus and air trapping, the goal of ventilation is to allow adequate expiratory time to prevent further air trapping and to avoid overdistending the lungs.

- **Low respiratory rate and short inspiratory time (A):** This setting allows for longer expiratory time, which is crucial for reducing air trapping and improving gas exchange.
- **High respiratory rate and short inspiratory time (B):** This would lead to rapid, shallow breaths, which can worsen air trapping.
- **Low respiratory rate and long inspiratory time (C):** This would increase peak airway pressures and risk of barotrauma.
- **High respiratory rate and long inspiratory time (D):** This combination would exacerbate air trapping and increase the risk of lung injury.

Therefore, a low respiratory rate and short inspiratory time are most appropriate to manage airflow obstruction and air trapping in a patient with status asthmaticus.

228. Answer: A. Beta-blockers
Explanation:

Beta-blockers are the cornerstone of long-term blood pressure control in patients with aortic dissection.

- **Beta-blockers (A):** These medications decrease heart rate and myocardial contractility, leading to reduced shear stress on the aorta. This is crucial in preventing aortic dissection progression and rupture.
- **Calcium channel blockers (B):** While they can lower blood pressure, they do not have the same beneficial effect on aortic wall stress as beta-blockers.
- **Angiotensin-converting enzyme (ACE) inhibitors (C):** These drugs can lower blood pressure but may increase afterload, which can be detrimental in aortic dissection.

- **Angiotensin II receptor blockers (ARBs) (D):** Similar to ACE inhibitors, ARBs can lower blood pressure but may also increase afterload.

In conclusion, beta-blockers are the preferred choice for long-term blood pressure management in patients with aortic dissection due to their ability to reduce aortic wall stress.

229. Answer: C. Echocardiogram
Explanation:
- **Echocardiogram (C):** This is the most sensitive and specific test for detecting pericardial effusion. It can visualize the fluid, measure its volume, and assess its hemodynamic impact.
- **Chest X-ray (A):** While it may show cardiomegaly or a water-bottle sign suggestive of pericardial effusion, it is less sensitive than echocardiography.
- **Electrocardiogram (ECG) (B):** Can show changes consistent with pericarditis, such as ST-segment elevation, but it is not specific for pericardial effusion.
- **Computed tomography (CT) scan of the chest (D):** Can detect pericardial effusion but is generally not the first-line test due to its higher cost, radiation exposure, and the need for contrast administration.

Therefore, echocardiography is the most reliable diagnostic test for detecting pericardial effusion in a patient with uremic pericarditis.

230. Answer: B. Change empiric antibiotic therapy
Explanation:
The patient is presenting with septic shock, a severe condition requiring prompt and effective antibiotic treatment. Given that blood cultures remain negative after 72 hours of broad-spectrum antibiotics, it is likely that the initial empiric therapy is not targeting the causative organism.
- **Discontinue antibiotics and observe (A):** This is not advisable as it increases the risk of the infection worsening.
- **Change empiric antibiotic therapy (B):** This is the most appropriate course of action. Based on the patient's clinical condition and potential pathogens, new antibiotics should be initiated.
- **Add antifungal therapy (C):** While fungal infections can cause sepsis, there is no indication for antifungal therapy at this point based on the given information.

- **Continue current therapy and re-evaluate in 48 hours (D):** Delaying antibiotic modification can increase the risk of treatment failure and worse outcomes.

It's crucial to reassess the patient's clinical status, obtain additional cultures (e.g., urine, sputum, wound), and consider other potential sources of infection while adjusting the antibiotic regimen.

231. Understanding the Question

The question presents a post-bariatric surgery patient who developed acute respiratory failure requiring reintubation. We are asked to identify the most likely cause of this respiratory failure among the given options.

Correct Answer: D. Obesity Hypoventilation Syndrome (OHS)

Explanation:

- **Obesity Hypoventilation Syndrome (OHS):** This is a chronic condition characterized by hypoventilation due to the excessive weight burden on the chest wall. It is often associated with sleep apnea, as in this case. Post-bariatric surgery, while aiming to improve overall health, can initially exacerbate respiratory issues due to the rapid fluid shifts and inflammatory response.
- **Risk factors** for OHS include severe obesity, sleep apnea, and polycythemia. Our patient has a history of both obesity and OSA, making OHS the most likely culprit for her acute respiratory failure.

Why Other Options Are Incorrect:

- **Pulmonary embolism (PE):** While PE is a serious concern in postoperative patients, it typically presents with tachypnea (rapid breathing), tachycardia, and chest pain, symptoms not specifically mentioned in the prompt.
- **Pneumonia:** Pneumonia can also cause respiratory failure, but it usually develops a few days post-operatively. The patient's rapid deterioration on postoperative day 2 is more consistent with OHS.
- **Atelectasis:** While atelectasis (collapse of lung tissue) is common after surgery, it typically doesn't lead to such rapid and severe respiratory failure as described.

Additional Considerations:

- **Rapid assessment and intervention** are crucial in managing patients with OHS and post-operative respiratory failure.

- **Non-invasive ventilation** may be considered as initial management before reintubation.
- **Long-term management** of OHS includes weight loss, sleep apnea treatment, and pulmonary rehabilitation.

Case Study: A similar case might involve a morbidly obese patient with OSA who undergoes gastric bypass surgery. Postoperatively, they develop increasing dyspnea, hypoxemia, and hypercapnia. A diagnosis of OHS is made, and the patient requires mechanical ventilation.

By understanding the pathophysiology of OHS and the clinical presentation of post-operative respiratory failure, healthcare providers can effectively identify and manage this potentially life-threatening condition.

232. Understanding the Question

We are asked to identify the scoring system used to assess the severity of alcoholic hepatitis and predict mortality in a patient with a history of alcohol abuse and acute alcoholic hepatitis.

Correct Answer: C. Glasgow Alcoholic Hepatitis Score (GAHS)

Explanation:

- **Glasgow Alcoholic Hepatitis Score (GAHS):** As the name suggests, this scoring system is specifically designed to assess the severity of alcoholic hepatitis and predict mortality. It incorporates clinical, laboratory, and imaging parameters to provide a comprehensive evaluation of the patient's condition.

Why Other Options Are Incorrect:

- **MELD score:** While MELD (Model for End-stage Liver Disease) is a crucial tool in assessing liver disease severity, it is more commonly used in patients with chronic liver disease, such as cirrhosis, rather than acute alcoholic hepatitis.
- **Child-Pugh score:** Similar to MELD, the Child-Pugh score is primarily used for chronic liver disease, not acute conditions like alcoholic hepatitis.
- **Maddrey Discriminant Function (DF):** This is an older scoring system that has been largely replaced by the GAHS due to its limitations in predicting mortality.

Additional Considerations:

- The GAHS is a valuable tool in guiding treatment decisions, such as the need for corticosteroid therapy.

- Other factors, such as the patient's overall health status and response to treatment, should also be considered in managing acute alcoholic hepatitis.

Case Study: A 52-year-old man with a history of heavy alcohol use is admitted with jaundice, abdominal pain, and ascites. Laboratory tests reveal elevated liver enzymes and bilirubin. A GAHS is calculated to be 15, indicating severe alcoholic hepatitis with a high risk of mortality. The patient is initiated on corticosteroid therapy and closely monitored in the ICU.

By accurately assessing the severity of alcoholic hepatitis using the GAHS, healthcare providers can optimize patient management and improve outcomes.

233. Understanding the Question

We are asked to identify a potential adverse effect of dobutamine, a medication used for inotropic support in a patient with cardiogenic shock.

Correct Answer: C. Tachyarrhythmias

Explanation:

- **Dobutamine** is a beta-adrenergic agonist that primarily increases heart contractility (inotropy). However, it also has some beta-1 and beta-2 receptor stimulating effects.
- **Tachyarrhythmias** are a common adverse effect of dobutamine due to its positive inotropic and chronotropic (increasing heart rate) properties. These arrhythmias can range from supraventricular tachycardias to ventricular arrhythmias.

Why Other Options Are Incorrect:

- **Bradycardia:** Dobutamine typically increases heart rate, not decreases it.
- **Hypotension:** Dobutamine is used to treat hypotension, not cause it.
- **Hyperkalemia:** Dobutamine does not directly affect potassium levels.

Additional Considerations:

- Close monitoring of heart rate and rhythm is essential when administering dobutamine.
- Beta-blockers can be used to manage tachycardia induced by dobutamine.
- Other inotropic agents, such as dopamine or epinephrine, might be considered if dobutamine is poorly tolerated or ineffective.

Case Study: A 72-year-old man with a recent myocardial infarction develops cardiogenic shock. Dobutamine is initiated to improve cardiac output. Within an hour, the patient develops atrial fibrillation with rapid ventricular response. The dobutamine dose is adjusted, and beta-blocker therapy is added to control the heart rate.

Understanding the potential adverse effects of dobutamine is crucial for safe and effective management of patients with cardiogenic shock.

234. Understanding the Question

We have a patient with septic shock secondary to pyelonephritis who remains hypotensive despite fluid resuscitation and norepinephrine. We are asked to determine the next appropriate intervention.

Correct Answer: A. Add vasopressin

Explanation:

- **Vasopressin** is a potent vasoconstrictor that can be added to norepinephrine to improve hemodynamic stability in patients with septic shock who remain hypotensive despite adequate fluid resuscitation and first-line vasopressors.
- It works by directly constricting blood vessels, increasing systemic vascular resistance, and consequently, raising blood pressure.

Why Other Options Are Incorrect:

- **Initiate hydrocortisone:** While hydrocortisone is recommended in septic shock patients with relative adrenal insufficiency, it is not the first-line treatment for refractory hypotension.
- **Start an epinephrine infusion:** Epinephrine is a stronger vasopressor than norepinephrine but is generally reserved for patients who do not respond to norepinephrine and vasopressin.
- **Increase the dose of norepinephrine:** Increasing the dose of norepinephrine might lead to increased risk of adverse effects without necessarily improving hemodynamic stability.

Additional Considerations:

- Continuous monitoring of blood pressure, heart rate, and urine output is essential when using vasopressin.
- Vasopressin can cause myocardial ischemia, so careful monitoring of cardiac biomarkers is necessary.
- Other adjunctive therapies, such as corticosteroids and early goal-directed therapy, should be considered in managing septic shock.

Case Study: A 32-year-old woman with pyelonephritis develops septic shock despite fluid resuscitation and increasing doses of norepinephrine. Vasopressin is added to the regimen, leading to a gradual improvement in blood pressure and hemodynamic stability.

By understanding the role of vasopressin in the management of septic shock, healthcare providers can optimize patient care and improve outcomes.

235. Understanding the Question

We have a patient with HFpEF who is refractory to diuretic therapy and we need to identify a medication to avoid due to the risk of worsening renal function.

Correct Answer: A. Nesiritide

Explanation:

- **Nesiritide** is a synthetic form of B-type natriuretic peptide. While it can be effective in reducing pulmonary congestion in acute decompensated heart failure, it has been associated with an increased risk of worsening renal function, particularly in patients with impaired renal function.

Why Other Options Are Incorrect:

- **Spironolactone:** This is an aldosterone antagonist often used in HFpEF to improve symptoms and survival. It actually has a protective effect on the kidneys.
- **Sacubitril/valsartan:** This is an angiotensin receptor-neprilysin inhibitor (ARNI) and is a cornerstone of HFpEF treatment. It has neutral or potentially beneficial effects on renal function.
- **Acetazolamide:** This is a diuretic that can be used in certain situations, but it's not the first-line treatment for HFpEF. It has a relatively low risk of worsening renal function.

Additional Considerations:

- Close monitoring of renal function is crucial when using nesiritide.
- Other options for managing refractory fluid overload in HFpEF include ultrafiltration and continuous renal replacement therapy.

Case Study: A 68-year-old woman with HFpEF is admitted with acute pulmonary edema. Despite high-dose diuretics, she remains severely dyspneic. Nesiritide is considered but ultimately avoided due to her baseline creatinine of 1.3 mg/dL. Instead, ultrafiltration is initiated with improvement in symptoms and renal function.

Understanding the potential risks of medications like nesiritide is crucial in optimizing care for patients with HFpEF and impaired renal function.

236. Understanding the Question

We have a patient with acute pancreatitis complicated by ARDS and are asked to determine the most important initial intervention to improve oxygenation.

Correct Answer: C. Intubation and mechanical ventilation with lung-protective strategy

Explanation:

- **ARDS** is a severe form of lung injury characterized by diffuse alveolar damage, leading to refractory hypoxemia.
- **Intubation and mechanical ventilation** are the cornerstone of ARDS management.
- A **lung-protective ventilation strategy** is essential to prevent further lung injury and improve oxygenation. This includes using low tidal volumes, low plateau pressures, and appropriate PEEP levels.

Why Other Options Are Incorrect:

- **High-flow nasal cannula (HFNC):** While HFNC can provide supplemental oxygen, it is generally not sufficient for patients with ARDS who require higher levels of oxygen support.
- **Noninvasive positive pressure ventilation (NIPPV):** NIPPV can be considered in selected patients with mild to moderate ARDS, but it is unlikely to be effective in severe cases like this.
- **Inhaled nitric oxide:** This is an adjunctive therapy for ARDS, not the initial treatment.

Additional Considerations:

- Early initiation of lung-protective ventilation is crucial to improve outcomes in ARDS.
- Other supportive measures, such as prone positioning and neuromuscular blockade, may be considered in severe cases.
- Prompt identification and management of the underlying cause of ARDS (in this case, acute pancreatitis) is essential.

Case Study: A 42-year-old man with severe acute pancreatitis develops progressive hypoxemia and respiratory distress. Despite increasing oxygen supplementation, his PaO2/FiO2 ratio deteriorates. The patient is intubated, placed on mechanical ventilation with lung-protective settings, and shows improvement in oxygenation.

By understanding the pathophysiology of ARDS and the importance of early, aggressive intervention, healthcare providers can optimize patient care and improve outcomes.

237. Understanding the Question

We have a patient with status asthmaticus who is intubated and mechanically ventilated. We need to identify a potential complication of this management.

Correct Answer: D. All of the above

Explanation:

- **Pneumothorax:** This is a potential complication of mechanical ventilation in any patient, but it can be particularly prevalent in patients with underlying lung disease like asthma. High airway pressures can cause alveolar rupture and air leakage into the pleural space.

- **Pneumomediastinum:** Similar to pneumothorax, high airway pressures can lead to air leakage into the mediastinum.

- **Hypotension:** This can occur due to several factors, including decreased venous return from positive pressure ventilation, reduced cardiac output, and the effects of medications used to manage the patient's condition.

Additional Considerations:

- Close monitoring of hemodynamics, respiratory status, and chest x-ray is essential to detect these complications early.

- Appropriate ventilator settings and careful management of airway pressures can help reduce the risk of these complications.

Case Study: A 28-year-old woman with severe asthma is intubated for status asthmaticus. During the course of mechanical ventilation, she develops sudden-onset hypotension and desaturation. A chest x-ray reveals a right-sided pneumothorax with mediastinal air. The patient requires urgent chest tube placement.

Understanding the potential complications of mechanical ventilation in patients with asthma is crucial for early detection and management.

238. Understanding the Question

We have a patient with a Stanford Type B aortic dissection who is hemodynamically stable and receiving medical management. We need to identify a medication that should be used with caution due to the risk of reflex tachycardia.

Correct Answer: A. Hydralazine

Explanation:

- **Hydralazine** is a direct-acting vasodilator that can cause a rapid drop in blood pressure. This abrupt decrease in blood pressure can trigger a reflex sympathetic response, leading to tachycardia. In a patient with an aortic dissection, this increased heart rate can exacerbate aortic shear stress and potentially worsen the dissection.

Why Other Options Are Incorrect:

- **Labetalol, Esmolol, and Metoprolol** are beta-blockers. They have both alpha and beta-blocking properties. Beta-blockade decreases heart rate and contractility, while alpha-blockade causes vasodilation. Therefore, they can effectively lower blood pressure without causing significant reflex tachycardia.

Additional Considerations:

- The choice of antihypertensive medication in aortic dissection should be based on the patient's hemodynamic status and the specific characteristics of the dissection.
- Other antihypertensive agents, such as calcium channel blockers (e.g., amlodipine) or angiotensin-converting enzyme (ACE) inhibitors, may also be considered depending on the clinical situation.

Case Study: A 58-year-old man with a Stanford Type B aortic dissection presents with mild hypertension. Initial treatment includes labetalol for blood pressure control. Hydralazine is considered but avoided due to the risk of reflex tachycardia.

Understanding the potential side effects of antihypertensive medications is crucial for optimal management of patients with aortic dissection.

239. Understanding the Question

We have a patient with chronic kidney disease who developed uremic pericarditis requiring pericardiocentesis. We are asked to determine the most likely cause of the bloody pericardial fluid.

Correct Answer: C. Uremia

Explanation:

- **Uremia** itself can lead to hemorrhagic pericarditis. The uremic environment contributes to platelet dysfunction, coagulation abnormalities, and increased vascular permeability, all of which can result in bleeding into the pericardial space.

Why Other Options Are Incorrect:

- **Trauma:** There is no indication of trauma in the patient's history.
- **Malignancy:** While malignancy can cause pericardial effusions, bloody pericardial fluid is more commonly associated with trauma or hemorrhagic diatheses, not malignancy.
- **Tuberculosis:** Although tuberculosis can cause pericarditis, it typically presents with a non-bloody effusion.

Additional Considerations:

- Despite the bloody nature of the fluid, the underlying cause is still uremic pericarditis.
- Management focuses on addressing the underlying renal dysfunction, often requiring dialysis.
- Pericardial effusion can recur, so close monitoring is necessary.

Case Study: A 72-year-old woman with end-stage renal disease presents with chest pain and pericarditis. Pericardiocentesis yields 400 mL of bloody fluid. Dialysis is initiated, and the patient's condition improves.

Understanding the complications of uremia, such as hemorrhagic pericarditis, is crucial for effective management of these patients.

240. **Understanding the Question**

We have a patient with septic shock secondary to pneumonia who has developed MRSA pneumonia. We need to identify the most appropriate antibiotic for this infection.

Correct Answer: A. Vancomycin

Explanation:

- **Vancomycin** is the drug of choice for the treatment of MRSA infections, including MRSA pneumonia. It is a glycopeptide antibiotic that effectively inhibits cell wall synthesis in MRSA.

Why Other Options Are Incorrect:

While other antibiotics might be effective against other bacterial infections, they are not the appropriate choice for MRSA.

Additional Considerations:

- The optimal duration of vancomycin therapy for MRSA pneumonia may vary depending on the patient's clinical response and other factors.
- Combination therapy with other antibiotics, such as an anti-pseudomonal beta-lactam, might be considered in certain cases.
- Close monitoring of renal function is necessary due to the potential nephrotoxicity of vancomycin.

Case Study: A 52-year-old woman with rheumatoid arthritis develops septic shock due to pneumonia. Initial empiric antibiotic coverage is initiated. After 72 hours, blood cultures grow MRSA. Vancomycin is added to the antibiotic regimen, and the patient's clinical condition improves.

Understanding the appropriate antibiotic choices for MRSA infections is crucial for optimizing patient outcomes.

241. **Understanding the Question**

We have a patient with new-onset atrial fibrillation with rapid ventricular response (RVR), hypotension, and multiple comorbidities including COPD, heart failure with reduced ejection fraction (HFrEF), hypertension, and coronary artery disease. We need to determine the priority intervention in addition to rate control.

Correct Answer: A. Anticoagulation

Explanation:

- **Anticoagulation** is the most critical intervention in this patient. Atrial fibrillation is a significant risk factor for stroke, and the patient's rapid ventricular response and underlying heart failure increase this risk further. Immediate anticoagulation is essential to prevent thromboembolic events.

Why Other Options Are Incorrect:

- **Cardioversion:** While cardioversion might be considered once the patient is hemodynamically stable, it is not the immediate priority. The focus should be on stabilizing the patient and preventing stroke.
- **Pulmonary artery catheter placement:** While this might be considered for hemodynamic monitoring in severe cases, it is not the initial priority. The

patient's hemodynamic instability is likely due to the rapid heart rate and low blood pressure, which need to be addressed first.

- **Renal replacement therapy:** Renal dysfunction might develop as a consequence of the patient's condition, but it is not the immediate priority.

Additional Considerations:

- The choice of anticoagulant (e.g., heparin, enoxaparin, or direct oral anticoagulants) will depend on the patient's specific clinical circumstances.
- Rapid rate control with beta-blockers or calcium channel blockers is crucial to improve hemodynamics.
- Once the patient is stabilized, further evaluation for cardioversion or rhythm control strategies can be considered.

Case Study: A 58-year-old man with a history of hypertension, coronary artery disease, COPD, and HFrEF presents with acute onset of palpitations, shortness of breath, and hypotension. He is found to be in atrial fibrillation with RVR. Immediate initiation of anticoagulation with intravenous heparin is started along with rapid rate control using beta-blockers.

Understanding the importance of timely anticoagulation in patients with atrial fibrillation and hemodynamic instability is crucial for preventing life-threatening complications.

242. Understanding the Question

We have a patient with SLE presenting with symptoms and imaging findings consistent with PRES. We need to identify the medication most commonly associated with PRES in SLE patients.

Correct Answer: A. Cyclophosphamide

Explanation:

- **Cyclophosphamide** is a cytotoxic agent commonly used in the treatment of lupus nephritis and severe SLE. It is strongly associated with the development of PRES, likely due to its effects on the vasculature and potential for inducing hypertension.

Why Other Options Are Incorrect:

- **Mycophenolate mofetil, hydroxychloroquine, and belimumab** are immunosuppressants used in the management of SLE but are less frequently associated with PRES compared to cyclophosphamide.

Additional Considerations:

- Other factors contributing to PRES in SLE patients include uncontrolled hypertension, rapid increases in blood pressure, and lupus flares.
- Prompt blood pressure control and supportive care are essential in managing PRES.
- In severe cases, plasma exchange or corticosteroids may be considered.

Case Study: A 45-year-old woman with SLE on cyclophosphamide for lupus nephritis develops sudden onset of headache, seizures, and altered mental status. Brain MRI reveals findings consistent with PRES. Cyclophosphamide is held, and blood pressure is aggressively managed. The patient's condition improves with supportive care.

Understanding the risk factors for PRES in SLE patients is crucial for early recognition, prevention, and management of this potentially serious complication.

243. Understanding the Question

We have a patient with COPD exacerbation and hypercapnic respiratory failure who is intubated and on mechanical ventilation. We need to identify the most important factor to consider when adjusting ventilator settings.

Correct Answer: D. Driving pressure

Explanation:

- **Driving pressure** is the difference between the plateau pressure and the positive end-expiratory pressure (PEEP). It is a more accurate indicator of the amount of pressure exerted on the lungs than peak inspiratory pressure.
- In patients with COPD, excessive driving pressure can lead to ventilator-induced lung injury (VILI), which can worsen the patient's condition.

Why Other Options Are Incorrect:

- **Peak inspiratory pressure:** While important, it is less reliable than driving pressure in predicting VILI. It can be influenced by factors other than lung mechanics, such as airway resistance.
- **Plateau pressure:** Reflects the pressure in the alveoli at the end of inspiration. It is important to monitor but not as crucial as driving pressure in preventing VILI.
- **PEEP:** While important for preventing alveolar collapse, excessive PEEP can also lead to VILI. The focus should be on optimizing driving pressure.

Additional Considerations:

- Lung-protective ventilation strategies, such as low tidal volumes and low driving pressures, are essential in managing patients with COPD exacerbation.
- Regular assessment of ventilator settings and patient response is crucial.

Case Study: A 72-year-old man with COPD is intubated for acute respiratory failure. Initial ventilator settings result in high driving pressure. By adjusting the tidal volume and PEEP, the driving pressure is reduced, leading to improved oxygenation and reduced risk of VILI.

Understanding the importance of driving pressure in ventilator management is crucial for preventing lung injury and optimizing patient outcomes in COPD exacerbation.

244. Understanding the Question

We have a patient with severe community-acquired pneumonia who has progressed to septic shock despite standard care. We are asked to identify the adjunctive therapy that can modulate the inflammatory response.

Correct Answer: D. All of the above

Explanation:

- **Sepsis** is characterized by a dysregulated inflammatory response. Several adjunctive therapies have shown potential benefits in modulating this response.
- **Vitamin C:** This antioxidant has been shown to reduce oxidative stress and inflammation in sepsis.
- **Thiamine:** Although primarily known for its role in energy metabolism, thiamine deficiency is common in critically ill patients and can exacerbate the inflammatory response. Thiamine supplementation has shown potential benefits in sepsis.
- **Hydrocortisone:** Corticosteroids have been used in sepsis for decades. While their role is still debated, they can be beneficial in specific patient populations, such as those with septic shock and relative adrenal insufficiency.

Additional Considerations:

- These adjunctive therapies should be considered as part of a comprehensive sepsis management protocol.
- The optimal dosing and duration of these therapies are still under investigation.
- Close monitoring of patient response is essential.

Case Study: A 32-year-old woman with severe pneumonia develops septic shock despite appropriate antibiotic therapy and fluid resuscitation. In addition to standard care, she receives vitamin C, thiamine, and low-dose hydrocortisone as part of a sepsis management bundle. Her inflammatory markers show a trend towards improvement, and she eventually recovers.

Understanding the potential benefits of adjunctive therapies in sepsis is crucial for optimizing patient care.

245. Understanding the Question

We have a patient with refractory cardiogenic shock despite inotropic and vasopressor support, who is also oliguric and has contraindications to other mechanical circulatory support devices. We are asked to identify the most appropriate intervention.

Correct Answer: A. Extracorporeal Membrane Oxygenation (ECMO)

Explanation:

- **Extracorporeal Membrane Oxygenation (ECMO)** is a life-support technique that provides both oxygenation and circulatory support. It is often considered a rescue therapy for patients with refractory cardiogenic shock who are not responding to conventional treatments.

- In this case, where the patient has contraindications to other mechanical circulatory support devices, ECMO would be the most appropriate option.

Why Other Options Are Not Applicable:

While other interventions might be considered in the management of cardiogenic shock, they are not suitable for this specific scenario:

- There are no other specific interventions mentioned in the options that directly address the patient's refractory cardiogenic shock and contraindications to other mechanical circulatory support devices.

Additional Considerations:

- ECMO is a complex procedure with significant risks and requires specialized expertise.

- Early initiation of ECMO in appropriate patients can improve outcomes.

- Close monitoring and management are essential during ECMO support.

Case Study: A 68-year-old man with HFrEF develops cardiogenic shock refractory to inotropic and vasopressor support. Due to contraindications for other mechanical circulatory support devices, ECMO is initiated. The patient's hemodynamics improve, and renal function recovers.

Understanding the indications and limitations of ECMO is crucial for managing complex cases of cardiogenic shock.

246. Understanding the Question

We have a patient with acute pancreatitis who has developed acute kidney injury (AKI) due to acute tubular necrosis (ATN). We need to determine the most appropriate initial management strategy.

Correct Answer: A. Aggressive fluid resuscitation

Explanation:

- **Acute tubular necrosis (ATN)** is often caused by ischemia, which is frequently related to hypovolemia.
- **Aggressive fluid resuscitation** is the cornerstone of initial management for AKI due to ATN. Adequate fluid volume is essential to restore renal perfusion and improve kidney function.

Why Other Options Are Incorrect:

- **Dopamine infusion:** While dopamine can be used to support blood pressure, it's not the primary treatment for AKI due to ATN. Aggressive fluid resuscitation is the initial focus.
- **Hemodialysis:** Hemodialysis is a life-saving treatment for severe AKI but is not the initial management strategy. It's typically reserved for patients with refractory fluid overload, hyperkalemia, or metabolic acidosis.
- **Renal biopsy:** A renal biopsy can help determine the underlying cause of AKI but is not the initial management strategy. In this case, the diagnosis of ATN is already suspected based on the clinical presentation.

Additional Considerations:

- Close monitoring of fluid balance, renal function, and electrolyte levels is essential.
- Other supportive measures, such as diuretics and vasopressors, may be considered based on the patient's clinical status.

Case Study: A 42-year-old man with acute pancreatitis develops AKI. Aggressive fluid resuscitation is initiated, leading to improvement in urine output and stabilization of renal function.

Understanding the importance of early and aggressive fluid resuscitation in the management of AKI due to ATN is crucial for improving patient outcomes.

247. Understanding the Question

We have a patient with status asthmaticus who is intubated and mechanically ventilated and potentially requiring prolonged neuromuscular blockade. We need to identify the potential complications of this intervention.

Correct Answer: D. All of the above

Explanation:

- **Prolonged weakness:** This is a direct consequence of neuromuscular blockade, as the patient's muscles are paralyzed.
- **Critical illness polyneuropathy (CIP):** This is a condition characterized by muscle weakness and atrophy that can develop in critically ill patients, especially those on prolonged neuromuscular blockade.
- **Increased risk of ventilator-associated pneumonia (VAP):** While not directly caused by neuromuscular blockade, prolonged immobility associated with paralysis can increase the risk of VAP.

Additional Considerations:

- Close monitoring of neuromuscular function is essential to minimize the duration of neuromuscular blockade.
- Early mobilization and physical therapy are crucial for preventing complications associated with prolonged immobility.

Case Study: A 28-year-old woman with severe asthma requires prolonged neuromuscular blockade for refractory status asthmaticus. Despite careful monitoring and management, she develops prolonged weakness and is diagnosed with CIP after extubation.

Understanding the potential complications of neuromuscular blockade is essential for optimizing patient care and preventing long-term sequelae.

248. Understanding the Question

We have a patient with a Stanford Type B aortic dissection who is stable and medically managed. We need to determine the most appropriate imaging modality for follow-up six months after the initial presentation.

Correct Answer: B. Computed tomography angiography (CTA) of the chest

Explanation:

- **Computed tomography angiography (CTA) of the chest** is the most appropriate imaging modality for follow-up assessment of aortic dissection. It provides excellent visualization of the aorta and its branches, allowing for accurate assessment of dissection progression, aneurysm formation, and potential complications.

Why Other Options Are Incorrect:

- **Chest X-ray:** While a chest X-ray can be useful for initial assessment, it lacks the detail required for follow-up of aortic dissections.

- **Transesophageal echocardiogram (TEE):** TEE is primarily used for evaluation of the ascending aorta and aortic arch. It is not ideal for assessing the descending aorta, which is typically involved in Type B dissections.

- **Magnetic resonance imaging (MRI) of the chest:** MRI can provide excellent image quality but is often time-consuming and not readily available in all settings. CTA is generally preferred for initial and follow-up assessments of aortic dissections.

Additional Considerations:

- The frequency of follow-up imaging may vary depending on the patient's clinical course and the severity of the initial dissection.

- Other imaging modalities, such as magnetic resonance angiography (MRA) or ultrasound, may be considered in specific circumstances.

Case Study: A 57-year-old man with a Stanford Type B aortic dissection is medically managed. A follow-up CTA six months later demonstrates stable dissection with no evidence of progression or complications.

Understanding the role of imaging in the management of aortic dissection is crucial for optimizing patient care and preventing adverse outcomes.

249. Understanding the Question

We have a patient with chronic kidney disease who developed uremic pericarditis requiring pericardiocentesis. We need to determine the most appropriate next step in management.

Correct Answer: B. Initiation of hemodialysis

Explanation:

- **Uremic pericarditis** is a serious complication of chronic kidney disease. While pericardiocentesis can relieve symptoms and improve hemodynamics, it is a temporary measure.

- **Initiation of hemodialysis** is the cornerstone of management for uremic pericarditis. It effectively removes uremic toxins, reduces pericardial inflammation, and prevents recurrence.

Why Other Options Are Incorrect:

- **Continued observation:** This is not appropriate as the patient has a serious complication of CKD that requires active intervention.
- **Administration of corticosteroids:** While corticosteroids may be considered in some cases of pericarditis, they are not the primary treatment for uremic pericarditis.
- **Pericardial window placement:** This procedure is reserved for recurrent pericardial effusions that do not respond to medical management and is not the initial treatment for uremic pericarditis.

Additional Considerations:

- Close monitoring of renal function and pericardial status is essential.
- Other supportive measures, such as diuretics and fluid management, may be necessary.

Case Study: A 72-year-old woman with end-stage renal disease develops uremic pericarditis requiring pericardiocentesis. Hemodialysis is initiated, and the patient's pericarditis resolves.

Understanding the importance of hemodialysis in managing uremic pericarditis is crucial for preventing complications and improving patient outcomes.

250. Understanding the Question

We have a patient with septic shock secondary to MRSA pneumonia. We need to determine the most appropriate duration of antibiotic therapy.

Correct Answer: C. 21 days

Explanation:

- **MRSA pneumonia** is a severe infection that typically requires prolonged antibiotic therapy to eradicate the organism and prevent relapse.
- The recommended duration of antibiotic therapy for MRSA pneumonia is generally **21 days**.

Why Other Options Are Incorrect:

- **Shorter durations** (7 or 14 days) are typically insufficient for treating MRSA pneumonia and may lead to treatment failure or recurrence.

- **Longer durations** (28 days) may not be necessary in all cases and could increase the risk of adverse drug reactions.

Additional Considerations:

- The actual duration of therapy may vary depending on the patient's clinical response, severity of illness, and other factors.
- Close monitoring of the patient's clinical status and laboratory parameters is essential.

Case Study: A 52-year-old woman with severe MRSA pneumonia is treated with vancomycin for 21 days. She shows clinical improvement, and follow-up cultures are negative for MRSA.

Understanding the appropriate duration of antibiotic therapy for MRSA pneumonia is crucial for optimizing patient outcomes and preventing treatment failures.

251. Understanding the Question

We have a patient with new-onset atrial fibrillation with rapid ventricular response (RVR), hypertension, type 2 diabetes mellitus, and chronic kidney disease (CKD). We need to determine the most appropriate medication for initial rate control.

Correct Answer: A. Diltiazem

Explanation:

- **Diltiazem** is a calcium channel blocker that effectively controls heart rate in atrial fibrillation with rapid ventricular response.
- It has a favorable side effect profile and is often preferred in patients with heart failure, which is common in patients with CKD.
- Diltiazem has a relatively neutral impact on renal function, making it a suitable choice for patients with CKD.

Why Other Options Are Less Appropriate:

- **Metoprolol:** While a beta-blocker can be effective for rate control, it may exacerbate hypotension and renal dysfunction in patients with CKD and heart failure.
- **Digoxin:** Although historically used for rate control, digoxin has a narrow therapeutic index and requires careful monitoring, making it less desirable as a first-line agent in this patient.

- **Amiodarone:** Amiodarone is primarily an antiarrhythmic agent used for rhythm control, not rate control. It also has significant side effects, including thyroid dysfunction and pulmonary toxicity, making it unsuitable for initial management.

Additional Considerations:

- Close monitoring of blood pressure and renal function is essential when using diltiazem.
- Other antiarrhythmic agents may be considered if diltiazem is ineffective or if the patient develops adverse effects.

Case Study: A 68-year-old woman with hypertension, type 2 diabetes mellitus, and CKD presents with new-onset atrial fibrillation with rapid ventricular response. Diltiazem is initiated, leading to effective rate control without significant hypotension or renal dysfunction.

Understanding the specific characteristics of different antiarrhythmic agents is crucial for optimal management of patients with atrial fibrillation and comorbidities.

252. Understanding the Question

We have a patient with a history of IV drug abuse presenting with fever, chills, a new murmur, and echocardiographic findings consistent with infective endocarditis caused by methicillin-sensitive Staphylococcus aureus (MSSA). We need to determine the most appropriate empiric antibiotic therapy.

Correct Answer: B. Nafcillin and gentamicin

Explanation:

- **Nafcillin** is the preferred beta-lactam antibiotic for the treatment of MSSA infections, including endocarditis.
- **Gentamicin** is added to provide synergistic coverage and to address potential intracellular bacterial burden.
- The combination of nafcillin and gentamicin is the standard of care for the initial treatment of MSSA endocarditis.

Why Other Options Are Incorrect:

- **Vancomycin and gentamicin:** While this combination is appropriate for methicillin-resistant Staphylococcus aureus (MRSA) endocarditis, it is not the first-line treatment for MSSA infections.

- **Daptomycin:** Daptomycin is effective against MSSA but is typically reserved for patients with penicillin allergies or those who fail initial therapy.
- **Ceftaroline:** This antibiotic has activity against MSSA but is not the preferred choice for endocarditis.

Additional Considerations:
- The duration of antibiotic therapy for endocarditis is typically 4-6 weeks.
- Surgical intervention may be required for patients with severe complications or persistent infection.
- Close monitoring of renal function is necessary due to the potential nephrotoxicity of gentamicin.

Case Study: A 35-year-old IV drug user presents with fever, chills, and a new heart murmur. Echocardiogram reveals aortic valve vegetation, and blood cultures grow MSSA. The patient is initiated on nafcillin and gentamicin. After 4 weeks of therapy, the patient becomes afebrile, and echocardiogram shows resolution of the vegetation.

Understanding the appropriate antibiotic therapy for infective endocarditis is crucial for optimizing patient outcomes.

253. **Understanding the Question**

We have a patient with COPD experiencing acute respiratory failure requiring mechanical ventilation. The question asks for the best strategy to reduce the risk of ventilator-induced lung injury (VILI).

Correct Answer: D. Lung-protective ventilation with low tidal volumes (6-8 mL/kg of predicted body weight) and PEEP titrated to maintain driving pressure < 15 cm H2O

Explanation:
- **Lung-protective ventilation** has been shown to significantly reduce the risk of VILI.
- **Low tidal volumes** prevent overdistension of the alveoli, which is a primary cause of VILI.
- **PEEP (Positive End-Expiratory Pressure)** helps to recruit and maintain open alveoli, improving oxygenation without excessive pressure.
- **Driving pressure** is the difference between the plateau pressure and PEEP, and keeping it low (<15 cm H2O) minimizes stress on the lungs.

Why Other Options Are Incorrect:

- **High tidal volume ventilation:** This is the opposite of lung-protective ventilation and increases the risk of VILI.
- **Low respiratory rate:** While important in some cases, it is not the primary determinant of VILI prevention.
- **High PEEP:** Excessive PEEP can also lead to VILI, so it must be titrated carefully.

Additional Considerations:
- Other strategies to reduce VILI include minimizing sedation, early mobilization, and proper patient positioning.
- Regular assessment of ventilator settings and lung mechanics is crucial.

Case Study: A 72-year-old COPD patient is intubated for acute respiratory failure. Lung-protective ventilation with low tidal volumes and PEEP is initiated. Regular adjustments are made to maintain driving pressure below 15 cm H2O. The patient shows improvement in oxygenation with minimal signs of lung injury.

By understanding the principles of lung-protective ventilation, healthcare providers can significantly reduce the risk of VILI in patients with acute respiratory failure.

254. Understanding the Question

We have a patient with SLE presenting with lupus nephritis and significant proteinuria. We need to identify the most effective medication for reducing proteinuria in this case.

Correct Answer: A. Mycophenolate mofetil (MMF)

Explanation:
- **Mycophenolate mofetil (MMF)** is a first-line immunosuppressant agent for the treatment of lupus nephritis. It effectively reduces proteinuria and improves renal function.
- MMF has a relatively favorable side effect profile compared to other immunosuppressive agents.

Why Other Options Are Incorrect:
- **Hydroxychloroquine:** While effective in managing mild SLE, hydroxychloroquine is not the primary treatment for lupus nephritis with significant proteinuria.

- **Cyclophosphamide:** Cyclophosphamide is a more potent immunosuppressant but carries a higher risk of side effects, including infertility and increased risk of malignancy. It is often used as induction therapy for severe lupus nephritis but not as a long-term maintenance treatment.
- **Belimumab:** This is a newer biologic agent used for SLE but its primary role is in treating active disease and is not specifically indicated for reducing proteinuria in lupus nephritis.

Additional Considerations:

- The choice of immunosuppressive therapy for lupus nephritis should be individualized based on the severity of the disease, patient comorbidities, and response to treatment.
- Close monitoring of renal function and complete blood count is essential during MMF therapy.

Case Study: A 32-year-old woman with SLE and lupus nephritis with significant proteinuria is initiated on mycophenolate mofetil. After several months of treatment, her proteinuria decreases, and renal function improves.

Understanding the role of different immunosuppressive agents in the management of lupus nephritis is crucial for optimizing patient outcomes.

255. Understanding the Question

We have a patient with cardiogenic shock secondary to acute myocardial infarction and severe aortic insufficiency. We need to identify the mechanical circulatory support device that is contraindicated in this patient.

Correct Answer: A. Impella

Explanation:

- **Impella** is a pump inserted into the left ventricle to augment cardiac output.
- In patients with **severe aortic insufficiency**, there is already a high left ventricular afterload due to blood regurgitating back into the left ventricle.
- Using Impella in this situation could worsen the afterload and further compromise cardiac function.

Why Other Options Are Not Contraindicated:

- **Intra-aortic balloon pump (IABP):** This device can be used in patients with aortic insufficiency. It improves coronary blood flow and reduces afterload.

- **TandemHeart:** This device provides additional circulatory support by pumping blood from the right atrium to the aorta. It can be used in patients with aortic insufficiency.
- **Extracorporeal membrane oxygenation (ECMO):** This is a life-support technique that provides both oxygenation and circulatory support. It can be used in complex cases, including those with aortic insufficiency.

Additional Considerations:
- The choice of mechanical circulatory support device depends on the specific clinical presentation, hemodynamic status, and patient-specific factors.
- Careful hemodynamic monitoring is essential during the use of any mechanical circulatory support device.

Case Study: A 68-year-old man with HFrEF and severe aortic insufficiency develops cardiogenic shock after an acute myocardial infarction. IABP is initially placed to improve hemodynamics. Due to persistent hypotension, ECMO is considered as a bridge to recovery or transplantation.

Understanding the contraindications and limitations of different mechanical circulatory support devices is crucial for optimal patient care.

256. Understanding the Question

We have a patient with severe acute pancreatitis complicated by pancreatic necrosis. The question asks for the most appropriate intervention for managing infected pancreatic necrosis.

Correct Answer: C. Surgical necrosectomy

Explanation:
- **Surgical necrosectomy** is the gold standard for the management of infected pancreatic necrosis.
- Despite advances in minimally invasive techniques, surgical debridement of infected necrotic pancreatic tissue remains the cornerstone of treatment.
- Early surgical intervention is associated with improved outcomes.

Why Other Options Are Incorrect:
- **Percutaneous drainage** and **endoscopic drainage** can be used for managing pancreatic necrosis, but they are primarily used for necrotic collections without infection.

- **Antibiotics alone** are not sufficient to treat infected pancreatic necrosis. While essential for controlling the infection, they cannot address the underlying necrotic tissue.

Additional Considerations:

- The timing of surgical intervention depends on the patient's clinical condition and the extent of necrosis.
- Minimally invasive techniques, such as video-assisted retroperitoneal debridement, may be considered in selected cases.
- Supportive care, including adequate fluid resuscitation, nutrition, and pain management, is crucial.

Case Study: A 42-year-old man with severe acute pancreatitis develops pancreatic necrosis with evidence of infection. Despite aggressive medical management, his condition deteriorates. Surgical necrosectomy is performed, and the patient eventually recovers.

Understanding the importance of timely surgical intervention in the management of infected pancreatic necrosis is crucial for improving patient outcomes.

257. Understanding the Question

We have a patient with severe sepsis due to community-acquired pneumonia who is intubated and mechanically ventilated. We need to determine the appropriate target for central venous oxygen saturation (ScvO2).

Correct Answer: B. ScvO2 > 60%

Explanation:

- **ScvO2** is a measure of oxygen content in mixed venous blood, reflecting tissue oxygenation.
- A target ScvO2 of **>60%** is generally recommended in patients with sepsis to ensure adequate tissue oxygen delivery.

Why Other Options Are Incorrect:

- **ScvO2 > 50%:** This value might be too low to ensure adequate tissue oxygenation in a patient with severe sepsis.
- **ScvO2 > 70% or > 80%:** These values are excessively high and might indicate over-resuscitation or other underlying issues.

Additional Considerations:

- ScvO2 is just one parameter for assessing tissue oxygenation and should be interpreted in conjunction with other clinical and laboratory findings.
- Other factors, such as lactate levels and mixed venous carbon dioxide tension (PvCO2), can also provide valuable information about tissue perfusion.

Case Study: A 28-year-old woman with severe sepsis is intubated and mechanically ventilated. ScvO2 monitoring is initiated, and the target is set at >60%. By optimizing fluid resuscitation and vasopressor therapy, the ScvO2 is maintained within the target range, indicating adequate tissue oxygenation.

Understanding the importance of ScvO2 monitoring and maintaining appropriate levels is crucial for optimizing the management of patients with sepsis.

258. Understanding the Question

We have a patient who underwent surgical repair for a Stanford Type A aortic dissection. We need to identify the most common postoperative complication.

Correct Answer: A. Stroke

Explanation:
- **Stroke** is the most common neurological complication following aortic dissection repair.
- This can occur due to embolic events, hypoperfusion, or vasospasm related to the surgical procedure or the underlying dissection process.

Why Other Options Are Less Common:
- **Renal failure**, **spinal cord ischemia**, and **myocardial infarction** can occur but are less common postoperative complications compared to stroke.

Additional Considerations:
- Early recognition and management of neurological symptoms are crucial to minimize stroke-related disability.
- Other potential complications include bleeding, infection, and arrhythmias.

Case Study: A 58-year-old man undergoes successful surgical repair of a Stanford Type A aortic dissection. On postoperative day 2, he develops sudden onset of weakness and slurred speech. A CT scan of the brain reveals a cerebral infarction.

Understanding the risk of stroke in patients undergoing aortic dissection repair is crucial for early detection and management.

259. Understanding the Question

We have a 70-year-old woman with chronic kidney disease (CKD) presenting with uremic encephalopathy. We need to identify the most appropriate treatment.

Correct Answer: A. Hemodialysis

Explanation:

- **Uremic encephalopathy** is a neurological syndrome caused by the accumulation of waste products in the blood due to kidney failure.
- **Hemodialysis** is the most effective treatment for removing these waste products and restoring normal brain function.

Why Other Options Are Incorrect:

- **Peritoneal dialysis** is an alternative to hemodialysis but is generally less efficient in removing waste products rapidly, making it less suitable for acute conditions like uremic encephalopathy.
- **Intravenous mannitol** and **hypertonic saline** are primarily used for managing cerebral edema, not for removing uremic toxins.

Additional Considerations:

- Early initiation of hemodialysis is crucial to prevent further neurological deterioration.
- Supportive care, including seizure prophylaxis and correction of electrolyte imbalances, is essential.

Case Study: A 72-year-old woman with CKD presents with confusion and lethargy. Blood tests reveal elevated creatinine and urea nitrogen levels. Hemodialysis is initiated, and the patient's mental status improves significantly within hours.

Understanding the importance of rapid intervention in uremic encephalopathy is crucial for optimizing patient outcomes.

260. Understanding the Question

We have a patient with septic shock secondary to pneumonia who is not improving despite 72 hours of broad-spectrum antibiotics and vasopressor support. Blood cultures remain negative. We need to determine the next steps in management.

Correct Answer: D. All of the above

Explanation:

- **This is a complex case where multiple possibilities should be considered.**
- **Add antifungal therapy:** Given the patient's clinical deterioration and negative blood cultures, it's essential to consider an alternative pathogen, such as a fungus.
- **Change to a different class of antibiotics:** While broad-spectrum antibiotics were initially appropriate, the lack of improvement suggests the possibility of antibiotic resistance or an alternative pathogen.
- **Search for a non-infectious cause of her symptoms:** Sepsis-like presentations can occur in the absence of infection. Conditions like adrenal insufficiency, myocardial infarction, or pulmonary embolism should be considered.

Additional Considerations:
- **Source control:** Ensuring adequate drainage of any underlying infection (e.g., lung abscess) is crucial.
- **Immunomodulatory therapies:** In refractory sepsis, therapies like corticosteroids or vitamin C may be considered.
- **Diagnostic evaluation:** Further investigations, such as echocardiogram, CT scan, or bronchoscopy, may be necessary to identify the underlying cause.

Case Study: A 52-year-old woman with rheumatoid arthritis develops septic shock with persistent fever and hypotension despite broad-spectrum antibiotics. Blood cultures remain negative. An echocardiogram reveals a vegetation on the mitral valve. The patient is started on antifungal therapy and undergoes surgical management of the endocarditis.

This case highlights the importance of considering multiple possibilities when a patient fails to respond to initial sepsis management.

261. Understanding the Question

We have a patient with atrial fibrillation presenting with symptoms of ischemic stroke and a negative head CT. We need to determine the appropriate time window for administering intravenous tissue plasminogen activator (tPA).

Correct Answer: B. Within 4.5 hours of symptom onset

Explanation:
- **Intravenous tissue plasminogen activator (tPA)** is a thrombolytic agent used to treat ischemic stroke.

- The recommended treatment window for tPA is **within 4.5 hours of symptom onset**.
- Adherence to this time window is crucial to maximize the chances of a good outcome.

Why Other Options Are Incorrect:
- **Within 3 hours of symptom onset:** While this was the initial treatment window, current guidelines have extended it to 4.5 hours.
- **Within 6 hours of symptom onset or within 24 hours of symptom onset:** These time windows are too long and decrease the likelihood of successful treatment with tPA.

Additional Considerations:
- Strict eligibility criteria must be met before administering tPA, including exclusion of hemorrhagic stroke, active bleeding, and other contraindications.
- Rapid assessment and treatment are crucial for optimal outcomes.

Case Study: A 68-year-old woman with atrial fibrillation presents with left-sided weakness and facial droop. A head CT is negative for hemorrhage. The patient receives tPA within 3 hours of symptom onset, and neurological function improves significantly.

Understanding the critical time window for tPA administration is essential for improving outcomes in patients with ischemic stroke.

262. **Understanding the Question**
We have a patient with infective endocarditis complicated by a perivalvular abscess who underwent surgical valve replacement and abscess debridement. We need to identify the most important factor in determining the duration of antibiotic therapy.

Correct Answer: D. All of the above
Explanation:
- **The type of organism isolated from blood cultures** is crucial as different organisms have varying antibiotic susceptibilities and required treatment durations.
- **The presence of complications**, such as heart failure or embolic events, can influence the overall severity of the infection and the duration of therapy needed.
- **The patient's immune status** can impact the body's ability to fight the infection and influence the length of treatment required.

All of these factors play a role in determining the optimal duration of antibiotic therapy for infective endocarditis, and they should be considered together when making treatment decisions.

263. Understanding the Question

We have a patient with COPD, ventilator-associated pneumonia caused by Pseudomonas aeruginosa, and a history of penicillin allergy. We need to select the most appropriate antibiotic.

Correct Answer: D. Aztreonam

Explanation:

- **Aztreonam** is a monobactam antibiotic with excellent activity against Pseudomonas aeruginosa.
- It is a good choice for patients with penicillin allergy as it is structurally unrelated to penicillins.

Why Other Options Are Incorrect:

- **Piperacillin/tazobactam, cefepime, and meropenem** are all beta-lactam antibiotics and would be contraindicated in a patient with a penicillin allergy due to the risk of cross-reactivity.

Additional Considerations:

- The choice of antibiotic should always be based on local susceptibility patterns.
- Combination therapy with an aminoglycoside might be considered in severe cases or for patients with risk factors for treatment failure.
- Close monitoring of renal function is necessary for patients receiving aminoglycosides.

Case Study: A 72-year-old COPD patient develops ventilator-associated pneumonia caused by Pseudomonas aeruginosa. Due to a history of penicillin allergy, aztreonam is initiated. The patient shows clinical improvement, and the infection resolves.

Understanding the antibiotic choices for patients with penicillin allergy is crucial for effective management of infections.

264. Understanding the Question

We have a patient with septic shock secondary to a pelvic abscess, with a history of chronic hypertension. We need to determine the appropriate MAP target for this patient.

Correct Answer: C. MAP > 70 mmHg

Explanation:

- **The general target for MAP in septic shock is >65 mmHg.** However, in patients with a history of **chronic hypertension**, a higher MAP target of **>70 mmHg** might be considered.
- This is because these patients have likely adapted to higher blood pressures, and a lower MAP might compromise cerebral and coronary perfusion.

Why Other Options Are Incorrect:

- **MAP > 60 mmHg:** This might be too low for a patient with septic shock and chronic hypertension.
- **MAP > 65 mmHg:** While this is the general target for septic shock, it might not be sufficient for patients with chronic hypertension.
- **MAP > 75 mmHg:** This is generally too high and could increase the risk of complications, such as myocardial ischemia or intracranial hemorrhage.

Additional Considerations:

- The MAP target should be individualized based on the patient's response to therapy and the presence of other comorbidities.
- Close monitoring of blood pressure and end-organ perfusion is essential.

Case Study: A 32-year-old woman with septic shock secondary to a pelvic abscess and a history of chronic hypertension is initiated on norepinephrine. The MAP target is set at >70 mmHg. The patient's blood pressure improves, and there are no signs of end-organ dysfunction.

Understanding the importance of individualized MAP targets in patients with septic shock and comorbidities is crucial for optimizing patient care.

265. Understanding the Question

We have a patient with HFpEF and renal insufficiency who is refractory to diuretics. We need to determine the most appropriate next step to improve diuresis.

Correct Answer: B. Ultrafiltration

Explanation:

- **Ultrafiltration** is a direct and effective method of removing excess fluid in patients with refractory fluid overload, especially those with renal insufficiency.
- It is a safe and efficient alternative to diuretics in patients with impaired kidney function.

Why Other Options Are Incorrect:
- **Continuous renal replacement therapy (CRRT):** While CRRT can remove fluid, it is generally indicated for patients with more severe renal dysfunction and electrolyte imbalances.
- **Low-dose dopamine infusion:** Dopamine is primarily used for hemodynamic support and has limited efficacy in promoting diuresis.
- **Metolazone:** This is a loop diuretic that would likely not be effective in a patient with refractory diuresis and renal insufficiency.

Additional Considerations:
- Ultrafiltration can be performed at the bedside, allowing for close monitoring of hemodynamic parameters.
- Other factors, such as underlying causes of fluid retention (e.g., hypoalbuminemia), should be addressed concurrently.

Case Study: A 68-year-old woman with HFpEF and chronic kidney disease is admitted with acute decompensated heart failure. Despite high-dose diuretics, she remains severely edematous. Ultrafiltration is initiated, leading to significant diuresis and improvement in symptoms.

Understanding the role of ultrafiltration in managing refractory fluid overload in patients with heart failure and renal insufficiency is crucial for optimizing patient care.

266. Understanding the Question

We have a patient with alcoholic hepatitis, acute liver failure, and developing hepatorenal syndrome (HRS). We need to identify the most appropriate medication to improve renal function and survival.

Correct Answer: C. Terlipressin

Explanation:
- **Hepatorenal syndrome (HRS)** is a renal dysfunction caused by severe liver disease. It is characterized by renal vasoconstriction and decreased renal blood flow.

- **Terlipressin** is a synthetic analogue of vasopressin with potent vasoconstrictive properties. It effectively increases systemic vascular resistance and renal perfusion, leading to improved renal function and increased urine output.
- Terlipressin has been shown to improve survival in patients with HRS.

Why Other Options Are Incorrect:
- **Octreotide:** Primarily used for management of variceal bleeding, it has limited role in HRS.
- **Midodrine:** An alpha-adrenergic agonist, it has a more limited effect on renal vasoconstriction compared to terlipressin.
- **Albumin:** While albumin is important in managing ascites and improving hemodynamic stability, it is not the primary treatment for HRS.

Additional Considerations:
- Early recognition and treatment of HRS are crucial for improving outcomes.
- Combination therapy with albumin may be considered in some cases.
- Liver transplantation is the definitive treatment for HRS but is often delayed until the patient stabilizes.

Case Study: A 42-year-old man with alcoholic hepatitis develops HRS. Terlipressin is initiated, leading to improvement in renal function and urine output. The patient's condition stabilizes, and he is eventually listed for liver transplantation.

Understanding the pathophysiology of HRS and the role of terlipressin in its management is crucial for improving patient outcomes.

267. **Understanding the Question**
We have a patient with status asthmaticus who is intubated and mechanically ventilated. We need to determine the most appropriate weaning strategy.

Correct Answer: D. T-piece trials
Explanation:
- **T-piece trials** involve disconnecting the patient from the ventilator for short periods to assess their ability to maintain adequate oxygenation and ventilation spontaneously.
- This is a gradual and controlled approach to weaning, which is particularly important in patients with asthma, as they may have rapid changes in respiratory status.

Why Other Options Are Incorrect:

- **Once-daily spontaneous breathing trial (SBT):** While SBT is a common weaning strategy, it might not be suitable for patients with unstable respiratory conditions like asthma.
- **Intermittent mandatory ventilation (IMV):** This mode is more appropriate for patients with stable respiratory conditions and does not gradually reduce ventilator support.
- **Pressure support ventilation (PSV):** While PSV is used in weaning, it is not the initial step and is typically used after successful T-piece trials.

Additional Considerations:

- Close monitoring of respiratory parameters, including oxygen saturation, heart rate, and respiratory rate, is essential during weaning.
- Reversing the underlying cause of respiratory failure (e.g., asthma exacerbation) is crucial for successful weaning.

Case Study: A 28-year-old woman with severe asthma is intubated for status asthmaticus. After initial stabilization, T-piece trials are initiated to assess readiness for extubation. The patient demonstrates adequate oxygenation and ventilation during the trials and is successfully extubated.

Understanding the appropriate weaning strategies for patients with asthma is crucial for preventing weaning failure and improving patient outcomes.

268. Understanding the Question

We have a patient with a Stanford Type B aortic dissection who is hemodynamically stable. We need to identify the medication that should be avoided due to the risk of worsening aortic wall stress.

Correct Answer: D. Nitroprusside

Explanation:

- **Nitroprusside** is a potent vasodilator that can rapidly decrease blood pressure. This abrupt reduction in blood pressure can increase shear stress on the aortic wall, potentially worsening the dissection.

Why Other Options Are Incorrect:

- **Beta-blockers, calcium channel blockers, and hydralazine** are generally considered safe for managing blood pressure in patients with aortic dissection. These medications help to reduce heart rate and blood pressure without causing excessive fluctuations that could increase aortic wall stress.

Additional Considerations:
• The choice of antihypertensive medication should be individualized based on the patient's hemodynamic status and the specific characteristics of the dissection.
• Careful monitoring of blood pressure and aortic dimensions is essential.

Case Study: A 57-year-old man with a Stanford Type B aortic dissection presents with hypertension. Nitroprusside is initially considered but avoided due to the risk of increased aortic wall stress. Labetalol is initiated instead to control blood pressure gradually.

Understanding the potential risks of different antihypertensive medications in the management of aortic dissection is crucial for optimizing patient care.

269. Understanding the Question

We have a patient with chronic kidney disease and uremic pericarditis who has undergone pericardiocentesis but continues to exhibit symptoms of cardiac tamponade. We need to determine the most appropriate next step in management.

Correct Answer: B. Pericardial window placement

Explanation:
• **Pericardial window placement** is a minimally invasive procedure that creates a one-way opening in the pericardium, allowing excess fluid to drain and preventing reaccumulation.
• It is indicated in patients with recurrent pericardial effusions or those who continue to have symptoms of cardiac tamponade despite pericardiocentesis.

Why Other Options Are Incorrect:
• **Repeat pericardiocentesis:** While it may temporarily relieve symptoms, it is unlikely to provide a long-term solution and carries the risk of complications.
• **Pericardiectomy:** This is a more invasive procedure and is generally reserved for patients with recurrent pericarditis or constrictive pericarditis.
• **Initiation of hemodialysis:** While essential for managing the underlying kidney disease, it does not directly address the cardiac tamponade.

Additional Considerations:
• Close monitoring of hemodynamic status is crucial after pericardial window placement.

- The underlying cause of the pericardial effusion (in this case, uremic pericarditis) should be addressed through dialysis and other supportive measures.

Case Study: A 72-year-old woman with CKD and uremic pericarditis undergoes pericardiocentesis but continues to have symptoms of cardiac tamponade. A pericardial window is placed, and the patient's symptoms resolve. Hemodialysis is initiated to manage the underlying kidney disease.

Understanding the different treatment options for pericardial effusion and selecting the appropriate intervention is crucial for improving patient outcomes.

270. Understanding the Question

We have a patient with septic shock due to MRSA pneumonia who has a complicated course with persistent bacteremia. We need to determine the appropriate duration of antibiotic therapy.

Correct Answer: D. 4-6 weeks

Explanation:

- **In cases of complicated MRSA pneumonia, especially with persistent bacteremia, a longer duration of antibiotic therapy is often required.**
- A treatment course of **4-6 weeks** is typically recommended to ensure complete eradication of the infection and prevent relapse.

Why Other Options Are Incorrect:

- Shorter durations of therapy (7, 14, or 21 days) are generally insufficient for treating complicated MRSA infections.

Additional Considerations:

- The specific duration of therapy should be individualized based on the patient's clinical response, the severity of the infection, and other factors.
- Close monitoring of the patient's clinical status and laboratory parameters is essential.

Case Study: A 52-year-old woman with severe MRSA pneumonia and persistent bacteremia is treated with vancomycin for 6 weeks. She shows gradual clinical improvement, and follow-up blood cultures become negative.

Understanding the need for prolonged antibiotic therapy in complicated MRSA infections is crucial for optimizing patient outcomes.

271. Understanding the Question

We have a patient with NSTEMI who has developed acute limb ischemia. We need to determine the most appropriate diagnostic test to confirm cholesterol embolism.

Correct Answer: B. Computed tomography angiography (CTA) of the lower extremities

Explanation:

• **Computed tomography angiography (CTA) of the lower extremities** is the most appropriate diagnostic test to confirm cholesterol embolism.

• CTA can visualize the blood vessels in the lower extremities and identify characteristic findings of cholesterol embolism, such as filling defects and distal arterial occlusions.

Why Other Options Are Incorrect:

• **Doppler ultrasound** can assess blood flow in the arteries but may not be sensitive enough to detect the specific findings of cholesterol embolism.

• **Magnetic resonance angiography (MRA)** can also visualize blood vessels but is generally less readily available and more time-consuming than CTA.

• **Skin biopsy** is not appropriate for diagnosing cholesterol embolism.

Additional Considerations:

• Early diagnosis and treatment of cholesterol embolism are crucial to prevent limb loss.

• Other diagnostic tests, such as blood tests for cholesterol emboli, may be considered to support the diagnosis.

Case Study: A 78-year-old woman with NSTEMI develops acute pain and swelling in her right leg. A CTA of the lower extremities reveals multiple filling defects in the popliteal and tibial arteries, consistent with cholesterol embolism.

Understanding the diagnostic approach to cholesterol embolism is essential for timely intervention and improved patient outcomes.

272. Understanding the Question

We have a patient who underwent surgical valve replacement for infective endocarditis. We need to identify the most common causative organism for prosthetic valve endocarditis within the first year post-surgery.

Correct Answer: B. Staphylococcus epidermidis

Explanation:

- **Staphylococcus epidermidis** is the most common cause of early prosthetic valve endocarditis (within the first year). It is a coagulase-negative staphylococcus that colonizes the skin and can adhere to prosthetic materials.

Why Other Options Are Incorrect:

- **Staphylococcus aureus**, while a common cause of native valve endocarditis, is less common in prosthetic valve endocarditis, especially early-onset infections.
- **Streptococcus species** and **Enterococcus species** are more commonly associated with native valve endocarditis rather than prosthetic valve endocarditis.

Additional Considerations:

- Prevention of prosthetic valve endocarditis includes appropriate antibiotic prophylaxis for high-risk procedures, meticulous surgical technique, and long-term anticoagulation in indicated patients.

273. **Understanding the Question**

We have a patient with COPD on mechanical ventilation and we're asked to identify the intervention most likely to reduce the risk of ventilator-induced diaphragm dysfunction (VIDD).

Correct Answer: D. All of the above

Explanation:

- **Ventilator-induced diaphragm dysfunction (VIDD)** is a condition where the diaphragm weakens due to prolonged inactivity on a ventilator.
- All of the listed options contribute to reducing the risk of VIDD:

o **Daily interruption of sedation:** This allows for spontaneous breathing and diaphragm activation.

o **Early mobilization:** Even if the patient is still intubated, passive range of motion exercises and early mobilization can help maintain muscle tone.

o **Neuromuscular electrical stimulation (NMES):** This directly stimulates the diaphragm muscles to prevent atrophy.

By implementing these interventions, we can significantly reduce the risk of VIDD and improve the patient's overall recovery.

274. **Understanding the Question**

We have a patient with septic shock secondary to a pelvic abscess who is on norepinephrine. We need to determine the appropriate target for central venous oxygen saturation (ScvO2).

Correct Answer: B. ScvO2 > 60%

Explanation:

- **ScvO2** is a measure of oxygen content in mixed venous blood, reflecting tissue oxygenation.
- A target ScvO2 of **>60%** is generally recommended in patients with sepsis to ensure adequate tissue oxygen delivery.

Why Other Options Are Incorrect:

- **ScvO2 > 50%:** This value might be too low to ensure adequate tissue oxygenation in a patient with severe sepsis.
- **ScvO2 > 70% or > 80%:** These values are excessively high and might indicate over-resuscitation or other underlying issues.

Additional Considerations:

- ScvO2 is just one parameter for assessing tissue oxygenation and should be interpreted in conjunction with other clinical and laboratory findings.
- Other factors, such as lactate levels and mixed venous carbon dioxide tension (PvCO2), can also provide valuable information about tissue perfusion.

Case Study: A 28-year-old woman with severe sepsis is intubated and mechanically ventilated. ScvO2 monitoring is initiated, and the target is set at >60%. By optimizing fluid resuscitation and vasopressor therapy, the ScvO2 is maintained within the target range, indicating adequate tissue oxygenation.

Understanding the importance of ScvO2 monitoring and maintaining appropriate levels is crucial for optimizing the management of patients with sepsis.

275. **Correct Answer: A. Continuous renal replacement therapy (CRRT)**

Explanation:

- **Continuous renal replacement therapy (CRRT)** is the most appropriate intervention in this case due to the patient's refractory fluid overload, renal insufficiency, and failure to respond to high-dose diuretics.
- CRRT offers precise fluid removal, electrolyte management, and acid-base balance correction, which are crucial in this patient.

Why other options are incorrect:

- **Ultrafiltration:** While effective for fluid removal, it might not be sufficient in patients with severe renal dysfunction and electrolyte imbalances.
- **Low-dose dopamine infusion:** Primarily used for hemodynamic support, it has limited efficacy in promoting diuresis.
- **Metolazone:** Another diuretic, unlikely to be effective in a patient with refractory diuresis and renal insufficiency.

Additional considerations:
- CRRT can be initiated gradually, allowing for careful monitoring of hemodynamic parameters.
- Other supportive measures, such as optimizing preload and afterload, should be considered concurrently.

By choosing CRRT, we address the patient's fluid overload, renal dysfunction, and electrolyte imbalances effectively.

276. Correct Answer: C. Model for End-Stage Liver Disease (MELD) score

Explanation:
- The **Model for End-Stage Liver Disease (MELD) score** is a widely used prognostic tool in patients with liver disease, including those with hepatorenal syndrome (HRS).
- It incorporates factors such as bilirubin, creatinine, and INR, which are all strongly associated with mortality in patients with liver disease.
- A higher MELD score indicates a more severe liver disease and a higher risk of mortality.

Why Other Options Are Incorrect:
- **Serum creatinine level:** While elevated creatinine is a hallmark of HRS, it is just one component of the MELD score and does not fully capture the overall severity of liver disease.
- **Serum bilirubin level:** Similar to creatinine, bilirubin is a component of the MELD score but does not provide a comprehensive assessment of the patient's prognosis.
- **Response to treatment with terlipressin:** While a positive response to terlipressin is associated with improved short-term outcomes, the MELD score remains the most reliable predictor of overall survival.

Additional Considerations:

- Other factors, such as the presence of complications (e.g., spontaneous bacterial peritonitis), can also influence the prognosis in patients with HRS.

The MELD score is a valuable tool for risk stratification and guiding treatment decisions in patients with HRS.

277. Correct Answer: A. Prolonged weakness
Explanation:

- **Prolonged weakness** is the most common complication associated with the use of neuromuscular blocking agents (NMBA) in patients with status asthmaticus. This is due to the paralysis induced by these agents.
- While **myopathy** and **hyperkalemia** can occur in critically ill patients, they are less commonly associated specifically with NMBA use in status asthmaticus.
Therefore, the most accurate answer is A. Prolonged weakness.

278. Correct Answer: A. Aortic aneurysm formation
Explanation:

- **Aortic aneurysm formation** is the most common long-term complication of type B aortic dissection. The weakened aortic wall due to the dissection process can lead to the formation of an aneurysm over time.
- Regular monitoring with imaging studies is crucial to detect the development of an aneurysm and to plan for potential interventions.

While other complications like stroke, renal failure, or aortic rupture can occur, aortic aneurysm formation is the most frequent long-term consequence of type B aortic dissection.

279. Understanding Uremic Pericarditis and Diagnostic Tests
Concept: Uremic pericarditis is a serious complication of advanced kidney disease. It occurs due to the accumulation of uremic toxins in the pericardial space, causing inflammation. Pericardiocentesis is a diagnostic and therapeutic procedure to remove excess fluid from the pericardial sac.

Correct Answer: C. Pericardial fluid triglyceride level

- **Explanation:** A high pericardial fluid triglyceride level is highly suggestive of uremic pericarditis. This is because uremic pericardial fluid often contains high levels of triglycerides due to the kidney's inability to clear lipids.
Why other options are incorrect:

- **A. Pericardial fluid culture:** While culture is important to rule out infectious pericarditis, it is unlikely to be helpful in differentiating uremic from other non-infectious pericarditis.
- **B. Pericardial fluid cytology:** Cytology can help identify malignant cells in pericardial fluid, but it is not specific for uremic pericarditis.
- **D. Pericardial fluid adenosine deaminase (ADA) level:** Elevated ADA levels are typically associated with tuberculous pericarditis, not uremic pericarditis.

Additional Considerations:
- Other diagnostic criteria for uremic pericarditis include a history of CKD, elevated BUN and creatinine levels, and characteristic ECG findings (e.g., electrical alternans).
- Management of uremic pericarditis focuses on improving kidney function (dialysis), controlling inflammation, and preventing recurrent pericarditis.

Case Study: A 72-year-old woman with a history of type 2 diabetes mellitus and CKD stage 4 presents with chest pain and shortness of breath. An echocardiogram reveals pericardial effusion. Pericardiocentesis is performed, and the fluid is sent for analysis. The pericardial fluid triglyceride level is found to be significantly elevated, confirming the diagnosis of uremic pericarditis.

By understanding the pathophysiology of uremic pericarditis and the diagnostic utility of different laboratory tests, the nurse practitioner can effectively diagnose and manage this potentially life-threatening condition.

280. Understanding Antibiotic Therapy Duration in Complicated MRSA Pneumonia

Concept: The duration of antibiotic therapy for MRSA pneumonia depends on several factors, including the severity of the infection, the patient's overall health status, and the presence of complications.

Correct Answer: D. 4-6 weeks
- **Explanation:** In patients with complicated MRSA pneumonia, such as those with septic shock, persistent bacteremia, or metastatic infection, a prolonged course of antibiotic therapy is typically required to eradicate the infection and prevent relapse. Guidelines recommend a duration of 4-6 weeks in these cases.

Why other options are incorrect:
- **A. 7 days:** This duration is too short for a complicated MRSA infection and is unlikely to achieve adequate treatment.

- **B. 14 days:** While longer than 7 days, a 14-day course may still be insufficient for complicated MRSA pneumonia.
- **C. 21 days:** Although longer than the previous options, a 21-day course might not be enough for severe cases with persistent bacteremia and metastatic infection.

Additional Considerations:

- The specific choice of antibiotic should be based on susceptibility testing and the patient's clinical condition.
- Close monitoring of the patient's clinical response, blood cultures, and inflammatory markers is essential to guide antibiotic therapy duration.
- Adjunctive therapies, such as supportive care and source control (if applicable), are crucial for improving outcomes.

Case Study: A 55-year-old man with diabetes and chronic obstructive pulmonary disease is admitted to the ICU with septic shock due to MRSA pneumonia. Despite initial improvement, the patient develops persistent bacteremia and endocarditis. In this case, a prolonged course of antibiotic therapy, likely in the range of 4-6 weeks, would be necessary.

By understanding the factors influencing antibiotic therapy duration and the potential consequences of inadequate treatment, the nurse practitioner can optimize patient outcomes in complicated MRSA pneumonia.

281. Understanding Cholesterol Emboli Syndrome

Concept: Cholesterol emboli syndrome (CES) is a rare condition characterized by the embolization of cholesterol crystals from atherosclerotic plaques into the microcirculation. It often occurs in patients with advanced atherosclerosis and is associated with significant morbidity and mortality.

Correct Answer: D. Supportive care and statin therapy

- **Explanation:** The mainstay of treatment for CES is supportive care, as there is no definitive curative therapy. This includes managing symptoms, preventing further embolization, and protecting vital organs. Statin therapy is recommended to lower cholesterol levels and potentially reduce the risk of future emboli.

Why other options are incorrect:

- **A. Systemic anticoagulation with heparin:** While anticoagulation might seem logical to prevent clot formation, it is generally not recommended for CES as it may increase the risk of bleeding without proven benefit.

- **B. Thrombolytic therapy with tissue plasminogen activator (tPA):** Thrombolytic therapy is primarily used for acute coronary syndromes, not CES. It is unlikely to be effective and carries a significant risk of bleeding.
- **C. Surgical revascularization:** Surgical intervention is not indicated for CES as it involves microvascular occlusion, which is not amenable to surgical repair.

Additional Considerations:

- Clinical manifestations of CES can be varied and include skin lesions (livedo reticularis, blue toes), renal dysfunction, gastrointestinal symptoms, and central nervous system involvement.
- Early recognition and diagnosis of CES are crucial for optimal management.
- Supportive care may include vasodilators, corticosteroids, and dialysis for renal impairment.

Case Study: A 75-year-old man with a history of coronary artery disease, peripheral arterial disease, and hypertension is hospitalized for an acute myocardial infarction. Several days later, he develops bilateral leg pain, livedo reticularis, and acute kidney injury. A skin biopsy confirms the diagnosis of CES. The patient is managed with supportive care, including intravenous fluids, vasodilators, and dialysis. Statin therapy is initiated to lower cholesterol levels.

By understanding the pathophysiology and clinical presentation of CES, the nurse practitioner can recognize the condition and provide appropriate management.

282. Understanding Factors Predicting Outcome in Infective Endocarditis

Concept: Infective endocarditis is a serious infection of the heart valves. When complicated by a perivalvular abscess, surgical intervention is often necessary. Several factors influence the outcome of surgery.

Correct Answer: D. All of the above

- **Explanation:** All of the mentioned factors - younger age, absence of a prosthetic valve, and early surgical intervention - are associated with a better prognosis after surgery for infective endocarditis complicated by a perivalvular abscess.
- **Younger age:** Younger patients generally have better overall health and reserve, which can improve their ability to tolerate surgery and recover.
- **Absence of a prosthetic valve:** Native valve endocarditis typically carries a better prognosis than prosthetic valve endocarditis, which is associated with higher rates of complications and mortality.

- **Early surgical intervention:** Prompt surgical intervention is crucial for controlling the infection, preventing further complications, and improving overall outcomes. Delayed surgery is associated with increased morbidity and mortality.

Additional Considerations:

- Other factors that can influence the outcome include the type of organism causing the infection, the extent of the infection, and the patient's overall health status.
- Postoperative management, including appropriate antibiotic therapy, anticoagulation, and close monitoring, is essential for preventing complications and optimizing recovery.

By understanding the factors that impact the outcome of surgery for infective endocarditis, the nurse practitioner can better counsel patients and their families, as well as optimize postoperative care.

283. Weaning Parameters for Successful Extubation in COPD

Concept: Weaning from mechanical ventilation is a critical step in the management of acute exacerbations of COPD. Several parameters are used to assess a patient's readiness for extubation.

Correct Answer: D. All of the above

- **Explanation:** All of the mentioned parameters - RSBI, NIF, and VC - are valuable predictors of successful extubation in COPD patients. They provide information about the patient's respiratory muscle strength, ventilatory capacity, and breathing pattern.
- **Rapid shallow breathing index (RSBI) less than 105:** RSBI is calculated by dividing the respiratory rate by the tidal volume. A lower RSBI indicates better respiratory muscle efficiency and is associated with a higher likelihood of successful extubation.
- **Negative inspiratory force (NIF) greater than -20 cmH2O:** NIF reflects respiratory muscle strength. A higher NIF indicates stronger muscles and a better ability to generate negative pressure to initiate inspiration.
- **Vital capacity (VC) greater than 10 mL/kg:** VC is a measure of lung volume. A higher VC indicates adequate lung function and is associated with a lower risk of post-extubation respiratory failure.

Additional Considerations:

- Other factors that influence the decision to extubate include hemodynamic stability, oxygenation status, and the presence of other organ dysfunction.
- A spontaneous breathing trial (SBT) is often performed to assess the patient's tolerance of breathing without ventilator support.
- Close monitoring of the patient after extubation is essential to identify and manage potential complications.

By considering multiple weaning parameters and carefully assessing the patient's overall clinical condition, the nurse practitioner can optimize the timing of extubation and improve patient outcomes.

284. Understanding Fluid Resuscitation in Septic Shock

Concept: Adequate fluid resuscitation is crucial in managing septic shock. The goal is to restore intravascular volume and improve tissue perfusion.

Correct Answer: D. Passive leg raise test resulting in an increase in stroke volume or pulse pressure

- **Explanation:** The passive leg raise test is a dynamic assessment of fluid responsiveness. It involves elevating the patient's legs for a short period and measuring the resulting changes in stroke volume or pulse pressure. A significant increase in these parameters suggests that the patient is fluid responsive, meaning they will benefit from additional fluid resuscitation.

Why other options are incorrect:

- **A. Central venous pressure (CVP) greater than 8 mmHg:** CVP is a static measurement that does not reliably predict fluid responsiveness. It can be influenced by many factors, including volume status, right ventricular function, and pulmonary vascular resistance.
- **B. Pulmonary capillary wedge pressure (PCWP) greater than 12 mmHg:** PCWP is primarily used in patients with left ventricular dysfunction and is not a reliable indicator of fluid responsiveness in septic shock.
- **C. Mean arterial pressure (MAP) greater than 65 mmHg:** While maintaining a MAP above 65 mmHg is important for tissue perfusion, it does not necessarily indicate adequate fluid resuscitation. A patient may require further fluid boluses even with a MAP above this threshold.

Additional Considerations:

- The passive leg raise test is a non-invasive and dynamic assessment of fluid responsiveness.

- Other factors to consider when evaluating fluid responsiveness include clinical assessment, urine output, and lactate levels.
- Excessive fluid resuscitation can lead to fluid overload and pulmonary edema, so it's important to monitor fluid balance closely.

By utilizing the passive leg raise test and considering other clinical factors, the nurse practitioner can optimize fluid resuscitation in patients with septic shock.

285. Understanding Diuretic Options in Acute Decompensated Heart Failure

Concept: Acute decompensated heart failure (ADHF) is a serious condition characterized by fluid overload. Diuretics are a cornerstone of treatment, but patients often require multiple agents or alternative strategies to achieve adequate diuresis.

Correct Answer: A. Tolvaptan

- **Explanation:** Tolvaptan is a vasopressin receptor antagonist that selectively blocks the V2 receptor in the collecting ducts of the kidney, increasing free water excretion. It is indicated for the treatment of ADHF in patients with hyponatremia and refractory fluid overload. Given the patient's history of renal insufficiency and failure to respond to metolazone, tolvaptan could be a suitable option.

Why other options are incorrect:

- **B. Conivaptan:** While also a vasopressin receptor antagonist, conivaptan blocks both V1 and V2 receptors. It is primarily used for the management of hyponatremia associated with ADHF, not specifically for diuresis.
- **C. Chlorothiazide:** Chlorothiazide is a thiazide diuretic, which is less potent than loop diuretics and is unlikely to be effective in a patient with refractory fluid overload.
- **D. Ultrafiltration:** Ultrafiltration is a mechanical method of fluid removal and is generally reserved for patients with severe refractory fluid overload who are at high risk for rapid deterioration. It is not typically the first-line treatment.

Additional Considerations:

- Tolvaptan has potential side effects, including increased serum sodium levels and worsening renal function, which require close monitoring.

- Other adjunctive therapies, such as ultrafiltration or continuous positive airway pressure (CPAP), may be considered in combination with diuretics for refractory fluid overload.
- The choice of diuretic and the need for additional interventions should be individualized based on the patient's clinical status, hemodynamic parameters, and response to initial therapy.

By understanding the different types of diuretics and their mechanisms of action, the nurse practitioner can select the most appropriate treatment for patients with ADHF and refractory fluid overload.

286. Hepatorenal Syndrome (HRS)

Concept: Hepatorenal syndrome (HRS) is a renal dysfunction that occurs in patients with advanced liver disease. It's characterized by a rapid decline in kidney function without intrinsic kidney damage.

Correct Answer: A. Type 1 HRS

- **Explanation:** Type 1 HRS is characterized by a rapid deterioration of renal function with a significant decrease in urine output (oliguria or anuria) over a few days. It is often precipitated by an acute insult such as an infection, gastrointestinal bleeding, or spontaneous bacterial peritonitis. Given the patient's presentation with acute liver failure and rapid development of renal dysfunction, Type 1 HRS is the most likely diagnosis.

Why other options are incorrect:

- **B. Type 2 HRS:** This type of HRS is characterized by a slower progression of renal dysfunction with persistent ascites despite diuretic therapy.
- **C. Type 3 HRS:** This term is not a recognized classification of HRS.
- **D. Type 4 HRS:** This term is also not a recognized classification of HRS.

Additional Considerations:

- HRS is a severe complication of liver disease with a high mortality rate.
- Early recognition and management are crucial for improving outcomes.
- Treatment options include vasoconstrictors (terlipressin or norepinephrine) and liver transplantation.

Understanding the different types of HRS is essential for accurate diagnosis and appropriate management.

287. Weaning from Mechanical Ventilation in Status Asthmaticus
Concept

Weaning a patient from mechanical ventilation requires careful assessment of several factors to minimize the risk of relapse. In the case of status asthmaticus, airway hyperresponsiveness and the degree of airflow obstruction are particularly critical.

Correct Answer: D. All of the above

- **Explanation:** All of the mentioned factors are crucial considerations when weaning a patient with status asthmaticus.
  - **Peak expiratory flow rate (PEFR):** This measures the maximum speed of air expelled from the lungs. A higher PEFR indicates improved airflow and is a positive sign for weaning.
  - **Forced expiratory volume in 1 second (FEV1):** This measures the volume of air forcefully exhaled in one second. An increasing FEV1 suggests improved lung function and is another important indicator.
  - **Airway responsiveness:** This refers to the degree of bronchoconstriction in response to stimuli. A decrease in airway responsiveness indicates improved asthma control and is essential for successful weaning.

Additional Considerations

- **Clinical assessment:** In addition to these parameters, a comprehensive clinical assessment, including oxygenation, ventilation, and hemodynamic stability, is essential.
- **Slow and gradual weaning:** Due to the risk of relapse, weaning should be performed slowly and gradually with close monitoring.
- **Bronchodilators:** Continued use of bronchodilators is crucial to maintain airway patency during the weaning process.

By carefully considering these factors and implementing a gradual weaning approach, the risk of relapse can be minimized, and successful extubation achieved.

288. Follow-up Imaging for Chronic Aortic Dissection
Concept

Aortic dissection is a serious condition where blood tears through the layers of the aorta. While acute dissections often require immediate intervention, chronic dissections can be managed medically. Follow-up imaging is essential to monitor the progression of the dissection and assess for complications.

Correct Answer: D. Magnetic resonance imaging (MRI) of the chest

- **Explanation:** MRI is the preferred imaging modality for follow-up assessment of chronic aortic dissection. It offers excellent soft tissue contrast, allowing for detailed visualization of the aortic wall, dissection flap, and any associated complications. MRI does not involve ionizing radiation, making it a safer option for long-term follow-up.

Why other options are incorrect:

- **A. Chest X-ray:** While useful for initial assessment, chest X-ray is not sensitive enough to detect subtle changes in aortic dissection.
- **B. Computed tomography angiography (CTA) of the chest:** While CTA provides good anatomical detail, it involves exposure to ionizing radiation, making it less desirable for long-term follow-up.
- **C. Transesophageal echocardiogram (TEE):** TEE is primarily used for acute aortic dissection or when surgical intervention is being considered. It is not ideal for long-term follow-up.

Additional Considerations

- The frequency of follow-up imaging depends on the stability of the dissection and the presence of any complications.
- Other factors to consider for follow-up include blood pressure control, heart rate management, and lifestyle modifications.

By using MRI for long-term follow-up, healthcare providers can monitor the progression of aortic dissection and intervene early if necessary.

289. Complications of Pericardiocentesis

Concept

Pericardiocentesis is a procedure to remove fluid from the pericardial sac. While generally safe, it carries certain risks.

Correct Answer: A. Pneumothorax

- **Explanation:** Pneumothorax, or collapsed lung, is the most common complication of pericardiocentesis. This occurs when the needle inadvertently punctures the lung during the procedure.

Why other options are incorrect:

- **B. Cardiac perforation:** While a serious complication, cardiac perforation is rare and usually occurs when the procedure is performed incorrectly.
- **C. Coronary artery laceration:** This is an extremely rare and life-threatening complication.
- **D. Infection:** Infection is a potential risk with any invasive procedure but is less common than pneumothorax in pericardiocentesis.

Additional Considerations

To minimize the risk of complications, pericardiocentesis should be performed by experienced clinicians using appropriate imaging guidance (such as echocardiography). Post-procedure monitoring of respiratory status is essential to detect early signs of pneumothorax.

Understanding the potential complications of pericardiocentesis is crucial for patient safety and effective management.

290. The duration of antibiotic therapy for MRSA pneumonia is influenced by several factors, including the severity of infection, presence of complications, and patient-specific factors.

Correct Answer: C. 8-12 weeks

- **Explanation:** In a patient with complicated MRSA pneumonia, such as this case with persistent bacteremia and metastatic infection to the spine, a prolonged course of antibiotic therapy is required. Guidelines generally recommend a duration of 8-12 weeks for such severe infections. This extended therapy is necessary to eradicate the infection and prevent relapse.

Why other options are incorrect:

- **A. 4-6 weeks:** This duration is typically sufficient for less severe MRSA pneumonia without complications.
- **B. 6-8 weeks:** While longer than 4-6 weeks, it may not be adequate for such a complex infection with metastatic involvement.
- **D. 12-16 weeks:** This duration is generally considered excessive for most cases of MRSA pneumonia, even in complicated settings.

Additional Considerations

- The specific antibiotic choice should be guided by susceptibility testing.
- Close monitoring of clinical response, blood cultures, and inflammatory markers is essential.

- Adjunctive therapies, such as surgical debridement of the spinal infection, may be necessary.

In cases of complicated MRSA pneumonia, a multidisciplinary approach involving infectious disease specialists is often recommended.

291. Understanding the Cause of Neurological Symptoms in SLE

Concept

Systemic lupus erythematosus (SLE) is an autoimmune disease that can affect multiple organs, including the central nervous system (CNS). Various neurological manifestations can occur in SLE patients.

Correct Answer: A. Posterior reversible encephalopathy syndrome (PRES)

- **Explanation:** PRES is a clinical syndrome characterized by headache, seizures, altered mental status, visual disturbances, and hypertension. It is often associated with rapid increases in blood pressure and is frequently seen in patients with underlying conditions such as SLE. The presence of hypertension, proteinuria, and hematuria in this patient supports the diagnosis of PRES.

Why other options are incorrect:

- **B. Lupus cerebritis:** While lupus cerebritis can cause neurological symptoms, it typically presents with more focal neurological deficits, such as hemiparesis or aphasia, rather than the global symptoms seen in PRES.

- **C. Cerebral vasculitis:** Cerebral vasculitis can lead to neurological symptoms, but it is less likely in this case given the absence of specific focal neurological findings and the presence of hypertension and renal involvement suggestive of PRES.

- **D. CNS infection:** While CNS infections can cause seizures and altered mental status, the patient's history of SLE, hypertension, proteinuria, and hematuria make PRES a more likely diagnosis.

Additional Considerations

- Early recognition and management of PRES are crucial to prevent permanent neurological damage.

- Blood pressure control is essential in the management of PRES.

- Other potential causes of neurological symptoms in SLE patients should be considered, such as lupus nephritis, thrombotic thrombocytopenic purpura (TTP), and hemolytic uremic syndrome (HUS).

Understanding the different neurological manifestations of SLE is essential for accurate diagnosis and appropriate management.

292. Choosing the Right Mechanical Circulatory Support Device

Concept

Cardiogenic shock is a life-threatening condition that requires immediate intervention. Mechanical circulatory support (MCS) devices can provide temporary support to the failing heart. The choice of device depends on several factors, including the patient's hemodynamic status, underlying condition, and comorbidities.

Correct Answer: A. Impella

- **Explanation:** An Impella device is a minimally invasive pump inserted via the femoral artery to provide circulatory support by augmenting cardiac output. It is particularly suitable for patients with severe peripheral arterial disease as it does not require cannulation of the venous system.

Why other options are incorrect:

- **B. Intra-aortic balloon pump (IABP):** While IABP can improve coronary blood flow and reduce afterload, it provides limited hemodynamic support compared to Impella and is less likely to be effective in severe cardiogenic shock.

- **C. TandemHeart:** This device provides additional circulatory support by pumping blood from the right ventricle to the aorta. However, it requires veno-arterial cannulation, which is contraindicated in patients with severe peripheral arterial disease.

- **D. Extracorporeal membrane oxygenation (ECMO):** ECMO is a highly invasive form of MCS that provides both respiratory and circulatory support. While it can be life-saving in refractory cases, it is generally considered a last resort due to its associated risks and complications.

Additional Considerations

- The decision to initiate MCS should be made promptly in patients with refractory cardiogenic shock.

- Other factors to consider include the patient's age, comorbidities, and the expected duration of MCS support.

- Close monitoring of hemodynamic parameters and organ perfusion is essential during MCS therapy.

By carefully selecting the appropriate MCS device, healthcare providers can improve outcomes for patients with cardiogenic shock.

293. Postoperative Respiratory Complications

Concept

Postoperative respiratory complications are common following bariatric surgery, especially in patients with underlying conditions such as obesity and obstructive sleep apnea.

Correct Answer: A. Pulmonary embolism

- **Explanation:** Given the patient's risk factors (obesity, postoperative immobilization) and the sudden onset of tachycardia, tachypnea, and hypoxia, pulmonary embolism is the most likely cause of her symptoms. This is a critical condition requiring immediate evaluation and treatment.

Why other options are incorrect:

- **B. Pneumonia:** While pneumonia is a possible complication, it usually develops more gradually and often presents with fever, cough, and sputum production.
- **C. Anastomotic leak:** An anastomotic leak would typically present with abdominal pain, fever, and signs of peritonitis.
- **D. Acute respiratory distress syndrome (ARDS):** ARDS usually develops later in the postoperative course and is associated with bilateral infiltrates on chest X-ray.

Additional Considerations

- Early diagnosis and treatment of pulmonary embolism are crucial to prevent complications such as pulmonary hypertension and right ventricular failure.
- Diagnostic tests such as D-dimer, CT pulmonary angiography, or ventilation-perfusion scan can be used to confirm the diagnosis.
- Supportive care, including oxygen therapy, anticoagulation, and fluid management, is essential.

Understanding the common postoperative complications in bariatric surgery patients is essential for early recognition and appropriate management.

294. Understanding ABG Values in COPD Exacerbation

Concept

In patients with COPD, the body compensates for chronic hypercapnia by retaining bicarbonate. Therefore, a normal or slightly alkaline pH is often seen. However, worsening respiratory acidosis (increased $PaCO_2$) with a declining pH indicates deteriorating respiratory function.

Correct Answer: B. pH 7.25, PaCO2 80 mmHg, PaO2 50 mmHg
- **Explanation:** This ABG result shows a severe acidosis (pH 7.25) with a markedly elevated PaCO2 (80 mmHg) and a low PaO2 (50 mmHg). This indicates a worsening respiratory failure and requires immediate intervention.

Why other options are incorrect:
- **A. pH 7.35, PaCO2 55 mmHg, PaO2 60 mmHg:** This ABG shows a compensated respiratory acidosis, which is typical in chronic COPD. While the PaCO2 is elevated, the pH is maintained within the normal range.
- **C. pH 7.45, PaCO2 35 mmHg, PaO2 80 mmHg:** This ABG is normal and does not reflect the expected findings in a patient with COPD exacerbation.
- **D. pH 7.30, PaCO2 40 mmHg, PaO2 70 mmHg:** This ABG shows mild respiratory acidosis with a relatively normal PaO2. While not ideal, it is not as critical as option B.

Additional Considerations
- The ABG results should be interpreted in conjunction with the patient's clinical status.
- Other factors, such as the patient's acid-base balance and electrolyte levels, should be considered when making treatment decisions.

A worsening ABG, as seen in option B, indicates a need for increased ventilator support or other interventions to improve gas exchange.

295. Assessing Tissue Oxygenation in Septic Shock
Concept

In septic shock, despite adequate fluid resuscitation and vasopressor support, tissue hypoperfusion can persist. Monitoring tissue oxygenation is crucial to guide further resuscitation efforts.

Correct Answer: B. Mixed venous oxygen saturation (SvO2)
- **Explanation:** SvO2 reflects the oxygen content of blood returning to the right heart. It provides valuable information about oxygen delivery and tissue oxygen extraction. A low SvO2 indicates inadequate oxygen delivery to the tissues, despite adequate oxygen content in arterial blood. This suggests the need for further interventions to improve tissue perfusion.

Why other options are incorrect:

- **A. Central venous oxygen saturation (ScvO2):** While ScvO2 can provide some information about oxygenation, it is less reliable than SvO2 in reflecting tissue oxygenation.
- **C. Arterial lactate:** Lactate is a marker of tissue hypoxia but is a retrospective indicator. It does not provide real-time information about tissue oxygenation and is less useful for guiding ongoing resuscitation.
- **D. Base deficit:** Base deficit is a component of metabolic acidosis and reflects the overall acid-base status. While it can provide information about the severity of shock, it is not as specific as SvO2 in assessing tissue oxygenation.

Additional Considerations

- A normal or elevated SvO2 despite adequate fluid resuscitation and vasopressor support may indicate increased oxygen consumption due to hypermetabolic state in sepsis.
- Other factors, such as hemoglobin concentration and oxygen delivery index, should be considered when interpreting SvO2.

By monitoring SvO2, clinicians can optimize fluid resuscitation, vasopressor support, and other interventions to improve tissue oxygenation in septic shock.

296. Understanding the Question

The question presents a scenario of a patient with heart failure with reduced ejection fraction (HFrEF) who has progressed to cardiogenic shock. We are asked to identify the most common cause of right ventricular (RV) failure in this context.

Correct Answer: C. Increased pulmonary vascular resistance

Explanation: In patients with left ventricular (LV) failure, the heart is unable to effectively pump blood out to the body. This leads to a backup of blood in the pulmonary circulation, causing increased pulmonary venous pressure. Over time, this increased pressure results in increased pulmonary vascular resistance (PVR).

Increased PVR places a greater workload on the right ventricle, as it must pump blood against higher resistance to perfuse the lungs. This increased afterload can lead to right ventricular dilation and dysfunction, ultimately resulting in right ventricular failure.

Why Other Options Are Incorrect:

- **A. Pulmonary embolism:** While a pulmonary embolism can cause acute RV failure, it is not the most common cause in the setting of chronic LV failure.
- **B. RV infarction:** This is an uncommon cause of RV failure and is usually associated with an acute coronary syndrome involving the right coronary artery.
- **D. Tricuspid regurgitation:** While tricuspid regurgitation can contribute to RV dysfunction, it is typically a consequence of RV dilation and increased pressure, rather than a primary cause.

Additional Considerations:

- The development of right ventricular failure in the setting of left ventricular failure is often referred to as biventricular failure.
- Early recognition and management of RV dysfunction are crucial for improving outcomes in patients with cardiogenic shock.
- Hemodynamic monitoring, including right atrial pressure, pulmonary artery pressure, and cardiac index, can help assess the severity of RV dysfunction.

Case Study: A 72-year-old man with a history of HFrEF presents with worsening dyspnea, orthopnea, and peripheral edema. He is admitted to the hospital with acute decompensated heart failure. On echocardiogram, he is found to have an ejection fraction of 25% and evidence of right ventricular dilation. This patient is at increased risk for developing RV failure due to the chronic LV dysfunction and increased pulmonary congestion.

By understanding the pathophysiology of biventricular failure, healthcare providers can implement appropriate interventions to optimize patient outcomes.

297. Understanding the Question

The question presents a patient with alcoholic hepatitis and acute liver failure who has developed hepatorenal syndrome (HRS). We are asked to identify the most common precipitating factor for HRS in patients with cirrhosis.

Correct Answer: A. Spontaneous Bacterial Peritonitis (SBP)

Explanation: Spontaneous Bacterial Peritonitis (SBP) is a common complication in patients with cirrhosis and ascites. It is a significant precipitating factor for hepatorenal syndrome (HRS). When SBP occurs, it triggers a systemic inflammatory response that can lead to vasoconstriction of the splanchnic circulation. This decreased blood flow to the kidneys, combined with the underlying liver dysfunction, contributes to the development of HRS.

Why Other Options Are Incorrect:

- **B. Gastrointestinal bleeding:** While gastrointestinal bleeding can worsen liver disease and precipitate acute kidney injury, it is generally less common as a precipitating factor for HRS compared to SBP.
- **C. Large-volume paracentesis:** While rapid removal of large volumes of ascitic fluid can lead to hemodynamic instability, it is generally not considered the most common precipitating factor for HRS.
- **D. Diuretic therapy:** Diuretics are often used to manage ascites in patients with cirrhosis, but excessive diuresis can lead to volume depletion and renal dysfunction. However, SBP is still considered the most common precipitating factor for HRS.

Additional Considerations:

- Early diagnosis and treatment of SBP are crucial in preventing the development of HRS.
- Prophylactic antibiotics are often used in patients with cirrhosis and ascites to reduce the risk of SBP.
- Other factors that can contribute to the development of HRS include sepsis, acute on chronic liver failure, and nephrotoxic medications.

Case Study: A 55-year-old woman with cirrhosis due to hepatitis C is admitted to the hospital with abdominal distension and fever. She is diagnosed with spontaneous bacterial peritonitis and initiated on appropriate antibiotic therapy. Despite treatment, her renal function deteriorates, and she develops HRS.

This case highlights the importance of early recognition and management of SBP to prevent complications such as HRS.

298. Understanding the Question

The question presents a patient with status asthmaticus requiring intubation and mechanical ventilation. We are asked to identify the most effective adjunctive therapy for reducing airway inflammation and improving bronchodilation.

Correct Answer: D. Inhaled Corticosteroids

Explanation: Inhaled corticosteroids are the cornerstone of long-term asthma management and are also essential in the treatment of acute severe asthma exacerbations, such as status asthmaticus. They have a potent anti-inflammatory effect, reducing airway edema, mucus production, and bronchial hyperresponsiveness. By targeting the underlying inflammation, inhaled corticosteroids help to improve bronchodilation, decrease airway resistance, and improve lung function.

Why Other Options Are Incorrect:
- **A. Magnesium sulfate:** While magnesium sulfate has bronchodilator properties, its primary role in status asthmaticus is to prevent bronchospasm, especially in patients with severe hypoxemia or hypercapnia. It is not as effective as inhaled corticosteroids in reducing airway inflammation.
- **B. Ketamine:** Ketamine is primarily used as a sedative or analgesic in the ICU setting. It has some bronchodilator effects but is not as effective as inhaled corticosteroids in reducing airway inflammation.
- **C. Heliox:** Heliox (a mixture of helium and oxygen) can improve gas exchange in patients with severe airflow obstruction. However, it does not directly address airway inflammation.

Additional Considerations:
- Inhaled corticosteroids should be administered early in the management of status asthmaticus to achieve optimal benefits.
- Other adjunctive therapies, such as beta-2 agonists, anticholinergics, and magnesium sulfate, may be used in combination with inhaled corticosteroids to achieve rapid bronchodilation.
- Close monitoring of respiratory function, including arterial blood gases and pulmonary function tests, is essential to assess the response to therapy.

Case Study: A 30-year-old woman with a history of severe asthma presents to the emergency department with worsening dyspnea, wheezing, and tachypnea. Despite aggressive treatment with beta-agonists and anticholinergics, her condition deteriorates, and she requires intubation. In addition to mechanical ventilation, inhaled corticosteroids are promptly administered to reduce airway inflammation and improve lung function.

By understanding the importance of inhaled corticosteroids in the management of status asthmaticus, healthcare providers can optimize patient outcomes and reduce the risk of complications.

299. Understanding the Question

The question presents a patient with a Stanford Type B aortic dissection who is hemodynamically stable. We are asked to identify the preferred antihypertensive medication for initial management.

Correct Answer: A. Labetalol

Explanation: Labetalol is the preferred initial antihypertensive agent for patients with acute Stanford Type B aortic dissection who are hemodynamically stable. It offers several advantages:

- **Combined alpha and beta-blockade:** Labetalol simultaneously blocks both alpha and beta receptors. This leads to a decrease in heart rate, blood pressure, and systemic vascular resistance, which are beneficial in reducing aortic shear stress and preventing dissection propagation.
- **Hemodynamic stability:** Labetalol typically produces a gradual and controlled reduction in blood pressure, minimizing the risk of hypotension and organ hypoperfusion.
- **Ease of titration:** Labetalol can be titrated intravenously to achieve desired blood pressure goals.

Why Other Options Are Incorrect:

- **B. Esmolol:** While esmolol is a beta-blocker, it lacks the alpha-blocking properties of labetalol. It primarily affects heart rate, and its effect on blood pressure may be less predictable.
- **C. Nitroprusside:** Nitroprusside is a potent vasodilator that can rapidly lower blood pressure. However, it can cause significant hypotension, cyanide toxicity, and increased intracranial pressure, making it less desirable for initial management of aortic dissection.
- **D. Nicardipine:** Nicardipine is a calcium channel blocker with vasodilatory effects. While it can lower blood pressure, it does not offer the combined alpha and beta-blocking properties of labetalol.

Additional Considerations:

- The goal of blood pressure management in aortic dissection is to reduce aortic shear stress without compromising organ perfusion.
- Continuous blood pressure monitoring is essential to guide antihypertensive therapy.
- Other medications, such as beta-blockers or calcium channel blockers, may be considered as adjunctive therapy if blood pressure control is not achieved with labetalol alone.

Case Study: A 60-year-old man presents with acute chest pain and is diagnosed with a Stanford Type B aortic dissection. He is hemodynamically stable with a blood pressure of 160/90 mmHg. Labetalol is initiated as the initial antihypertensive agent, and the blood pressure is gradually reduced to a target range.

By understanding the rationale for using labetalol in the management of aortic dissection, healthcare providers can optimize patient outcomes and minimize the risk of complications.

300. **Understanding the Question**

The question presents a patient with chronic kidney disease and uremic pericarditis who undergoes pericardiocentesis. We are asked to identify the most suggestive finding in pericardial fluid analysis for uremic pericarditis.

Correct Answer: D. All of the above

Explanation: Uremic pericarditis is characterized by an inflammatory process within the pericardium due to the accumulation of uremic toxins. As a result, the pericardial fluid often exhibits several abnormal characteristics:

• **High protein content:** The increased permeability of the inflamed pericardial membranes allows for the leakage of proteins into the pericardial space.

• **Low glucose concentration:** The inflammatory process consumes glucose, leading to a lower glucose concentration in the pericardial fluid compared to serum.

• **Elevated lactate dehydrogenase (LDH) level:** LDH is an enzyme released from damaged cells, including those in the inflamed pericardium. Therefore, elevated LDH levels in pericardial fluid are indicative of pericardial inflammation.

While each of these findings individually supports the diagnosis of uremic pericarditis, the combination of all three is highly suggestive of this condition.

Why Other Options Are Incorrect:

Since all of the listed options contribute to the diagnosis of uremic pericarditis, there is no single best answer other than "all of the above."

Additional Considerations:

• Other diagnostic tests, such as echocardiography and electrocardiography, are essential for assessing the severity of pericarditis and the presence of complications like cardiac tamponade.

• Prompt initiation of dialysis is crucial in managing uremic pericarditis and preventing further complications.

Case Study: A 65-year-old man with end-stage renal disease presents with chest pain and dyspnea. An echocardiogram reveals pericardial effusion, and pericardiocentesis is performed. The pericardial fluid analysis shows high protein content, low glucose concentration, and elevated LDH levels, consistent with uremic pericarditis. The patient is immediately started on dialysis, and his symptoms improve.

By understanding the characteristic findings of pericardial fluid analysis in uremic pericarditis, healthcare providers can make an accurate diagnosis and initiate appropriate treatment.

301. Understanding the Question

The patient has severe ARDS with a PaO2/FiO2 ratio of 100, indicating severe hypoxemia despite high oxygen levels. The goal is to improve oxygenation.

Correct Answer: D. Administer prone positioning

Explanation: Prone positioning has been shown to significantly improve oxygenation in patients with ARDS. By placing the patient face down, it redistributes lung and alveolar pressures, improving ventilation and perfusion matching. This leads to increased oxygenation and improved lung compliance.

Why Other Options Are Incorrect:

• **A. Increase PEEP:** While increasing PEEP can improve oxygenation, it's often limited by the risk of barotrauma and volutrauma. In this case, the patient is already severely hypoxemic, and increasing PEEP might not be sufficient.

• **B. Initiate neuromuscular blockade:** Neuromuscular blockade can improve oxygenation by reducing oxygen consumption, but it's a high-risk intervention with potential complications. It's not the first-line treatment for severe hypoxemia in ARDS.

• **C. Start inhaled nitric oxide therapy:** Inhaled nitric oxide can improve oxygenation by pulmonary vasodilation, but it is not as effective as prone positioning in severe ARDS. Additionally, it has potential side effects, including methemoglobinemia.

Additional Considerations:

• Prone positioning should be considered early in the management of severe ARDS.

- Other supportive measures, such as adequate fluid management, low tidal volumes, and lung recruitment maneuvers, should be combined with prone positioning.
- Careful monitoring of hemodynamic parameters and oxygenation is essential during prone positioning.

Case Study: A 60-year-old male with sepsis-induced ARDS is intubated and on maximal ventilator support, including high PEEP and FiO2. Despite these measures, his PaO2/FiO2 ratio remains low. Prone positioning is initiated, and within a few hours, his oxygenation improves significantly.

By understanding the benefits of prone positioning in severe ARDS, healthcare providers can optimize patient care and improve outcomes.

302. **Understanding the Question**

A patient with DKA presents with a low serum potassium level. We are asked to determine the most appropriate next step in management.

Correct Answer: B. Administer intravenous potassium chloride

Explanation: Hypokalemia is a common complication of DKA due to osmotic diuresis, intracellular potassium shift, and vomiting. Despite the low potassium level, it is crucial to correct it gradually and cautiously. **Administering intravenous potassium chloride** is the most appropriate next step.

Why Other Options Are Incorrect:

- **A. Start an insulin drip at 0.1 units/kg/hour:** While insulin is essential in managing DKA, it can exacerbate hypokalemia by driving potassium intracellularly. It should be initiated after adequate potassium replacement has begun.
- **C. Administer intravenous bicarbonate:** Bicarbonate is generally not recommended in the management of DKA unless the pH is critically low (<7.1) and there is evidence of severe acidosis affecting cardiac function.
- **D. Start an isotonic saline infusion:** Fluid resuscitation with isotonic saline is crucial in DKA, but it does not directly address the hypokalemia.

Additional Considerations:

- Potassium replacement should be administered under close monitoring of serum potassium levels and electrocardiogram (ECG) changes.
- The rate of potassium infusion should be adjusted based on the severity of hypokalemia and the patient's renal function.

- Other electrolytes, such as magnesium and phosphate, should also be monitored and replaced as needed.

Case Study: A 55-year-old man with type 1 diabetes presents with severe dehydration, polyuria, and altered mental status. Laboratory results confirm DKA with a serum potassium of 2.5 mEq/L. An ECG shows changes consistent with hypokalemia. Intravenous potassium chloride is initiated while insulin therapy is started cautiously.

By understanding the importance of potassium replacement in the management of DKA, healthcare providers can prevent life-threatening arrhythmias and improve patient outcomes.

303. Understanding the Question

A patient with acute pancreatitis and alcohol abuse has developed acute kidney injury (AKI) with oliguria. We need to determine the most likely mechanism of AKI in this context.

Correct Answer: A. Prerenal Azotemia

Explanation: The most common cause of AKI in patients with acute pancreatitis is **prerenal azotemia**. This occurs due to decreased renal perfusion secondary to:

- **Hypovolemia:** Severe pancreatitis can lead to significant fluid shifts into the peritoneal cavity (third spacing), resulting in decreased intravascular volume and reduced renal blood flow.
- **Splanchnic vasoconstriction:** The inflammatory response associated with pancreatitis can cause systemic vasoconstriction, including in the renal vasculature, reducing renal perfusion.

Why Other Options Are Incorrect:

- **B. Acute tubular necrosis (ATN):** While ATN can occur in severe pancreatitis, it is less common than prerenal azotemia as the initial cause of AKI.
- **C. Interstitial nephritis:** This is an inflammatory condition of the kidney tubules, typically caused by drug reactions or infections. It is less likely in the acute setting of pancreatitis.
- **D. Glomerulonephritis:** This is an inflammatory condition of the glomeruli, usually associated with systemic diseases or infections. It is not a common cause of AKI in acute pancreatitis.

Additional Considerations:

- Early recognition and management of prerenal azotemia are crucial to prevent progression to more severe forms of AKI.
- Aggressive fluid resuscitation is often necessary to improve renal perfusion and prevent further kidney injury.
- Other factors that can contribute to AKI in pancreatitis include direct renal injury from pancreatic enzymes, sepsis, and multiple organ dysfunction syndrome (MODS).

Case Study: A 40-year-old man with a history of alcohol abuse is admitted with severe pancreatitis. He develops hypotension and oliguria. Laboratory tests reveal elevated creatinine and BUN with a urine sodium concentration <20 mEq/L, consistent with prerenal azotemia. Aggressive fluid resuscitation is initiated, and renal function gradually improves.

Understanding the pathophysiology of AKI in pancreatitis is essential for timely intervention and improved patient outcomes.

304. Understanding the Question

A patient with atrial fibrillation and chronic kidney disease has had an ischemic stroke and is ineligible for thrombolysis or thrombectomy. We need to select the most appropriate medication for secondary stroke prevention.

Correct Answer: D. Apixaban

Explanation: Apixaban is the most appropriate choice for secondary stroke prevention in this patient. Here's why:

- **Efficacy:** Apixaban has been shown to be effective in reducing the risk of stroke and systemic embolism in patients with atrial fibrillation.
- **Safety:** Compared to warfarin, apixaban carries a lower risk of intracranial hemorrhage, which is particularly important in patients with chronic kidney disease who are at increased bleeding risk.
- **Convenience:** Apixaban has a fixed dosing regimen and does not require routine INR monitoring, making it easier to manage compared to warfarin.
- **Renal adjustment:** Apixaban dosing can be adjusted based on renal function, making it suitable for patients with chronic kidney disease.

Why Other Options Are Incorrect:

- **A. Aspirin:** While aspirin can reduce the risk of ischemic stroke, it is less effective than anticoagulants in preventing stroke in patients with atrial fibrillation.

- **B. Clopidogrel:** Clopidogrel is an antiplatelet agent primarily used for coronary artery disease prevention. It is not as effective as anticoagulants for stroke prevention in atrial fibrillation.
- **C. Warfarin:** While warfarin is effective in preventing stroke, it has a narrow therapeutic index, requires frequent INR monitoring, and carries a higher risk of bleeding compared to newer anticoagulants like apixaban.

Additional Considerations:
- The choice of anticoagulant should be individualized based on the patient's specific risk factors, comorbidities, and bleeding risk.
- Regular monitoring of renal function is important in patients taking apixaban, especially those with chronic kidney disease.
- Other anticoagulants, such as dabigatran or rivaroxaban, may also be considered depending on individual patient factors.

Case Study: A 72-year-old woman with atrial fibrillation and chronic kidney disease stage 3 experiences an ischemic stroke. Given her renal function and the need for effective stroke prevention with a lower bleeding risk, apixaban is initiated. Regular monitoring of renal function and clinical assessment for bleeding complications are performed.

By understanding the advantages of apixaban in this patient population, healthcare providers can optimize stroke prevention and minimize the risk of adverse events.

305. Understanding the Question

A patient with systemic lupus erythematosus (SLE) is admitted to the ICU with acute lupus pneumonitis. We are asked to identify the most common presenting symptom.

Correct Answer: C. Dyspnea

Explanation: Dyspnea, or shortness of breath, is the most common presenting symptom of lupus pneumonitis. This is due to the inflammatory process affecting the lungs, leading to impaired gas exchange and reduced oxygenation.

Why Other Options Are Incorrect:
- **A. Pleuritic chest pain:** While pleuritic chest pain can occur in lupus pneumonitis due to inflammation of the pleural lining, it is not the most common presenting symptom.

- **B. Cough:** Cough is a common symptom of many lung conditions, but it may not be the predominant symptom in lupus pneumonitis.
- **D. Hemoptysis:** Hemoptysis (coughing up blood) is a serious symptom but is less common in lupus pneumonitis compared to dyspnea.

Additional Considerations:
- Lupus pneumonitis can range from mild to severe and can progress rapidly.
- Early recognition and treatment are crucial to prevent respiratory failure.
- Other symptoms of lupus pneumonitis may include fever, fatigue, and non-productive cough.

Case Study: A 32-year-old woman with SLE presents with increasing shortness of breath over the past week. Chest X-ray reveals bilateral pulmonary infiltrates consistent with lupus pneumonitis. She is admitted to the ICU for close monitoring and treatment.

Understanding the common presenting symptoms of lupus pneumonitis is essential for early diagnosis and management.

306. **Understanding the Question**

A patient with cardiogenic shock secondary to myocardial infarction is refractory to inotropic and vasopressor support. We need to select the most appropriate mechanical circulatory support device given the patient's severe peripheral arterial disease and ineligibility for ECMO.

Correct Answer: B. Intra-aortic balloon pump (IABP)

Explanation: An **Intra-aortic balloon pump (IABP)** is the most appropriate choice for this patient. Here's why:

- **Improved coronary perfusion:** The IABP augments coronary blood flow by increasing coronary perfusion pressure during diastole.
- **Reduced afterload:** The IABP decreases afterload by reducing aortic pressure during systole, improving cardiac output.
- **Enhanced oxygen delivery:** By improving coronary perfusion and reducing afterload, the IABP enhances oxygen delivery to the myocardium.
- **Less invasive:** Compared to other mechanical circulatory support devices, the IABP is less invasive and requires a smaller arterial incision. This is crucial for patients with peripheral arterial disease.

Why Other Options Are Incorrect:

- **A. Impella:** While Impella can provide significant hemodynamic support, it requires placement in the left ventricle and involves higher risks, including bleeding and infection. This is not ideal for patients with severe peripheral arterial disease.
- **C. TandemHeart:** This device provides partial circulatory support but is generally used as a bridge to transplantation or recovery. It is not the first-line option for patients with acute cardiogenic shock.
- **D. Ventricular assist device (VAD):** VADs are complex devices requiring major surgery and are typically reserved for patients with end-stage heart failure who are candidates for transplantation. They are not suitable for acute, reversible conditions like cardiogenic shock.

Additional Considerations:
- The IABP is a temporary measure to support cardiac function while other therapies, such as percutaneous coronary intervention (PCI) or coronary artery bypass graft (CABG), are being considered.
- Careful monitoring of hemodynamic parameters and device-related complications is essential during IABP therapy.

Case Study: A 68-year-old man with a history of coronary artery disease presents with cardiogenic shock after an acute myocardial infarction. Despite maximal medical therapy, his cardiac index remains low. Due to severe peripheral arterial disease, an IABP is inserted. The patient's hemodynamics improve, allowing for successful PCI and subsequent recovery.

By understanding the indications and benefits of IABP in the management of cardiogenic shock, healthcare providers can optimize patient care and improve outcomes.

307. Understanding the Question

A patient with severe alcoholic hepatitis and encephalopathy requires a medication to reduce ammonia levels. We need to identify the most effective option.

Correct Answer: A. Lactulose

Explanation: Lactulose is the most effective medication for reducing ammonia levels in patients with hepatic encephalopathy, including those with alcoholic hepatitis. It works by acidifying the colon, which traps ammonia and converts it into ammonium ions. These ions are then excreted in the stool.

Why Other Options Are Incorrect:

- **B. Rifaximin:** Rifaximin is a non-absorbable antibiotic that reduces intestinal bacteria, thereby decreasing ammonia production. It is often used as an adjunct to lactulose, but it is not as effective as lactulose alone in reducing ammonia levels.
- **C. Neomycin:** Neomycin is another non-absorbable antibiotic with ammonia-reducing properties. However, it has a higher risk of systemic absorption and nephrotoxicity compared to rifaximin, making it less preferred.
- **D. L-ornithine L-aspartate (LOLA):** LOLA is a synthetic amino acid combination that supports liver function but does not directly reduce ammonia levels.

Additional Considerations:

- Lactulose can cause osmotic diarrhea, which can lead to electrolyte imbalances. Monitoring of electrolytes is essential.
- Combination therapy with lactulose and rifaximin may be considered in refractory cases.
- Other supportive measures, such as protein restriction and adequate hydration, are important in managing hepatic encephalopathy.

Case Study: A 45-year-old man with alcoholic hepatitis develops confusion and asterixis. Ammonia levels are elevated.Lactulose is initiated, and his mental status gradually improves.

By understanding the mechanism of action of lactulose and its role in managing hepatic encephalopathy, healthcare providers can effectively treat this condition and improve patient outcomes.

308. Understanding the Question

A patient with status asthmaticus is on mechanical ventilation. We need to identify the intervention most likely to reduce the risk of ventilator-induced lung injury (VILI) and barotrauma.

Correct Answer: C. Permissive hypercapnia

Explanation: Permissive hypercapnia involves allowing a higher-than-normal level of carbon dioxide in the blood to prevent ventilator-induced lung injury. By allowing a slightly higher $PaCO_2$, we can use lower tidal volumes and plateau pressures, reducing the risk of barotrauma and volutrauma.

Why Other Options Are Incorrect:

- **A. High tidal volume ventilation:** High tidal volumes are associated with increased risk of VILI and barotrauma.
- **B. High plateau pressure:** High plateau pressure indicates overdistension of the lungs and is a major contributor to VILI.
- **D. High respiratory rate:** A high respiratory rate can increase tidal volume and mean airway pressure, leading to increased risk of VILI.

Additional Considerations:

- Permissive hypercapnia should be used cautiously and monitored closely to prevent severe acidosis.
- Other strategies to reduce VILI include using low tidal volumes, recruiting maneuvers, and minimizing sedation.

Case Study: A 30-year-old patient with severe asthma is intubated for status asthmaticus. To prevent VILI, the ventilator settings are adjusted to allow a slightly higher PaCO2 while maintaining adequate oxygenation. This allows for lower tidal volumes and plateau pressures, reducing the risk of lung injury.

By understanding the principles of permissive hypercapnia, healthcare providers can optimize ventilator management in patients with ARDS and reduce the risk of complications.

309. Understanding the Question

We are asked to determine the most important factor influencing the long-term prognosis of a patient with a stable Stanford Type B aortic dissection.

Correct Answer: B. Extent of the dissection

Explanation: The **extent of the dissection** is the most critical factor in determining the long-term prognosis of a patient with a Stanford Type B aortic dissection. A longer dissection with involvement of distal aortic branches carries a higher risk of complications, such as aortic rupture, malperfusion syndromes, and aneurysm formation.

Why Other Options Are Incorrect:

- **A. Age:** While age can be a risk factor for aortic dissection, it is not as crucial as the extent of the dissection in determining long-term prognosis.
- **C. Presence of complications:** Complications certainly impact the patient's condition, but they are often a result of the dissection's extent.

- **D. Blood pressure control:** Effective blood pressure management is essential for acute management but does not directly influence the long-term prognosis as much as the dissection's extent.

Additional Considerations:

- Regular imaging follow-up is essential to monitor the progression of the dissection and detect any complications.
- Lifestyle modifications, such as blood pressure control and smoking cessation, are important in preventing complications.
- Surgical intervention may be considered in cases of progressive aortic enlargement, impending rupture, or refractory complications.

Case Study: A 58-year-old man with a Stanford Type B aortic dissection involving the descending thoracic aorta and left subclavian artery is treated medically. Due to the extensive nature of the dissection, he is at increased risk for complications and requires close monitoring and potential intervention.

By understanding the significance of dissection extent, healthcare providers can accurately assess the patient's risk and develop an appropriate management plan.

310. **Understanding the Question**

A patient with chronic kidney disease (CKD) and uremic pericarditis has undergone pericardiocentesis for cardiac tamponade but is experiencing recurrence. We are asked to determine the most appropriate next step.

Correct Answer: B. Pericardial window placement

Explanation: A **pericardial window** is the most appropriate next step in a patient with recurrent cardiac tamponade despite pericardiocentesis. This procedure involves creating a persistent opening in the pericardium to allow for drainage of excess fluid and prevent reaccumulation.

Why Other Options Are Incorrect:

- **A. Repeat pericardiocentesis:** Repeated pericardiocentesis is a temporary measure and is not effective in preventing recurrent tamponade.
- **C. Pericardiectomy:** Pericardiectomy is a surgical procedure to remove the pericardium. It is considered for patients with recurrent tamponade refractory to other treatments and is generally reserved for more severe cases.
- **D. Initiation of hemodialysis:** While hemodialysis is crucial in managing CKD, it does not directly address the recurrent cardiac tamponade.

Additional Considerations:

• The decision to proceed with a pericardial window should be made in consultation with a cardiothoracic surgeon.

• Other potential complications of uremic pericarditis, such as constrictive pericarditis, should be considered.

Case Study: A 72-year-old woman with CKD and uremic pericarditis undergoes pericardiocentesis for cardiac tamponade, but the fluid rapidly reaccumulates. A pericardial window is placed, and the patient's symptoms resolve without recurrence.

By understanding the limitations of pericardiocentesis in recurrent tamponade and the benefits of a pericardial window, healthcare providers can optimize patient management.

311. Understanding the Question

A 72-year-old woman presents with altered mental status, agitation, visual hallucinations, tachycardia, and hypertension. We are asked to identify the most likely cause of her symptoms given her medication history.

Correct Answer: A. Delirium due to anticholinergic toxicity

Explanation:

The key to this question lies in the patient's medication history. Diphenhydramine, a first-generation antihistamine, has significant anticholinergic properties. Anticholinergic toxicity can manifest with symptoms such as:

• Altered mental status
• Agitation
• Delirium
• Visual hallucinations
• Tachycardia
• Hypertension

The patient's recent initiation of diphenhydramine, combined with her presenting symptoms, strongly suggests anticholinergic toxicity as the most likely cause.

Why Other Options Are Incorrect:

• **B. Acute stroke:** While stroke can cause altered mental status, the rapid onset of symptoms and the presence of anticholinergic side effects make this less likely.

- **C. Sepsis:** Sepsis often presents with fever, hypotension, and tachycardia. The patient's symptoms are more consistent with anticholinergic toxicity.
- **D. Worsening dementia:** While dementia can cause cognitive decline, the acute onset of symptoms and the presence of anticholinergic side effects make this less likely.

Additional Considerations:

- It's important to discontinue the diphenhydramine immediately and monitor the patient closely.
- Supportive care, including hydration and possibly medication to manage agitation, may be necessary.
- Other anticholinergic medications should be reviewed and discontinued if possible.

Case Study: A 75-year-old woman with mild dementia starts diphenhydramine for seasonal allergies. Within a few days, she develops confusion, agitation, and visual hallucinations. Her physical exam reveals dry mucous membranes, dilated pupils, and tachycardia. The diagnosis of anticholinergic toxicity is made, and the diphenhydramine is discontinued. Her symptoms improve over the next few days.

By understanding the common side effects of anticholinergic medications, healthcare providers can quickly identify and treat anticholinergic toxicity.

312. Understanding the Question

A patient with end-stage renal disease on hemodialysis presents with fever, chills, and an infected arteriovenous fistula (AVF). We are asked to identify the most likely causative organism.

Correct Answer: A. Staphylococcus aureus

Explanation:

- **Staphylococcus aureus** is the most common organism causing infections related to hemodialysis access, including AVF infections. It is a common skin colonizer and has a propensity for causing skin and soft tissue infections.

Why Other Options Are Incorrect:

- **B. Streptococcus viridans:** While a common cause of endocarditis, Streptococcus viridans is less likely to cause AVF infections.

- **C. Pseudomonas aeruginosa:** Pseudomonas aeruginosa is often associated with hospital-acquired infections and can cause various infections, but it's less common in AVF infections compared to Staphylococcus aureus.
- **D. Candida albicans:** Candida albicans is a fungal organism more commonly associated with candidemia and other systemic infections rather than AVF infections.

Additional Considerations:

- Prompt diagnosis and treatment of AVF infections are crucial to prevent complications such as sepsis.
- Blood cultures should be obtained to identify the specific causative organism.
- The infected AVF may require surgical intervention or removal in severe cases.

Case Study: A 48-year-old man with end-stage renal disease on hemodialysis presents with fever, chills, and redness around his AVF. Blood cultures grow Staphylococcus aureus. The patient is initiated on intravenous vancomycin and undergoes surgical debridement of the infected AVF.

By understanding the common causative organisms of AVF infections, healthcare providers can initiate appropriate antimicrobial therapy and prevent complications.

313. Understanding the Question

A patient with COPD and obesity hypoventilation syndrome is in acute respiratory failure requiring mechanical ventilation. We need to select the most appropriate ventilation mode.

Correct Answer: C. Synchronized intermittent mandatory ventilation (SIMV)

Explanation: SIMV is the most appropriate ventilation mode for this patient. It allows for patient-triggered breaths in addition to mandatory ventilator breaths. This mode provides a balance of ventilator support while allowing the patient to participate in breathing, which is crucial for patients with COPD.

Why Other Options Are Incorrect:

- **A. Assist-control ventilation (ACV):** ACV delivers a preset tidal volume for every breath, whether patient-initiated or ventilator-delivered. This can lead to overventilation and lung injury in patients with COPD.

- **B. Pressure-controlled ventilation (PCV):** PCV delivers a set inspiratory pressure, which may not be suitable for patients with COPD, as it can lead to overdistension of the lungs.
- **D. Pressure support ventilation (PSV):** PSV provides pressure support for spontaneous breaths but does not guarantee a minimum tidal volume. This may not be sufficient for a patient in acute respiratory failure.

Additional Considerations:
- Low tidal volumes and permissive hypercapnia are often used in patients with COPD to minimize lung injury.
- Other ventilator settings, such as PEEP and inspiratory time, should be adjusted based on the patient's specific needs and response to therapy.

Case Study: A 72-year-old man with COPD and obesity hypoventilation syndrome is intubated for acute respiratory failure. SIMV is initiated with low tidal volumes and permissive hypercapnia. The patient's oxygenation and ventilation gradually improve.

By understanding the advantages of SIMV in patients with COPD, healthcare providers can optimize ventilator management and improve patient outcomes.

314. Understanding the Question

A young patient with no significant medical history has developed septic shock secondary to community-acquired pneumonia and is on mechanical ventilation with a PaO2/FiO2 ratio of 80, indicating moderate to severe hypoxemia. We need to identify the most appropriate intervention to improve oxygenation.

Correct Answer: A. Increase PEEP

Explanation: Increasing **Positive End-Expiratory Pressure (PEEP)** is the most appropriate initial step to improve oxygenation in this patient. PEEP helps to recruit and stabilize alveoli, improve oxygenation, and reduce lung edema.

Why Other Options Are Incorrect:
- **B. Initiate neuromuscular blockade:** While neuromuscular blockade can improve oxygenation by reducing oxygen consumption, it is generally reserved for refractory hypoxemia and should not be the first-line intervention.
- **C. Start inhaled nitric oxide therapy:** Inhaled nitric oxide is a vasodilator used in specific cases of pulmonary hypertension and is not typically the first-line treatment for hypoxemia in ARDS.

- **D. Administer prone positioning:** Prone positioning is effective in improving oxygenation in severe ARDS but is generally reserved for patients with more severe hypoxemia (PaO2/FiO2 ratio < 100) and after other interventions have failed.

Additional Considerations:

- The optimal level of PEEP should be determined based on the patient's response and the balance between improving oxygenation and reducing the risk of barotrauma.
- Other supportive measures, such as adequate fluid management and low tidal volumes, are essential in managing ARDS.

Case Study: A 32-year-old woman with community-acquired pneumonia develops septic shock and requires mechanical ventilation. Her initial PaO2/FiO2 ratio is 80. Increasing PEEP leads to improvement in oxygenation, and her condition stabilizes.

By understanding the role of PEEP in managing ARDS, healthcare providers can optimize ventilator management and improve patient outcomes.

315. Understanding the Question

We are asked to identify the complication of cardiogenic shock associated with the highest mortality rate.

Correct Answer: A. Acute Kidney Injury (AKI)

Explanation: Acute Kidney Injury (AKI) is a common and severe complication of cardiogenic shock, and it is associated with the highest mortality rate. The decreased cardiac output in cardiogenic shock leads to reduced renal perfusion, resulting in AKI. This vicious cycle further exacerbates the patient's condition and increases the risk of death.

Why Other Options Are Incorrect:

- **B. Multi-organ failure:** While multi-organ failure is a serious complication of cardiogenic shock, it is often a consequence of AKI and other organ hypoperfusion.
- **C. Ventricular arrhythmias:** Ventricular arrhythmias are a common complication of myocardial infarction and can contribute to cardiogenic shock but do not typically carry the same level of mortality as AKI.

- **D. Stroke:** Stroke can occur in cardiogenic shock due to embolization or hypoperfusion, but it is generally less common and has a lower mortality rate compared to AKI.

Additional Considerations:

Early recognition and management of AKI in cardiogenic shock are crucial for improving patient outcomes. Aggressive fluid resuscitation, vasopressor support, and renal replacement therapy may be necessary.

Case Study: A 68-year-old man with cardiogenic shock develops oliguria and rising creatinine levels, indicating AKI. Despite aggressive treatment, his renal function continues to deteriorate, leading to multi-organ failure and death.

Understanding the high mortality associated with AKI in cardiogenic shock emphasizes the importance of early detection and intervention.

316. **The Correct Answer:**

A. Elevated ammonia levels

Explanation:

Hepatic encephalopathy is a neuropsychiatric syndrome that develops in patients with severe liver disease. The most critical factor in its pathogenesis is the **elevation of ammonia levels** in the blood.

- **Normal liver function:** The liver plays a crucial role in converting ammonia, a toxic byproduct of protein metabolism, into urea, which is then excreted by the kidneys.
- **Liver failure:** When the liver is severely damaged, as in alcoholic hepatitis and acute liver failure, its ability to process ammonia is impaired. This leads to a buildup of ammonia in the bloodstream.
- **Ammonia toxicity:** High levels of ammonia cross the blood-brain barrier and cause brain dysfunction, resulting in the symptoms of hepatic encephalopathy, which can range from mild confusion to coma.

Why Other Options Are Incorrect:

- **B. Increased inflammatory cytokines:** While inflammation is a common feature of liver disease and can contribute to various complications, it is not the primary cause of hepatic encephalopathy.
- **C. Cerebral edema:** Cerebral edema can occur in severe liver disease, but it is a consequence of hepatic encephalopathy rather than a primary cause.

- **D. Oxidative stress:** Oxidative stress is involved in the pathogenesis of liver disease, but it is not the primary factor responsible for the development of hepatic encephalopathy.

Additional Considerations:

- Other factors can precipitate hepatic encephalopathy in patients with liver disease, including gastrointestinal bleeding, infections, electrolyte imbalances, and certain medications.
- The management of hepatic encephalopathy focuses on reducing ammonia levels through measures such as lactulose, rifaximin, and dietary protein restriction.
- Early recognition and treatment of hepatic encephalopathy are essential to prevent complications and improve patient outcomes.

Case Study: A 55-year-old man with cirrhosis develops increasing confusion and lethargy. Laboratory tests reveal elevated ammonia levels. He is diagnosed with hepatic encephalopathy and started on lactulose to reduce ammonia production.

By understanding the critical role of ammonia in the pathogenesis of hepatic encephalopathy, healthcare providers can effectively diagnose and manage this condition in patients with liver disease.

317. Pseudomonas aeruginosa Infection in Cystic Fibrosis

Understanding the Question

The question is asking about the most suitable antibiotic to treat a Pseudomonas aeruginosa infection in a cystic fibrosis patient experiencing a pulmonary exacerbation.

The Correct Answer:

D. Ciprofloxacin

Explanation:

Pseudomonas aeruginosa is a common and problematic pathogen in patients with cystic fibrosis, often leading to severe pulmonary exacerbations. The choice of antibiotic depends on several factors, including the patient's clinical condition, the severity of the infection, and the organism's susceptibility patterns.

- **Ciprofloxacin** is a fluoroquinolone antibiotic with excellent activity against Pseudomonas aeruginosa, including many multidrug-resistant strains. It is often the first-line choice for treating pulmonary exacerbations in cystic fibrosis patients due to its oral bioavailability, allowing for continued treatment at home after hospitalization.

Why Other Options Are Incorrect:

• **A. Cefepime:** While cefepime is a broad-spectrum cephalosporin with activity against Pseudomonas aeruginosa, it is often reserved for more severe infections or when other options are not suitable.

• **B. Meropenem:** Meropenem is a carbapenem antibiotic with broad-spectrum activity, including against Pseudomonas aeruginosa. However, it is typically used for severe infections or when other antibiotics have failed.

• **C. Piperacillin/tazobactam:** This combination antibiotic has good activity against Pseudomonas aeruginosa, but it is often associated with higher rates of adverse effects compared to ciprofloxacin.

Additional Considerations:

• The choice of antibiotic may need to be adjusted based on the results of culture and sensitivity testing.

• Combination therapy with other antibiotics may be necessary for severe infections or when there is evidence of mixed bacterial infections.

• Prophylactic antibiotics are often used in cystic fibrosis patients to prevent pulmonary exacerbations.

• Adherence to antibiotic therapy is crucial to prevent the development of antibiotic resistance.

Case Study: A 22-year-old woman with cystic fibrosis presents with increased sputum production, cough, and shortness of breath. A sputum culture grows Pseudomonas aeruginosa. Ciprofloxacin is initiated as initial therapy.

By selecting appropriate antibiotics for the treatment of Pseudomonas aeruginosa infections, healthcare providers can improve patient outcomes and prevent complications in cystic fibrosis patients.

318. **The Correct Answer:**

C. Spinal cord ischemia

Explanation:

Spinal cord ischemia is a unique and severe complication associated with aortic dissection repair. It occurs due to impaired blood flow to the spinal cord, often resulting from decreased perfusion pressure or occlusion of the spinal arteries during the surgical procedure.

- **The aorta:** The aorta is the main artery supplying blood to the body, including the spinal cord.
- **Dissection and surgery:** The dissection itself can disrupt blood flow to the spinal arteries, and the surgical repair process can further compromise blood flow to this critical region.
- **Consequences:** Spinal cord ischemia can lead to a range of neurological deficits, from mild sensory disturbances to complete paralysis.

Why Other Options Are Incorrect:
- **A. Stroke:** While stroke is a potential complication after any major surgery, it is not specific to aortic dissection repair.
- **B. Renal failure:** Renal failure is a common complication in critically ill patients, including those undergoing aortic dissection repair, but it is not specific to this procedure.
- **D. Postoperative delirium:** Delirium is a common postoperative complication in elderly patients and those with underlying medical conditions, but it is not specifically associated with aortic dissection repair.

Additional Considerations:
- Early recognition and management of spinal cord ischemia are crucial to prevent permanent neurological damage.
- Measures to optimize spinal cord perfusion, such as maintaining adequate blood pressure and avoiding hypotension, are essential during and after surgery.
- Other potential complications of aortic dissection repair include:
  - Heart failure
  - Arrhythmias
  - Organ dysfunction
  - Infection
  - Bleeding

Case Study: A 60-year-old man undergoes successful surgical repair of an acute type A aortic dissection. Postoperatively, he develops weakness and numbness in his legs. An MRI confirms spinal cord ischemia.

By understanding the risk of spinal cord ischemia in patients undergoing aortic dissection repair, healthcare providers can implement preventive measures and promptly recognize and manage this potentially devastating complication.

319. Uremic Pericarditis and Echocardiography

Understanding the Question

The question asks about the most likely echocardiographic finding in a 70-year-old woman with chronic kidney disease (CKD) and uremic pericarditis.

The Correct Answer:

A. Pericardial effusion

Explanation:

Uremic pericarditis is an inflammation of the pericardium (the sac surrounding the heart) caused by the buildup of uremic toxins in the blood due to kidney failure. One of the most common echocardiographic findings in this condition is a **pericardial effusion**, which is the accumulation of fluid within the pericardial sac.

- **Uremia and inflammation:** The uremic toxins irritate the pericardium, leading to inflammation and fluid buildup.
- **Echocardiographic appearance:** A pericardial effusion appears as an anechoic (black) space between the heart and the pericardium on echocardiography.

Why Other Options Are Incorrect:

- **B. Left ventricular hypertrophy:** This is a thickening of the heart muscle due to increased workload, often seen in conditions like hypertension or aortic stenosis. It is not typically associated with uremic pericarditis.
- **C. Mitral valve prolapse:** This is a condition where the mitral valve bulges into the left atrium during heartbeats. It is unrelated to kidney disease or pericarditis.
- **D. Aortic stenosis:** This is a narrowing of the aortic valve, which can lead to left ventricular hypertrophy. It is not associated with uremic pericarditis.

Additional Considerations:

- While pericardial effusion is common in uremic pericarditis, other echocardiographic findings may include pericardial thickening and even constrictive pericarditis in severe cases.
- The presence of a pericardial effusion should prompt prompt evaluation and management to prevent cardiac tamponade, a life-threatening complication.

Case Study: A 72-year-old woman with end-stage renal disease presents with chest pain. An echocardiogram reveals a moderate pericardial effusion. The diagnosis of uremic pericarditis is made, and hemodialysis is initiated.

Early diagnosis and management of uremic pericarditis through echocardiography are essential to prevent complications and improve patient outcomes.

320. Identifying a Persistent Source of Infection in Septic Shock

Understanding the Question

The question presents a case of a 50-year-old woman with septic shock secondary to pneumonia who is not responding to treatment. The goal is to determine the most appropriate diagnostic test to identify a potential ongoing source of infection.

The Correct Answer:

D. All of the above

Explanation:

Given the patient's clinical presentation and lack of improvement despite appropriate therapy, it is crucial to investigate potential alternative sources of infection. All of the mentioned diagnostic tests can provide valuable information:

- **A. Computed tomography (CT) scan of the abdomen and pelvis:** This can identify intra-abdominal infections such as abscesses, pancreatitis, or urinary tract infections, which can be sources of sepsis.
- **B. Transthoracic echocardiogram (TTE):** This can detect endocarditis, a potential source of persistent infection in patients with sepsis.
- **C. Magnetic resonance imaging (MRI) of the spine:** This can identify spinal epidural abscesses, a rare but potentially life-threatening complication.

Why Other Options Are Incorrect:

Since each of these tests offers unique diagnostic possibilities for different types of infections, it is not appropriate to choose only one. A comprehensive evaluation is necessary to identify the underlying cause of persistent sepsis.

Additional Considerations:

- Other diagnostic tests, such as ultrasound-guided aspiration of potential abscesses or bone marrow cultures, may also be considered based on clinical findings.
- It is essential to re-evaluate the initial antibiotic choice and consider the possibility of antibiotic resistance.
- Supportive care, including adequate fluid resuscitation, vasopressor support, and organ dysfunction management, remains crucial.

Case Study: A 55-year-old man with sepsis develops worsening renal function despite appropriate antibiotic therapy. A CT scan of the abdomen reveals a perinephric abscess. Successful drainage of the abscess leads to clinical improvement.

By considering multiple diagnostic possibilities and conducting a thorough evaluation, healthcare providers can increase the chances of identifying the underlying cause of persistent sepsis and improving patient outcomes.

321. Prioritizing Management in Atrial Fibrillation with Rapid Ventricular Response

Understanding the Question

The patient is a 72-year-old with multiple comorbidities presenting with atrial fibrillation and rapid ventricular response (RVR) leading to hemodynamic instability (hypotension). The question asks for the immediate priority after rate control.

The Correct Answer:

B. Immediate electrical cardioversion

Explanation:

The patient is in a critical condition due to hemodynamic instability secondary to rapid ventricular response. In such cases, **immediate restoration of normal sinus rhythm** is paramount.

• **Electrical cardioversion** is the most rapid and effective method to achieve this goal.

• Once hemodynamic stability is restored, other management strategies can be implemented.

Why Other Options Are Incorrect:

• **A. Anticoagulation with warfarin:** While anticoagulation is crucial to prevent stroke in patients with atrial fibrillation, it is not the immediate priority in a hemodynamically unstable patient.

• **C. Initiation of amiodarone for rhythm control:** Amiodarone is an antiarrhythmic drug that can be used for rhythm control, but it takes time to work and is not as effective as immediate cardioversion in this setting.

• **D. Assessment of reversible causes of atrial fibrillation:** Identifying the underlying cause of atrial fibrillation is important, but it should not delay immediate life-saving interventions.

Additional Considerations:

- After successful cardioversion, anticoagulation should be initiated promptly to prevent stroke.
- The choice of anticoagulant depends on the patient's risk factors and contraindications.
- Rate control medications may be needed to prevent recurrence of rapid ventricular response.
- Underlying causes of atrial fibrillation should be investigated once the patient is stabilized.

Case Study: A 75-year-old man with a history of heart failure and atrial fibrillation presents to the emergency department with acute shortness of breath and hypotension. An electrocardiogram confirms atrial fibrillation with a rapid ventricular response. The patient undergoes immediate electrical cardioversion, which successfully restores sinus rhythm. He is subsequently started on anticoagulation and beta-blocker therapy.

In conclusion, rapid ventricular response leading to hemodynamic instability in atrial fibrillation requires immediate intervention with electrical cardioversion to restore normal sinus rhythm and improve patient outcomes.

322. PRES and Medication Management in SLE

Understanding the Question

The patient is a 42-year-old woman with SLE presenting with symptoms consistent with PRES. The question asks which medication is most likely to be held or discontinued to facilitate recovery.

The Correct Answer:

D. Cyclophosphamide

Explanation:

PRES is often associated with rapid increases in blood pressure, renal dysfunction, and immunosuppressive medications. Cyclophosphamide is a potent immunosuppressant with a well-established association with PRES. Therefore, it is the most likely culprit in this case.

- **Cyclophosphamide and PRES:** This medication can induce endothelial injury and vasoconstriction, leading to the development of PRES.
- **Management:** In patients with SLE and PRES, holding or reducing the dose of cyclophosphamide is often necessary to facilitate recovery.

Why Other Options Are Incorrect:

- **A. Hydroxychloroquine:** While a mainstay in SLE treatment, hydroxychloroquine has a low risk of causing PRES.
- **B. Belimumab:** This is a newer biologic agent used for SLE, and there is insufficient evidence to link it directly to PRES.
- **C. Mycophenolate mofetil:** Although an immunosuppressant, it is less strongly associated with PRES compared to cyclophosphamide.

Additional Considerations:

- **Blood pressure control:** Aggressive blood pressure management is essential in treating PRES.
- **Supportive care:** Adequate hydration, seizure control, and monitoring of renal function are crucial.
- **Other potential causes:** It's important to consider other potential causes of PRES, such as preeclampsia, eclampsia, and sepsis.

Case Study: A 45-year-old woman with SLE on cyclophosphamide develops severe headaches, seizures, and visual disturbances. Brain MRI confirms PRES. Cyclophosphamide is held, and blood pressure is aggressively managed. The patient gradually recovers.

By recognizing the association between cyclophosphamide and PRES and taking prompt action to address the underlying cause, healthcare providers can improve outcomes for patients with SLE and PRES.

323. Monitoring Parameters in a Ventilated COPD Patient

Understanding the Question

The question asks about the most important parameters to monitor in a COPD patient with acute exacerbation and hypercapnic respiratory failure who is on mechanical ventilation.

The Correct Answer:

D. All of the above

Explanation:

All of the listed parameters are crucial for assessing the effectiveness of ventilation and guiding ventilator adjustments in a patient with COPD and acute respiratory failure.

- **A. End-tidal carbon dioxide (EtCO2):** This provides a continuous, non-invasive measure of carbon dioxide levels at the end of each exhalation. It reflects alveolar ventilation and is useful for monitoring trends and making rapid adjustments to ventilator settings.

- **B. Arterial blood gas (ABG):** ABG analysis provides a comprehensive assessment of oxygenation, ventilation, and acid-base balance. It is essential for verifying the effectiveness of ventilation, evaluating oxygenation status, and determining acid-base disturbances.
- **C. Peak inspiratory pressure (PIP):** This parameter reflects the pressure required to deliver a breath to the patient. Monitoring PIP helps to assess lung compliance and the risk of ventilator-induced lung injury (VILI).

Additional Considerations:

- Other important parameters to monitor include tidal volume, respiratory rate, minute ventilation, plateau pressure, and oxygen saturation.
- Dynamic compliance can be calculated from PIP and plateau pressure to assess lung elasticity.
- Regular assessment of the patient's clinical status, including level of sedation, hemodynamic stability, and oxygenation, is essential.

By closely monitoring these parameters, healthcare providers can optimize ventilator settings, minimize complications, and improve patient outcomes in patients with COPD and acute respiratory failure.

324. Improving Oxygenation in ARDS

Understanding the Question

The patient is a 30-year-old with septic shock and acute respiratory distress syndrome (ARDS) as evidenced by the PaO2/FiO2 ratio of 80. The question asks about potential interventions to recruit collapsed alveoli and improve oxygenation.

The Correct Answer:

D. All of the above

Explanation:

All of the listed interventions are commonly used strategies to improve oxygenation in patients with ARDS by recruiting collapsed alveoli and improving lung compliance.

- **A. Increasing PEEP:** Positive end-expiratory pressure (PEEP) helps to prevent alveolar collapse at the end of expiration, thus improving oxygenation.

- **B. Prone positioning:** Placing the patient prone can redistribute lung fluids and improve ventilation-perfusion matching, leading to increased oxygenation.
- **C. Recruitment maneuvers:** These involve applying high levels of positive pressure to open collapsed alveoli. They can be performed using various techniques, including sustained inflations and oscillatory ventilation.

Additional Considerations:

- The optimal level of PEEP and the frequency of prone positioning should be individualized based on patient-specific factors and monitoring of hemodynamic and respiratory parameters.
- Recruitment maneuvers should be performed cautiously to avoid barotrauma.
- Other supportive measures, such as adequate fluid management and lung-protective ventilation strategies, are essential in the management of ARDS.

By combining these interventions, healthcare providers can improve oxygenation, reduce the risk of ventilator-induced lung injury, and enhance patient outcomes in ARDS.

325. End-Organ Hypoperfusion in Cardiogenic Shock

Understanding the Question

The patient is a 65-year-old with HFrEF in cardiogenic shock despite inotropic and vasopressor support. The question asks for the laboratory finding most indicative of end-organ hypoperfusion.

The Correct Answer:

D. All of the above

Explanation:

All of the listed laboratory findings are indicative of end-organ hypoperfusion in a patient with cardiogenic shock.

- **A. Elevated serum creatinine:** This indicates impaired kidney function, a common manifestation of end-organ hypoperfusion.
- **B. Elevated lactate levels:** Lactate is produced in tissues under hypoxic conditions. Elevated lactate levels reflect tissue hypoxia and inadequate oxygen delivery.
- **C. Decreased urine output:** Reduced urine output is a classic sign of renal hypoperfusion and decreased glomerular filtration rate.

Additional Considerations:

- Other markers of end-organ hypoperfusion include elevated liver enzymes, increased bilirubin, and altered mental status.
- Early recognition and management of end-organ hypoperfusion are crucial to prevent irreversible organ damage.

By monitoring these laboratory parameters, healthcare providers can assess the severity of end-organ hypoperfusion and adjust treatment accordingly.

326. Hepatorenal Syndrome (HRS) and First-Line Therapy

Understanding the Question

The question pertains to a patient with alcoholic hepatitis, acute liver failure, and subsequently developing hepatorenal syndrome (HRS) type 1. It asks for the first-line medication for this condition.

The Correct Answer:

A. Terlipressin

Explanation:

Hepatorenal syndrome (HRS) is a renal dysfunction caused by severe liver disease. It is divided into two types:

- **Type 1 HRS:** Rapidly progressive renal failure with a marked reduction in renal blood flow.
- **Type 2 HRS:** More gradual renal dysfunction with a slower decline in renal function.

Terlipressin is a synthetic analogue of vasopressin, which acts as a potent vasoconstrictor. It is the first-line therapy for type 1 HRS. By constricting the splanchnic vasculature, terlipressin helps to increase renal blood flow and improve renal function.

Why Other Options Are Incorrect:

- **B. Midodrine:** While midodrine is a peripheral alpha-adrenergic agonist used to treat orthostatic hypotension, it is not as effective as terlipressin in improving renal function in type 1 HRS.
- **C. Octreotide:** Octreotide is a somatostatin analogue used for various conditions, but it is not indicated for the treatment of type 1 HRS.
- **D. Albumin:** Albumin is used in the management of HRS, but it is considered an adjunctive therapy rather than the first-line treatment.

Additional Considerations:

- Along with terlipressin, albumin administration is often used to expand plasma volume and improve renal perfusion.
- Dialysis may be required in refractory cases of HRS.
- Liver transplantation is the definitive treatment for HRS.

By understanding the pathophysiology of HRS and the role of terlipressin in its management, healthcare providers can improve patient outcomes.

327. Adjunctive Therapy for Status Asthmaticus
Understanding the Question

The patient is a 25-year-old with status asthmaticus refractory to standard therapy. The question asks about potential adjunctive therapies to reduce airway inflammation and improve bronchodilation.

The Correct Answer:

B. Inhaled helium-oxygen mixture (heliox)

Explanation:

- **Inhaled helium-oxygen mixture (heliox):** This is a gas mixture with a lower density than air. It reduces airway resistance, allowing for easier airflow. In severe asthma exacerbations, heliox can improve gas exchange and reduce the work of breathing.

Why Other Options Are Incorrect:

- **A. Ketamine infusion:** While ketamine has bronchodilator properties and has been studied in asthma, it's not a first-line treatment for status asthmaticus.
- **C. Bronchial thermoplasty:** This is a long-term treatment for severe asthma, involving thermal ablation of airway smooth muscle. It's not appropriate for acute exacerbations.
- **D. Extracorporeal membrane oxygenation (ECMO):** ECMO is a life-saving therapy for severe respiratory failure, but it's indicated when other treatments have failed and the patient is at imminent risk of death. It's not a first-line therapy for status asthmaticus.

Additional Considerations:

- Other potential adjunctive therapies for refractory status asthmaticus include magnesium sulfate, inhaled nitric oxide, and extracorporeal carbon dioxide removal (ECCO2R).
- Early identification and aggressive management of status asthmaticus are crucial to prevent severe complications and improve outcomes.

By understanding the pathophysiology of asthma and the available treatment options, healthcare providers can optimize the management of severe asthma exacerbations.

328. Aortic Dissection and Lifestyle Modifications

Understanding the Question

The question pertains to a 55-year-old man with a Stanford type B aortic dissection and asks about the most important lifestyle modification to prevent progression.

The Correct Answer:

A. Smoking cessation

Explanation:

Smoking is a significant risk factor for aortic dissection. Nicotine increases blood pressure and heart rate, placing additional stress on the aorta. It also damages blood vessel walls, contributing to aortic weakening. Therefore, **smoking cessation** is the most critical lifestyle modification for this patient.

Why Other Options Are Incorrect:

• **B. Weight loss:** While weight loss is generally beneficial for cardiovascular health, it is not as directly linked to aortic dissection progression as smoking.

• **C. Dietary sodium restriction:** Sodium reduction is important for blood pressure control, but it is not as potent as smoking cessation in preventing aortic dissection progression.

• **D. Exercise:** While exercise is generally recommended, it's crucial to avoid strenuous activities that can increase blood pressure and stress the aorta.

Additional Considerations:

• Other lifestyle modifications, such as stress management and adequate sleep, can also be beneficial in overall cardiovascular health.

• Regular blood pressure monitoring and medication adherence are essential for managing hypertension.

By prioritizing smoking cessation, this patient can significantly reduce the risk of aortic dissection progression and improve overall cardiovascular health.

329. Purulent Pericarditis and Common Microorganisms
Understanding the Question

The question pertains to a 70-year-old woman with CKD and uremic pericarditis who underwent pericardiocentesis with drainage of bloody fluid. It asks about the most common microorganism associated with purulent pericarditis.

The Correct Answer:

A. Staphylococcus aureus

Explanation:

While the patient in the scenario presented has a bloody pericardial effusion, which is more typical of uremic pericarditis, the question specifically asks about the most common microorganism associated with *purulent* pericarditis.

- **Staphylococcus aureus** is a common cause of purulent pericarditis. It is a gram-positive bacterium that can cause severe infections.

Why Other Options Are Incorrect:

- **B. Streptococcus pneumoniae, C. Haemophilus influenzae, and D. Escherichia coli:** These organisms are more commonly associated with other types of infections and are less likely to cause purulent pericarditis.

Additional Considerations:

- Purulent pericarditis is a serious condition requiring prompt diagnosis and treatment with appropriate antibiotics.
- Other microorganisms that can cause purulent pericarditis include Streptococcus species, Pseudomonas aeruginosa, and various anaerobes.
- The specific causative organism should be identified through culture and sensitivity testing of the pericardial fluid.

It's important to note that the patient in the scenario has a bloody pericardial effusion, which is more consistent with uremic pericarditis than purulent pericarditis. However, the question specifically asked about the most common organism associated with purulent pericarditis.

330. Non-Infectious Causes of Persistent Septic Shock
Understanding the Question

The patient is a 50-year-old woman with rheumatoid arthritis and septic shock refractory to antibiotic therapy. The question asks about potential management strategies if a non-infectious cause is suspected.

The Correct Answer:

D. All of the above

Explanation:

Given the persistent septic shock despite appropriate antibiotic therapy, it is essential to consider non-infectious causes. All of the listed options should be considered in the management of this patient.

- **A. Discontinuation of antibiotics:** If a non-infectious cause is suspected, continuing antibiotics may be unnecessary and could potentially increase the risk of adverse effects.
- **B. Initiation of immunosuppressive therapy:** In certain autoimmune conditions, an overactive immune response can mimic sepsis. Immunosuppressive therapy may be considered in these cases, but it should be done cautiously and under close monitoring.
- **C. Evaluation for underlying malignancy:** Malignancies can present with symptoms similar to sepsis, such as fever, weight loss, and fatigue. Therefore, an evaluation for underlying malignancy is warranted.

Additional Considerations:

- Other potential non-infectious causes of persistent septic shock include drug reactions, connective tissue diseases, and endocrine disorders.
- A comprehensive diagnostic workup, including imaging studies, laboratory tests, and consultations with specialists, may be necessary to identify the underlying cause.

By considering all potential causes and implementing appropriate management strategies, healthcare providers can improve patient outcomes.

331. Empiric Antibiotic Therapy for Urosepsis

Understanding the Question

The patient is a 62-year-old with hypertension and type 2 diabetes mellitus experiencing septic shock secondary to urosepsis. The question asks for the most appropriate empiric antibiotic regimen.

The Correct Answer:

A. Vancomycin and piperacillin-tazobactam

Explanation:

Urosepsis is a severe infection originating from the urinary tract that leads to systemic inflammation and organ dysfunction. Empiric antibiotic therapy should cover a broad spectrum of potential pathogens, including gram-positive, gram-negative organisms, and anaerobes.

- **Vancomycin:** This is a glycopeptide antibiotic effective against gram-positive organisms, including methicillin-resistant Staphylococcus aureus (MRSA), which can be a cause of urosepsis.
- **Piperacillin-tazobactam:** This is a combination antibiotic effective against both gram-positive and gram-negative bacteria, including common uropathogens like Escherichia coli and Pseudomonas aeruginosa.

Why Other Options Are Incorrect:

- **B. Cefepime and metronidazole:** While cefepime covers gram-negative organisms, it may not be adequate for MRSA coverage. Metronidazole covers anaerobes but lacks coverage for gram-positive organisms.
- **C. Meropenem and vancomycin:** While this combination provides broad coverage, it might be considered overkill for initial empiric therapy and could increase the risk of antimicrobial resistance.
- **D. Ceftriaxone and azithromycin:** This combination is not appropriate for severe infections like septic shock due to limited coverage against gram-negative organisms and potential resistance.

Additional Considerations:

- The choice of empiric antibiotics should be based on local epidemiology and resistance patterns.
- Once culture and sensitivity results are available, the antibiotic regimen should be de-escalated accordingly.
- Early initiation of appropriate antibiotic therapy is crucial for improving patient outcomes in sepsis.

By choosing a broad-spectrum antibiotic combination like vancomycin and piperacillin-tazobactam, healthcare providers can effectively treat urosepsis until definitive culture results are available.

332. **Most Likely Diagnosis: B. Lupus Pericarditis**
Explanation:

- **Lupus pericarditis** is an inflammation of the pericardium caused by systemic lupus erythematosus (SLE).
- The patient's history of SLE, combined with the presenting symptoms of fever, chest pain, and friction rub, strongly supports this diagnosis.

- A pericardial effusion, as detected by echocardiogram, is a common finding in lupus pericarditis.

Why Other Options Are Less Likely:

- **A. Acute myocardial infarction (MI):** While chest pain is a common symptom of MI, the presence of a friction rub and pericardial effusion is more characteristic of pericarditis than MI.
- **C. Dressler's syndrome:** This is a post-myocardial infarction syndrome, which is unlikely in this patient with no history of MI.
- **D. Pulmonary embolism (PE):** Chest pain and dyspnea are common symptoms of PE, but a friction rub and pericardial effusion are not typical findings.

In conclusion, given the patient's history of SLE and the presenting symptoms, lupus pericarditis is the most likely diagnosis.

333. Improving Chances of Successful Extubation in COPD

The Correct Answer:

D. All of the above

Explanation:

All of the listed strategies are crucial for improving the chances of successful extubation in a patient with COPD and acute respiratory failure.

- **A. Early mobilization and physical therapy:** These help to maintain muscle strength, prevent deconditioning, and improve overall respiratory function.
- **B. Daily spontaneous awakening trial (SAT) and spontaneous breathing trial (SBT):** These assess the patient's readiness for extubation and help to minimize the duration of mechanical ventilation.
- **C. Use of noninvasive ventilation (NIV) as a bridge to extubation:** NIV can be used to support respiratory function while weaning the patient from invasive ventilation.

A comprehensive approach that incorporates all of these strategies is essential for optimizing patient outcomes.

334. The Correct Answer: A. Mean Arterial Pressure (MAP)

Explanation:

- **Mean arterial pressure (MAP)** is the primary parameter used to guide the titration of norepinephrine in a patient with septic shock.

- MAP reflects the average arterial pressure during one cardiac cycle and is a crucial indicator of tissue perfusion.
- The goal of norepinephrine therapy is to maintain adequate MAP to ensure sufficient blood flow to vital organs.

Why Other Options Are Less Appropriate:
- **B. Central venous pressure (CVP):** While CVP can provide information about fluid status, it is not a reliable indicator of tissue perfusion and should not be the primary guide for norepinephrine titration.
- **C. Cardiac index (CI):** CI is a measure of cardiac output relative to body size. While it can provide information about cardiac function, it is not as directly related to tissue perfusion as MAP and should not be the sole determinant of norepinephrine dose.
- **D. Systemic vascular resistance (SVR):** SVR reflects the resistance to blood flow offered by the blood vessels. While it can be monitored to assess the effects of vasopressors, it is not the primary target for norepinephrine therapy.

By focusing on maintaining an adequate MAP, clinicians can optimize tissue perfusion and improve patient outcomes in septic shock.

335. **The Correct Answer: B. Nesiritide**
Explanation:
- **Nesiritide** is a recombinant form of the B-type natriuretic peptide (BNP). It acts as a potent vasodilator, reducing preload and afterload, and promoting diuresis. It is particularly useful in patients with acute decompensated heart failure (ADHF) who have not responded adequately to diuretics.

Why Other Options Are Less Appropriate:
- **A. Low-dose dopamine:** While dopamine can increase renal blood flow, it has limited efficacy in enhancing diuresis in patients with HFpEF. It also carries the risk of increasing myocardial oxygen demand.
- **C. Tolvaptan:** Tolvaptan is a vasopressin receptor antagonist that promotes aquaresis. However, it is primarily used in patients with hyponatremia due to heart failure and is not the first-line treatment for diuresis in ADHF.
- **D. Conivaptan:** Similar to tolvaptan, conivaptan is a vasopressin receptor antagonist, but it has a higher affinity for the V2 receptor. It is used in the management of hyponatremia in patients with cirrhosis, not in ADHF for diuresis.

Therefore, nesiritide is the most appropriate adjunctive therapy to enhance diuresis in this patient with HFpEF and refractory ADHF.

336. The Correct Answer: D. All of the above
Explanation:
All of the listed laboratory parameters are crucial for monitoring the response to therapy in a patient with hepatorenal syndrome (HRS) treated with terlipressin.
- **Serum creatinine:** This is a direct marker of kidney function and is used to assess the progression or improvement of renal failure.
- **Urine output:** Monitoring urine output helps to evaluate the effectiveness of terlipressin in improving renal perfusion and increasing diuresis.
- **Serum sodium:** Changes in serum sodium levels can occur in patients with HRS and can influence the management of fluid balance.

By closely monitoring these parameters, healthcare providers can assess the patient's response to therapy and adjust treatment accordingly.

337. The Correct Answer: A. Inhaled helium-oxygen mixture (heliox)
Explanation:
The patient is experiencing severe status asthmaticus despite maximal medical therapy, as evidenced by high peak airway pressures and worsening oxygenation. Inhaled helium-oxygen mixture (heliox) is a valuable adjunctive therapy in this situation.
- **Heliox** is a gas mixture with lower density than air, which reduces airway resistance and improves airflow. This can lead to decreased peak airway pressures and improved oxygenation.

Why Other Options Are Less Appropriate:
- **B. Intravenous ketamine:** While ketamine has bronchodilator properties, its use in severe status asthmaticus is limited and not a first-line treatment.
- **C. Bronchial thermoplasty:** This is a long-term treatment for severe asthma and is not indicated for acute exacerbations.
- **D. Extracorporeal membrane oxygenation (ECMO):** ECMO is a life-saving therapy for severe respiratory failure but is considered a last resort and not the initial approach for this patient.

By using heliox, clinicians can potentially improve the patient's respiratory status and avoid further escalation of therapy.

338. The Correct Answer: C. Presence of complications, such as malperfusion or impending rupture

Explanation:

The decision to proceed with surgical or endovascular repair for a Stanford Type B aortic dissection is primarily based on the presence of complications or the risk of imminent complications.

• **Presence of complications:** Factors such as malperfusion (decreased blood flow to vital organs), impending rupture, or rapidly expanding aortic diameter indicate a high risk of adverse outcomes and often necessitate intervention.

• **Age of the patient, size of the aortic aneurysm, and patient's preference:** While these factors can influence the decision-making process, they are secondary to the presence or absence of complications.

By prioritizing the management of complications and preventing life-threatening events, healthcare providers can improve patient outcomes.

339. The Correct Answer: D. All of the above

Explanation:

All of the listed complications are potential outcomes of uremic pericarditis and require close monitoring:

• **A. Cardiac tamponade:** This is a life-threatening condition where fluid accumulates in the pericardial sac, compressing the heart.

• **B. Pericardial constriction:** This is a chronic condition where the pericardium becomes thickened and scarred, restricting the heart's ability to fill with blood.

• **C. Pericardial effusion:** While often present in uremic pericarditis, it can worsen and lead to cardiac tamponade if not monitored closely.

Early detection and management of these complications are crucial for improving patient outcomes.

340. Understanding the Question

The patient is a 50-year-old woman with rheumatoid arthritis who has developed septic shock due to pneumonia. Despite aggressive treatment, her condition is worsening. The question asks which diagnostic test should be considered to explore a non-infectious cause for her persistent symptoms.

Correct Answer: A. Autoantibody testing

Explanation:

Given the patient's history of rheumatoid arthritis, an autoimmune condition, and the lack of improvement despite appropriate antibiotic therapy, it is crucial to consider an autoimmune flare-up as a potential cause of her persistent septic shock. Autoantibody testing can help identify underlying autoimmune processes contributing to her condition.

• **Autoantibody testing** can reveal the presence of antibodies that target the body's own tissues. In the context of rheumatoid arthritis, these antibodies can contribute to systemic inflammation and potentially worsen the patient's septic shock.

Why other options are incorrect:

• **Bone marrow biopsy:** While this test can be valuable in diagnosing certain infections or hematological disorders, it is less likely to be the most appropriate initial step in this case given the patient's known autoimmune condition.

• **Abdominal ultrasound:** This test is primarily used to evaluate abdominal organs and is not directly relevant to investigating an autoimmune cause of septic shock.

• **All of the above:** This option is incorrect as only autoantibody testing is directly relevant to investigating a non-infectious cause in this specific patient.

Additional Considerations:

• It's essential to differentiate between sepsis induced by an infection and sepsis induced by an autoimmune flare.

• Other autoimmune conditions, such as lupus or vasculitis, can mimic or exacerbate sepsis.

• Early recognition and management of autoimmune flares are crucial for improving patient outcomes.

• Collaborating with a rheumatologist can be beneficial in managing patients with overlapping infectious and autoimmune conditions.

By considering autoantibody testing, the healthcare provider can gain valuable insights into the underlying pathophysiology of the patient's condition and potentially guide further treatment decisions.

341. Understanding the Question

A 58-year-old man with a history of hypertension and alcoholic cirrhosis presents with active upper gastrointestinal bleeding (hematemesis and melena).

He is currently hemodynamically stable. The question asks for the most appropriate next step in management.

Correct Answer: C. Perform upper endoscopy

Explanation:

The most critical step in managing acute upper gastrointestinal bleeding, especially in a patient with known risk factors like cirrhosis, is to identify the source of bleeding. **Upper endoscopy** is the gold standard for diagnosing and treating the underlying cause of upper gastrointestinal bleeding.

• **Upper endoscopy** allows direct visualization of the esophagus, stomach, and duodenum, enabling identification of the bleeding source (e.g., esophageal varices, peptic ulcer disease, Mallory-Weiss tear).

• Once the source is identified, appropriate therapeutic interventions can be initiated during the endoscopy, such as variceal band ligation, sclerotherapy, or hemostasis of an active ulcer.

Why other options are incorrect:

• **Transfuse packed red blood cells (PRBCs):** While blood transfusion may be necessary to maintain hemodynamic stability, it is a supportive measure and not the primary treatment for active bleeding.

• **Initiate octreotide infusion:** Octreotide is a vasoactive medication that can reduce portal pressure and slow bleeding from esophageal varices. However, it should be used as an adjunct to endoscopy, not as a primary treatment.

• **Administer intravenous proton pump inhibitor (PPI):** PPIs are used to prevent ulcer recurrence but do not address active bleeding.

Additional Considerations:

• Rapid assessment and resuscitation are crucial in managing acute upper gastrointestinal bleeding.

• Other diagnostic tests (e.g., CT angiography) may be considered if endoscopy is unsuccessful or contraindicated.

• Interventional radiology procedures (e.g., embolization) can be used as salvage therapy for refractory bleeding.

• Close monitoring of hemodynamic status, coagulation parameters, and electrolyte balance is essential.

By performing an early upper endoscopy, the healthcare team can effectively diagnose and treat the underlying cause of bleeding, improving patient outcomes.

342. Understanding the Question

A 35-year-old woman with SLE presents with AKI and thrombocytopenia. The question asks for the most important laboratory test to evaluate for TTP.

Correct Answer: C. ADAMTS13 activity

Explanation:

Thrombotic thrombocytopenic purpura (TTP) is a rare but life-threatening disorder characterized by a pentad of symptoms: thrombocytopenia, microangiopathic hemolytic anemia, neurological abnormalities, fever, and renal dysfunction. It is primarily caused by a deficiency or dysfunction of ADAMTS13, a metalloprotease enzyme responsible for cleaving von Willebrand factor (VWF) multimers.

• **ADAMTS13 activity** is a direct measure of the enzyme's function and is the most specific test for diagnosing TTP. Low ADAMTS13 activity is strongly suggestive of TTP.

Why other options are incorrect:

• **Anti-nuclear antibody (ANA) titer:** While ANA is a marker for autoimmune diseases like SLE, it is not specific for TTP.

• **Anti-dsDNA antibody titer:** This test is specifically for monitoring disease activity in SLE and is not relevant for diagnosing TTP.

• **Complement levels (C3 and C4):** Complement levels can be abnormal in various conditions, including SLE and TTP, but they are not specific for TTP diagnosis.

Additional Considerations:

• Other laboratory tests, such as peripheral blood smear (showing schistocytes), lactate dehydrogenase (LDH), and bilirubin, can support the diagnosis of TTP.

• Rapid diagnosis and initiation of plasma exchange are crucial for managing TTP.

• Differentiating TTP from other microangiopathic hemolytic anemias (e.g., hemolytic uremic syndrome) is essential for appropriate treatment.

By measuring ADAMTS13 activity, healthcare providers can quickly confirm or exclude the diagnosis of TTP and initiate timely treatment.

343. Understanding the Question

A 75-year-old patient with COPD is experiencing a severe exacerbation with hypercapnic respiratory failure despite optimal medical management. The question asks for the intervention most likely to improve survival.

Correct Answer: C. Noninvasive ventilation (NIV)

Explanation:

Noninvasive ventilation (NIV) has been shown to significantly improve survival and reduce the need for invasive mechanical ventilation in patients with acute exacerbations of COPD and hypercapnic respiratory failure.

• **NIV** provides respiratory support by delivering positive pressure via a mask, improving oxygenation and reducing carbon dioxide retention.

• By preventing or delaying the need for intubation, NIV can reduce the risk of complications associated with invasive ventilation, such as ventilator-associated pneumonia and muscle weakness.

Why other options are incorrect:

• **Inhaled corticosteroids:** While corticosteroids are essential in managing COPD exacerbations, they are primarily anti-inflammatory agents and do not address the immediate respiratory failure.

• **Inhaled bronchodilators:** Bronchodilators are also crucial in COPD management, but their primary role is to relax airway smooth muscle and improve airflow. They are less effective in addressing severe hypercapnia and respiratory failure.

• **Tracheostomy:** Tracheostomy is an invasive procedure typically reserved for patients who fail NIV and require prolonged mechanical ventilation. It is not the initial treatment of choice for acute exacerbation with hypercapnic respiratory failure.

Additional Considerations:

• Early initiation of NIV is crucial for optimal outcomes.

• Patient-physician communication and shared decision-making are essential in determining the appropriateness of NIV.

• Close monitoring of patient's clinical status, blood gases, and ventilator settings is required.

By implementing NIV promptly, healthcare providers can improve the chances of survival and recovery for patients with severe COPD exacerbations and hypercapnic respiratory failure.

344. Understanding the Question

A 30-year-old woman with community-acquired pneumonia develops septic shock and requires mechanical ventilation. Despite conventional ventilation, her PaO2/FiO2 ratio is 80, indicating severe hypoxemia. The question asks for the most likely strategy to improve oxygenation.

Correct Answer: B. Extracorporeal membrane oxygenation (ECMO)

Explanation:

Extracorporeal membrane oxygenation (ECMO) is a life-saving therapy for patients with severe refractory hypoxemia who fail to respond to conventional ventilation. It provides direct oxygenation and carbon dioxide removal by circulating the patient's blood through an artificial lung.

- **ECMO** is indicated in cases of severe ARDS with persistent hypoxemia despite maximal ventilator support, as seen in this patient.
- It allows for complete lung rest and recovery while providing essential gas exchange.

Why other options are incorrect:

- **High-frequency oscillatory ventilation (HFOV):** While HFOV can be beneficial in certain respiratory failure conditions, it is generally less effective than ECMO in severe ARDS with refractory hypoxemia.
- **Inhaled nitric oxide:** Inhaled nitric oxide can improve oxygenation in some patients with ARDS, but its effect is often limited and unpredictable.
- **Prone positioning:** Prone positioning can improve oxygenation in ARDS patients but is typically used as an adjunct to other therapies, not as a primary treatment for refractory hypoxemia.

Additional Considerations:

- ECMO is a complex and high-risk therapy that requires specialized expertise and equipment.
- Patient selection for ECMO is crucial, and careful consideration of risks and benefits must be made.
- Other supportive measures, such as lung protective ventilation strategies and appropriate fluid management, are essential in managing ARDS patients.

ECMO offers a lifeline for patients with severe ARDS and refractory hypoxemia when conventional therapies fail.

345. Understanding the Question

A 65-year-old man with coronary artery disease is in cardiogenic shock despite multiple inotropic and vasopressor agents. The question asks for the most important factor determining prognosis.

Correct Answer: D. Time to reperfusion therapy

Explanation:

The most critical factor influencing prognosis in cardiogenic shock secondary to myocardial infarction is the **time to reperfusion therapy**. Early reperfusion of the infarcted myocardium is essential to limit myocardial damage and improve survival.

- **Reperfusion therapy**, such as primary percutaneous coronary intervention (PCI) or fibrinolytic therapy, aims to restore blood flow to the ischemic heart muscle.

- Rapid reperfusion can salvage viable myocardial tissue, improve cardiac function, and decrease the risk of complications like ventricular arrhythmias and heart failure.

Why other options are incorrect:

- **Age:** While age is a risk factor for cardiovascular disease, it is not as directly impactful on prognosis as time to reperfusion in this acute setting.

- **Extent of myocardial damage:** The extent of myocardial damage is influenced by the time to reperfusion, so while it impacts prognosis, it is not the primary determinant.

- **Presence of comorbidities:** Comorbidities can contribute to the overall risk, but they are not as directly tied to the immediate outcome as time to reperfusion.

Additional Considerations:

- Other factors influencing prognosis include the patient's overall hemodynamic stability, response to treatment, and development of complications.

- Timely initiation of supportive measures, such as mechanical circulatory support (e.g., intra-aortic balloon pump, ventricular assist device), can improve outcomes.

- Early recognition and management of cardiogenic shock are crucial for optimizing patient care.

By emphasizing the importance of rapid reperfusion, healthcare providers can significantly improve the chances of survival and recovery for patients with cardiogenic shock.

346. Understanding the Question

A 40-year-old man with alcoholic hepatitis and acute liver failure develops hepatorenal syndrome (HRS). The question asks for the most important prognostic factor for survival in HRS.

Correct Answer: A. Severity of liver disease

Explanation:

The **severity of liver disease** is the most critical prognostic factor for survival in hepatorenal syndrome (HRS). HRS is a renal dysfunction that occurs as a complication of advanced liver disease. The underlying liver disease progression directly impacts the patient's overall prognosis.

- **Advanced liver disease** leads to portal hypertension, splanchnic vasodilation, and decreased effective circulating blood volume, contributing to the development of HRS.
- Patients with severe liver disease have a higher risk of complications, such as hepatic encephalopathy and spontaneous bacterial peritonitis, which further worsen prognosis.

Why other options are incorrect:

- **Response to volume expansion:** While volume expansion is a cornerstone of HRS management, it does not directly predict long-term survival.
- **Response to terlipressin therapy:** Terlipressin is a vasoconstrictor used in HRS management, but its effectiveness in improving long-term survival is limited.
- **Baseline renal function:** While baseline renal function is important, it is a reflection of the severity of liver disease and not an independent prognostic factor.

Additional Considerations:

- Early recognition and management of HRS are crucial for improving outcomes.
- Liver transplantation is the definitive treatment for HRS in patients with end-stage liver disease.
- Supportive care, including dialysis and electrolyte management, is essential in managing HRS.

Understanding the severity of liver disease helps clinicians assess the patient's overall prognosis and guide treatment decisions accordingly.

347. Understanding the Question

A 25-year-old woman with asthma is in severe respiratory distress (status asthmaticus) requiring intubation. The question asks for the medication most likely to improve bronchodilation and reduce airway inflammation.

Correct Answer: D. All of the above

Explanation:

All of the listed medications play a crucial role in managing status asthmaticus and contribute to bronchodilation and reduced airway inflammation.

- **Inhaled corticosteroids:** These are potent anti-inflammatory agents that reduce airway inflammation and edema, improving lung function over time.
- **Intravenous magnesium sulfate:** While the exact mechanism is not fully understood, magnesium sulfate has bronchodilator properties and can help relax airway smooth muscle.
- **Inhaled beta-agonists:** These are the first-line treatment for acute bronchospasm, rapidly relaxing airway smooth muscle and improving airflow.

Additional Considerations:

- The combination of these medications is often necessary to achieve optimal control of severe asthma exacerbations.
- Other medications, such as anticholinergics (e.g., ipratropium bromide) and intravenous beta-agonists (e.g., albuterol), may also be used in refractory cases.
- Early and aggressive treatment is essential to prevent respiratory failure and improve patient outcomes.

By utilizing a combination of inhaled corticosteroids, intravenous magnesium sulfate, and inhaled beta-agonists, healthcare providers can effectively address both the bronchoconstriction and inflammation associated with status asthmaticus.

348. Understanding the Question

A 55-year-old man with a history of hypertension and hyperlipidemia has a Stanford Type B aortic dissection. He is stable and managed medically. The question asks for the best diagnostic test for long-term surveillance.

Correct Answer: A. Computed tomography angiography (CTA) of the chest

Explanation:

Computed tomography angiography (CTA) of the chest is the most appropriate imaging modality for long-term surveillance of a Stanford Type B aortic dissection.

• **CTA** provides excellent visualization of the aorta and its branches, allowing for accurate assessment of aortic dissection progression, aneurysm formation, and potential complications.

• It offers high spatial resolution and can detect even subtle changes in aortic dimensions and morphology.

Why other options are incorrect:

• **Transthoracic echocardiogram (TTE):** While useful for evaluating cardiac function, TTE has limited ability to assess the thoracic aorta and its branches.

• **Magnetic resonance imaging (MRI) of the chest:** Although MRI can provide excellent soft tissue detail, it is generally less accessible and time-consuming compared to CTA for aortic dissection surveillance.

• **Chest X-ray:** Chest X-ray is not sensitive enough for detecting aortic dissection or monitoring its progression.

Additional Considerations:

• Surveillance frequency depends on the patient's clinical status and the initial extent of the dissection.

• Other imaging modalities, such as transesophageal echocardiography (TEE) or magnetic resonance angiography (MRA), may be considered in specific cases.

• Close clinical monitoring for symptoms of aortic dissection progression is essential.

CTA is the preferred imaging study for long-term surveillance of Stanford Type B aortic dissection due to its accuracy, accessibility, and ability to assess aortic changes over time.

349. Understanding the Question

A 70-year-old woman with chronic kidney disease (CKD) has developed uremic pericarditis. The question asks for the most common ECG finding in this condition.

Correct Answer: A. ST-segment elevation

Explanation:

The most common ECG finding in uremic pericarditis is **ST-segment elevation**. This is similar to the ECG changes seen in acute pericarditis.

- **ST-segment elevation** in uremic pericarditis is typically diffuse and concave upward, with reciprocal ST depression in lead aVR.
- It's important to differentiate uremic pericarditis from acute coronary syndrome (ACS), as both can present with ST-segment elevation.

Why other options are incorrect:

- **PR depression:** While PR depression can occur in pericarditis, it's not the most common finding.
- **Electrical alternans:** This ECG finding is associated with cardiac tamponade, a complication of pericarditis, but it's not the initial or most common finding.
- **Diffuse ST-segment depression and T-wave inversions:** These changes are more suggestive of myocardial ischemia or injury, not pericarditis.

Additional Considerations:

- Other ECG findings in uremic pericarditis may include sinus tachycardia, low voltage QRS complexes, and PR interval prolongation.
- Echocardiography is essential to confirm the diagnosis of pericarditis and to assess for pericardial effusion or tamponade.
- Prompt treatment of the underlying renal failure is crucial for managing uremic pericarditis.

Recognizing the classic ECG findings of uremic pericarditis is important for early diagnosis and appropriate management.

350. Understanding the Question

A 50-year-old woman with rheumatoid arthritis has developed septic shock secondary to pneumonia. Despite antibiotic therapy, her condition is worsening. The question asks for the appropriate diagnostic test to evaluate for a fungal infection.

Correct Answer: D. All of the above

Explanation:

Given the patient's severe illness and lack of response to antibiotics, it is crucial to consider a fungal infection as a potential cause. All of the listed tests can be helpful in diagnosing invasive fungal infections:

- **Serum galactomannan:** This test detects a cell wall component of Aspergillus species, which is a common cause of invasive fungal infections.
- **Beta-D-glucan:** This test detects a cell wall component of many different fungal species, making it a broader screening tool.

- **Fungal blood cultures:** While less sensitive than galactomannan or beta-D-glucan, positive fungal blood cultures confirm invasive fungal infection.

Additional Considerations:

- The choice of specific tests may depend on the patient's clinical presentation, risk factors, and available resources.
- It's important to interpret test results in the context of the patient's clinical condition and other laboratory findings.
- Early diagnosis and initiation of antifungal therapy are crucial for improving outcomes in invasive fungal infections.

By considering all of these tests, healthcare providers can increase the likelihood of diagnosing a fungal infection and initiating appropriate treatment.

351. Understanding the Question

A 72-year-old woman with multiple comorbidities including CKD and atrial fibrillation presents with rapid ventricular response (RVR). The question asks for the most appropriate initial management strategy.

Correct Answer: A. Intravenous diltiazem

Explanation:

Intravenous diltiazem is the most appropriate initial management strategy for this patient with RVR.

- **Diltiazem** is a calcium channel blocker that effectively slows ventricular rate in atrial fibrillation without causing significant hypotension.
- It is particularly suitable for patients with impaired renal function, as it is primarily metabolized in the liver.

Why other options are incorrect:

- **Intravenous metoprolol:** While beta-blockers are effective in controlling heart rate, they can cause hypotension and bradycardia, particularly in patients with impaired renal function.
- **Intravenous digoxin:** Digoxin has a narrow therapeutic index and requires careful monitoring, especially in patients with renal impairment. It is not the first-line treatment for rapid ventricular response.
- **Electrical cardioversion:** Electrical cardioversion is indicated for hemodynamic instability or refractory RVR. However, in this patient who is relatively stable, medical management should be attempted first.

Additional Considerations:

- Continuous monitoring of blood pressure, heart rate, and rhythm is essential during diltiazem infusion.
- If diltiazem is ineffective, other agents such as beta-blockers or amiodarone can be considered.
- The underlying cause of atrial fibrillation should be investigated and treated accordingly.

By choosing diltiazem as the initial management strategy, the healthcare provider can effectively control the patient's heart rate while minimizing the risk of hypotension and other adverse effects.

352. Understanding the Question

A 45-year-old man with a history of intravenous drug use underwent successful surgery for infective endocarditis and perivalvular abscess. Six weeks later, he presents with recurrent fever, chills, and fatigue. The question asks for the most likely cause of these symptoms.

Correct Answer: A. Recurrent infective endocarditis

Explanation:

Given the patient's history of infective endocarditis, recent surgery, and persistent infectious symptoms, **recurrent infective endocarditis** is the most likely cause.

- Despite successful surgery, residual infected tissue or vegetation may have been left behind, leading to persistent bacteremia and recurrent infection.
- The patient's risk factors, such as intravenous drug use, continue to predispose him to endocarditis.

Why other options are incorrect:

- **Postoperative infection:** While postoperative infections are possible, the timing of the symptoms (six weeks post-surgery) is more consistent with recurrent endocarditis.
- **Drug fever:** Drug fever typically presents with a characteristic rash and is usually accompanied by other symptoms like eosinophilia.
- **Deep vein thrombosis (DVT):** While DVT can cause fever, it's less likely to be the primary cause of the patient's symptoms given the history of endocarditis.

Additional Considerations:

- Blood cultures and echocardiogram are essential for diagnosing recurrent endocarditis.

- Prompt initiation of appropriate antibiotic therapy is crucial for managing the infection.
- Repeat surgery may be necessary in cases of persistent or recurrent infection.

The patient's history and clinical presentation strongly suggest recurrent infective endocarditis, warranting further investigation and treatment.

353. Understanding the Question

A 75-year-old man with COPD is in acute respiratory failure requiring mechanical ventilation. The question asks for adjunctive therapies to improve oxygenation and reduce ventilator-induced lung injury (VILI).

Correct Answer: D. All of the above

Explanation:

All of the listed options can be considered as adjunctive therapies to improve oxygenation and reduce VILI in patients with acute respiratory distress syndrome (ARDS), a common complication of severe COPD exacerbations.

- **Inhaled nitric oxide:** This gas can selectively dilate pulmonary vasculature, improving oxygenation.
- **High-frequency oscillatory ventilation (HFOV):** This ventilation mode can improve oxygenation and reduce lung injury by providing smaller tidal volumes and higher respiratory rates.
- **Prone positioning:** This has been shown to significantly improve oxygenation and reduce mortality in ARDS patients by improving lung aeration.

Additional Considerations:

- The choice of adjunctive therapy depends on the severity of the patient's condition, the available resources, and the expertise of the healthcare team.
- It's important to note that these therapies are often used in combination with other lung-protective ventilation strategies, such as low tidal volumes and permissive hypercapnia.
- Continuous monitoring of the patient's clinical status and hemodynamic parameters is essential when using these adjunctive therapies.

By considering all of these options, healthcare providers can optimize patient care and improve outcomes in patients with severe COPD exacerbations and ARDS.

354. Understanding the Question

A 30-year-old woman with severe pneumonia and septic shock is on mechanical ventilation with a low PaO2/FiO2 ratio. The question asks which ventilatory strategy is most likely to worsen oxygenation.

Correct Answer: C. High tidal volume ventilation (10-12 mL/kg of predicted body weight)

Explanation:

High tidal volume ventilation has been shown to increase the risk of ventilator-induced lung injury (VILI) and worsen oxygenation in patients with acute respiratory distress syndrome (ARDS).

- **VILI** occurs when excessive tidal volumes cause overdistension of the alveoli, leading to damage and decreased lung compliance.
- This damage impairs gas exchange and worsens hypoxemia.

Why other options are incorrect:

- **Lung-protective ventilation with low tidal volumes (6-8 mL/kg of predicted body weight):** This strategy is the cornerstone of ARDS management and has been shown to improve oxygenation and reduce mortality.
- **High PEEP (15-20 cm H2O):** Positive end-expiratory pressure (PEEP) helps to prevent alveolar collapse and improve oxygenation. While excessive PEEP can lead to barotrauma, the given range is generally considered safe.
- **Recruitment maneuvers:** These maneuvers involve applying high levels of PEEP to open collapsed lung units and improve oxygenation.

Additional Considerations:

- Lung-protective ventilation strategies, including low tidal volumes, PEEP, and limiting plateau pressures, are essential in managing patients with ARDS.
- Other factors affecting oxygenation include appropriate fluid management, prone positioning, and addressing underlying causes of hypoxemia.

By avoiding high tidal volume ventilation and implementing lung-protective strategies, healthcare providers can improve patient outcomes in ARDS.

355. Understanding the Question

A 65-year-old man with heart failure is in cardiogenic shock after an acute myocardial infarction. Despite treatment, his cardiac index remains low. The question asks for the biomarker most strongly associated with mortality in this condition.

Correct Answer: C. Lactate

Explanation:

Lactate is the most strongly associated with mortality in cardiogenic shock. It is a sensitive marker of tissue hypoperfusion and anaerobic metabolism.

- **Elevated lactate levels** indicate inadequate oxygen delivery to tissues, which is a hallmark of cardiogenic shock.
- Serial lactate measurements can help monitor the patient's response to treatment and predict outcomes.

Why other options are incorrect:

- **Brain natriuretic peptide (BNP) and N-terminal pro-brain natriuretic peptide (NT-proBNP):** These biomarkers are primarily associated with heart failure and can be elevated in cardiogenic shock but are less specific for predicting mortality compared to lactate.
- **Troponin I:** While troponin is a marker of myocardial injury and is elevated in acute myocardial infarction, it is less predictive of short-term mortality in the setting of cardiogenic shock compared to lactate.

Additional Considerations:

- Other factors influencing mortality in cardiogenic shock include the extent of myocardial damage, time to reperfusion, and the patient's overall hemodynamic status.
- Early recognition and aggressive management of cardiogenic shock are crucial for improving outcomes.

Lactate is a valuable tool for assessing tissue perfusion and guiding treatment decisions in patients with cardiogenic shock.

356. Understanding the Question

The question presents a patient with severe liver disease (alcoholic hepatitis and acute liver failure) complicated by hepatorenal syndrome (HRS), a kidney dysfunction caused by liver failure. The goal is to identify the most crucial factor in determining if this patient requires a liver transplant.

The Correct Answer: A. MELD score

MELD (Model for End-stage Liver Disease) score is the most accurate predictor of short-term mortality in patients with advanced liver disease, including those with HRS. It incorporates factors like bilirubin, creatinine, INR, and sodium levels. A higher MELD score indicates more severe liver disease and a higher risk of imminent death.

In the context of liver transplantation, the MELD score is used to prioritize patients on the waiting list. Patients with higher MELD scores are prioritized because they have a higher risk of death without a transplant.

Why Other Options are Incorrect:

• **Child-Pugh score:** While it assesses liver function, it is less predictive of short-term mortality compared to MELD. It is more useful for long-term prognosis and management.

• **Response to terlipressin therapy:** Terlipressin is a vasoconstrictor used to manage HRS. While a good response can improve kidney function, it does not predict the overall severity of liver disease or the need for transplantation.

• **Presence of ascites:** Ascites is a common complication of liver disease but is not as strong a predictor of short-term mortality as MELD.

Additional Considerations:

• **Other factors** besides MELD can influence the decision for liver transplantation, such as the patient's overall health status, age, and social support.

• **Early recognition and management of HRS** are crucial to improve patient outcomes and potentially delay the need for transplantation.

• **Liver transplantation** is a complex procedure with significant risks and benefits, and the decision should be made in collaboration with the patient, family, and a multidisciplinary transplant team.

Case Study: A patient with a MELD score of 30 is at significantly higher risk of death within three months compared to a patient with a MELD score of 15. This patient would likely be prioritized for liver transplantation.

357. Understanding the Question

The question describes a young woman with severe asthma requiring intubation and mechanical ventilation. It asks about the most likely complication arising from prolonged mechanical ventilation in this context.

The Correct Answer: D. All of the above

All of the listed complications - pneumonia, barotrauma, and diaphragmatic dysfunction - are commonly associated with prolonged mechanical ventilation.

- **Pneumonia:** Patients on mechanical ventilation are at increased risk of developing pneumonia, often referred to as ventilator-associated pneumonia (VAP). This is due to a combination of factors, including the presence of an endotracheal tube, impaired cough and mucociliary clearance, and the patient's underlying condition (in this case, severe asthma).
- **Barotrauma:** This refers to lung injury caused by excessive pressure during mechanical ventilation. It can lead to pneumothorax, pneumomediastinum, or even pulmonary bullae. The risk of barotrauma is higher in patients with underlying lung disease, such as asthma.
- **Diaphragmatic dysfunction:** Prolonged immobilization of the diaphragm due to mechanical ventilation can lead to weakness and atrophy of the muscle. This can contribute to weaning difficulties and prolonged ventilation time.

Why Other Options are Incorrect:

Given the high risk of all three complications in this patient, none of the individual options can be considered the most likely.

Additional Considerations:

- **Prevention strategies** for these complications include meticulous oral care, elevation of the head of the bed, careful monitoring of ventilator settings, and early mobilization.
- **Regular assessment** of the patient's respiratory status and ventilator settings is crucial to minimize the risk of complications.
- **Close collaboration** between the respiratory therapist, pulmonologist, and critical care team is essential in managing patients on prolonged mechanical ventilation.

Case Study: A patient with status asthmaticus on prolonged mechanical ventilation develops a fever, increased respiratory secretions, and a new infiltrate on chest X-ray, suggestive of VAP. Additionally, the patient experiences sudden-onset chest pain and desaturation, raising suspicion for a pneumothorax (barotrauma).

358. Understanding the Question

The patient has a Stanford Type B aortic dissection, meaning the tear in the aorta starts distal to the left subclavian artery. The question asks which medication is contraindicated due to the risk of increasing aortic wall stress.

The Correct Answer: C. Hydralazine

Hydralazine is a vasodilator that primarily decreases peripheral vascular resistance. While it can effectively lower blood pressure, it can also increase cardiac output. This increased cardiac output can lead to increased aortic wall stress, which is undesirable in a patient with an aortic dissection.

Why Other Options are Incorrect:

- **Beta-blockers:** These medications decrease heart rate and contractility, reducing aortic wall stress. They are a cornerstone of treatment for aortic dissection.
- **Calcium channel blockers:** These can lower blood pressure and heart rate, helping to reduce aortic wall stress. They are often used in combination with beta-blockers.
- **Nitroprusside:** This is a potent vasodilator that can rapidly lower blood pressure. It is used in hypertensive emergencies, including aortic dissection, to control blood pressure quickly.

Additional Considerations:

- The goal of medical management for aortic dissection is to reduce aortic wall stress by lowering blood pressure and heart rate.
- Careful monitoring of blood pressure and aortic dimensions is essential during treatment.
- Surgical intervention may be necessary in certain cases, such as uncontrolled hypertension, rapidly expanding aortic diameter, or impending or completed rupture.

Case Study: A patient with a Stanford Type B aortic dissection is started on beta-blockers and calcium channel blockers. Blood pressure is initially well controlled. However, the patient develops worsening chest pain and increasing aortic diameter. Hydralazine is considered but is avoided due to the risk of increased aortic wall stress. Instead, nitroprusside is initiated to rapidly lower blood pressure.

359. Understanding the Question

A patient with chronic kidney disease (CKD) has developed uremic pericarditis leading to cardiac tamponade, requiring pericardiocentesis. Despite this procedure, the patient is experiencing recurrent tamponade. The question asks for the most appropriate next step in management.

The Correct Answer: B. Pericardial window placement

Pericardial window placement is the most appropriate next step in managing recurrent cardiac tamponade despite pericardiocentesis. This procedure creates a persistent opening in the pericardium, allowing fluid to drain continuously and preventing reaccumulation.

Why Other Options are Incorrect:

- **Repeat pericardiocentesis:** While effective in temporarily relieving cardiac tamponade, it is not a durable solution and is likely to result in recurrent tamponade.

- **Pericardiectomy:** This is a more invasive procedure and is generally reserved for recurrent tamponade that is refractory to other treatments or in cases of constrictive pericarditis.

- **Initiation of hemodialysis:** While dialysis is essential in managing CKD, it is not a direct treatment for cardiac tamponade. It may help improve overall uremic status but will not address the underlying issue of fluid accumulation in the pericardium.

Additional Considerations:

- **Underlying cause:** Addressing the underlying cause of uremic pericarditis, which is the CKD itself, is crucial for preventing recurrence.

- **Other treatment options:** In some cases, medications like corticosteroids or colchicine may be considered to reduce pericardial inflammation.

- **Complications:** Pericardial window placement can be associated with complications such as bleeding, infection, and pneumothorax.

Case Study: A patient with CKD and recurrent cardiac tamponade undergoes pericardial window placement. After the procedure, the patient's symptoms resolve, and there is no recurrence of tamponade. Dialysis is continued to manage the underlying CKD.

360. Understanding the Question

A patient with rheumatoid arthritis develops septic shock but doesn't respond to standard treatment. The question asks for potential alternative diagnoses.

The Correct Answer: D. All of the above

All of the listed conditions can mimic sepsis and complicate the management of patients with rheumatoid arthritis.

- **Macrophage Activation Syndrome (MAS):** This is a rare but life-threatening complication of autoimmune diseases like rheumatoid arthritis. It's characterized by fever, cytopenias, hepatosplenomegaly, and elevated ferritin levels. MAS can mimic sepsis and is often resistant to standard antibiotic therapy.

- **Drug-induced lupus:** Certain medications used to treat rheumatoid arthritis can induce lupus-like symptoms. While less likely to cause septic shock, it can contribute to a complex clinical picture and delay diagnosis.
- **Adult-onset Still's disease:** This is a rare inflammatory condition that can mimic sepsis. It often presents with fever, rash, arthritis, and elevated inflammatory markers.

Why Other Options are Incorrect:

Given the complexity of the case and the overlapping features of these conditions, it's essential to consider all of them as potential diagnoses.

Additional Considerations:

- **Prompt recognition** of these conditions is crucial for optimal patient management.
- **Interdisciplinary collaboration** between rheumatologists and critical care specialists is essential in these complex cases.
- **Specific diagnostic tests** may be necessary to differentiate between these conditions, such as ferritin levels, liver enzymes, and antinuclear antibodies.

Case Study: A patient with rheumatoid arthritis develops fever, hypotension, and elevated inflammatory markers. Despite broad-spectrum antibiotics, the patient's condition worsens. Laboratory tests reveal cytopenias and elevated ferritin levels, consistent with macrophage activation syndrome.

361. Understanding the Question

A 78-year-old woman with multiple comorbidities presents with new-onset atrial fibrillation with rapid ventricular response (RVR) and hemodynamic instability. The question asks for the most appropriate next step in management after rate control.

The Correct Answer: A. Perform electrical cardioversion

Given the patient's hemodynamic instability (blood pressure 100/60 mmHg) despite rapid ventricular response, immediate electrical cardioversion is the most appropriate next step. Rapid ventricular response in the setting of hypotension can lead to decreased cardiac output and tissue perfusion.

Why Other Options are Incorrect:

- **Initiate amiodarone for rhythm control:** While amiodarone can be used for rhythm control in atrial fibrillation, it is not the first-line treatment in hemodynamically unstable patients.
- **Assess and correct underlying causes of atrial fibrillation:** This is an important step in the management of atrial fibrillation, but it should be done after stabilizing the patient's hemodynamic status.
- **Start intravenous heparin infusion:** While anticoagulation is important to prevent stroke in atrial fibrillation, it is not indicated in this patient who is already on apixaban.

Additional Considerations:
- **Rapid cardioversion:** Due to the patient's hemodynamic instability, synchronized cardioversion should be performed as soon as possible.
- **Risk of embolization:** Given the patient's history of atrial fibrillation, the risk of embolization should be considered before cardioversion. Transesophageal echocardiogram (TEE) may be indicated to assess for left atrial thrombus.
- **Post-cardioversion management:** After successful cardioversion, anticoagulation should be continued to prevent recurrent atrial fibrillation and embolization.

Case Study: A 78-year-old woman with atrial fibrillation and hypotension undergoes immediate synchronized cardioversion, which successfully restores sinus rhythm. Blood pressure improves after cardioversion. Anticoagulation is continued, and further evaluation for the underlying cause of atrial fibrillation is initiated.

362. Understanding the Question

A patient with a history of intravenous drug use and a recent history of infective endocarditis with perivalvular abscess is presenting with recurrent fever, chills, and fatigue despite successful surgical treatment. The question asks for the most likely diagnostic test to identify the source of the recurrent infection.

The Correct Answer: C. 18F-FDG PET/CT scan

An **18F-FDG PET/CT scan** is the most likely test to identify the source of recurrent infection in this patient. This imaging modality can detect areas of increased metabolic activity, which is characteristic of infection. It can identify occult abscesses, persistent infection, or new foci of infection that may not be apparent on other imaging studies.

Why Other Options are Incorrect:

• **Transthoracic echocardiogram (TTE):** While useful for evaluating cardiac structures and function, TTE is less likely to detect extracardiac foci of infection.

• **Transesophageal echocardiogram (TEE):** Although more sensitive than TTE for detecting cardiac abnormalities, TEE is primarily used for evaluating the heart and is less likely to identify extracardiac infections.

• **Gallium scan:** While gallium scans can be used to detect infection, they are less specific than PET/CT and may have false-positive results.

Additional Considerations:

• **Other diagnostic tests:** Depending on the clinical suspicion, other tests such as bone marrow biopsy, MRI, or CT scans of specific areas may be considered.

• **Antibiotic therapy:** While definitive diagnosis is crucial, empirical antibiotic therapy may be initiated based on clinical suspicion.

• **Surgical intervention:** If a new focus of infection is identified, surgical intervention may be required.

Case Study: A patient with recurrent fever after infective endocarditis surgery undergoes an 18F-FDG PET/CT scan which reveals a hepatic abscess. The patient undergoes percutaneous drainage of the abscess, and the fever resolves.

363. Understanding the Question

A patient with COPD, acute exacerbation, and hypercapnic respiratory failure is on mechanical ventilation. After developing Pseudomonas aeruginosa pneumonia, the question asks for the most appropriate antibiotic considering the patient's history of acute kidney injury (AKI).

The Correct Answer: C. Ceftazidime/avibactam

Ceftazidime/avibactam is the most appropriate antibiotic choice for this patient.

• **Ceftazidime** is an active cephalosporin against Pseudomonas aeruginosa.

• **Avibactam** is a beta-lactamase inhibitor that enhances the activity of ceftazidime against many beta-lactamase-producing organisms, including Pseudomonas aeruginosa.

• This combination is particularly suitable for patients with renal impairment as it does not require dose adjustments based on renal function.

Why Other Options are Incorrect:

- **Cefepime:** While active against Pseudomonas aeruginosa, it requires dose adjustments in patients with renal impairment, making it less ideal for this patient.
- **Meropenem:** Although effective against Pseudomonas aeruginosa, it has a renal elimination pathway and requires dose adjustments in patients with AKI.
- **Imipenem/cilastatin:** While broad-spectrum, it also undergoes renal elimination and requires dose adjustments in renal impairment.

Additional Considerations:
- **Antibiotic selection:** The choice of antibiotic should always be guided by local susceptibility patterns.
- **Duration of therapy:** The duration of antibiotic therapy typically depends on the clinical response and the patient's overall condition.
- **Monitoring:** Close monitoring of renal function and antibiotic levels is essential in patients with AKI.

Case Study: A patient with COPD, on mechanical ventilation, develops Pseudomonas aeruginosa pneumonia and has a history of AKI. Ceftazidime/avibactam is initiated. The patient's renal function is monitored closely, and the antibiotic therapy is adjusted as needed based on clinical response and culture results.

364. Understanding the Question

A young woman with septic shock secondary to a pelvic abscess is receiving norepinephrine. The question asks for the most reliable indicator of adequate fluid resuscitation.

The Correct Answer: D. Stroke Volume Variation (SVV)

Stroke volume variation (SVV) is the most reliable indicator of fluid responsiveness in this patient. It measures the change in stroke volume during the respiratory cycle. A high SVV (typically >13%) indicates fluid responsiveness, meaning the patient is likely to benefit from fluid resuscitation.

Why Other Options are Incorrect:
- **Central venous pressure (CVP):** While CVP can be used to assess fluid status, it is less reliable than SVV, especially in patients with sepsis. CVP can be affected by many factors, including vasomotor tone, intrathoracic pressure, and right ventricular function.

- **Pulmonary capillary wedge pressure (PCWP):** PCWP is an invasive measure of left ventricular filling pressure. It is not as reliable as SVV in determining fluid responsiveness, especially in patients with sepsis.
- **Mean arterial pressure (MAP):** MAP is a measure of blood pressure but does not directly assess fluid responsiveness. It can be affected by vasoconstrictors like norepinephrine, making it less reliable in this context.

Additional Considerations:

- **Dynamic parameters:** SVV is a dynamic parameter that reflects the body's response to fluid challenge. Static parameters like CVP and PCWP may not accurately reflect fluid responsiveness in dynamic conditions.
- **Other factors:** Factors such as blood loss, ongoing fluid losses, and the patient's overall clinical condition should also be considered when assessing fluid responsiveness.
- **Fluid challenge:** A fluid challenge can be performed to assess the patient's response to fluid resuscitation and to confirm fluid responsiveness.

Case Study: A patient with septic shock and a high SVV receives a bolus of crystalloid fluid. After the fluid challenge, the SVV decreases significantly, indicating that the patient was fluid responsive.

365. Understanding the Question

A patient with HFpEF and acute decompensated heart failure is refractory to diuretics and has a history of anuria. The question asks which adjunctive therapy is contraindicated.

The Correct Answer: B. Ultrafiltration

Ultrafiltration is contraindicated in a patient with anuria. Ultrafiltration relies on a pressure gradient to remove fluid, and if there is no urine output (anuria), it can lead to severe electrolyte imbalances and hemodynamic instability.

Why Other Options are Incorrect:

- **Continuous renal replacement therapy (CRRT):** This is a suitable option for patients with acute kidney injury, including those with anuria. It can remove fluids, electrolytes, and waste products while providing acid-base balance.
- **Low-dose dopamine infusion:** While its efficacy in acute heart failure is debated, it is not contraindicated in anuria. It may have some vasodilatory and diuretic effects.

- **Metolazone:** This is a loop diuretic that can be used in conjunction with other diuretics to increase diuresis. It is not contraindicated in anuria but may not be effective if there is no urine output.

Additional Considerations:

- **Cautious fluid management:** Patients with HFpEF and acute decompensated heart failure are often fluid overloaded. However, excessive fluid removal can lead to hypotension and impaired renal function.
- **Hemodynamic monitoring:** Close monitoring of hemodynamic parameters is crucial during fluid management and the use of adjunctive therapies.
- **Other treatment options:** Depending on the patient's clinical status, other therapies such as inotropes or vasodilators may be considered.

Case Study: A patient with HFpEF, acute decompensated heart failure, and anuria is initiated on CRRT to manage fluid overload and electrolyte imbalances. Low-dose dopamine and metolazone are also considered as adjunctive therapies.

366. Understanding the Question

A patient with alcoholic hepatitis and acute liver failure has developed hepatic encephalopathy. The question asks for the most effective intervention to prevent recurrent episodes.

The Correct Answer: B. Rifaximin

Rifaximin is the most effective medication for the primary prevention of hepatic encephalopathy in patients with cirrhosis. It works by reducing the intestinal bacterial load, thereby decreasing the production of ammonia and other toxic substances that contribute to hepatic encephalopathy.

Why Other Options are Incorrect:

- **Lactulose:** While lactulose is a mainstay treatment for acute episodes of hepatic encephalopathy, it is less effective for long-term prevention compared to rifaximin.
- **Neomycin:** Neomycin is an older antibiotic used for hepatic encephalopathy, but it has significant side effects, including nephrotoxicity and ototoxicity. It is generally considered a second-line agent.
- **Dietary protein restriction:** While protein restriction can be helpful in managing hepatic encephalopathy, it is often difficult to adhere to and may lead to malnutrition. It is not as effective as pharmacological interventions like rifaximin.

Additional Considerations:
- **Combination therapy:** In some cases, a combination of rifaximin and lactulose may be used for optimal management.
- **Non-pharmacological measures:** Other measures to prevent hepatic encephalopathy include adequate hydration, avoiding constipation, and managing underlying liver disease.
- **Patient education:** Patient education about the importance of medication adherence and dietary modifications is crucial for preventing recurrent episodes.

Case Study: A patient with cirrhosis and a history of hepatic encephalopathy is started on rifaximin for primary prevention. The patient remains encephalopathy-free for several months, demonstrating the effectiveness of the medication.

367. Understanding the Question

A patient with severe asthma (status asthmaticus) is intubated and on mechanical ventilation. The question asks for an adjunctive therapy to reduce airway inflammation given the patient's lack of response to standard treatment.

The Correct Answer: A. Intravenous magnesium sulfate

Intravenous magnesium sulfate can be considered as an adjunctive therapy for severe asthma refractory to standard treatments. It has bronchodilator and anti-inflammatory properties, which may help to improve lung function in these patients.

Why Other Options are Incorrect:
- **Inhaled helium-oxygen mixture (heliox):** While heliox can improve gas exchange in patients with severe airflow obstruction, it does not directly address airway inflammation.
- **Bronchial thermoplasty:** This is a long-term treatment for severe asthma and is not indicated in acute exacerbations like status asthmaticus.
- **Extracorporeal membrane oxygenation (ECMO):** ECMO is a life-saving therapy for severe respiratory failure but is indicated when other treatments have failed and the patient is at imminent risk of death. It is not a first-line therapy for airway inflammation.

Additional Considerations:
- **Other adjunctive therapies:** Other potential adjunctive therapies for severe asthma include inhaled nitric oxide and inhaled corticosteroids.

- **Early goal-directed therapy:** Aggressive management of severe asthma, including early intubation and mechanical ventilation, is crucial to improve outcomes.
- **Continuous monitoring:** Close monitoring of hemodynamic parameters, arterial blood gases, and clinical status is essential during the management of status asthmaticus.

Case Study: A patient with status asthmaticus on mechanical ventilation is unresponsive to standard therapy. Intravenous magnesium sulfate is administered as an adjunct to other treatments. The patient shows improvement in lung function and requires lower ventilator support.

368. Understanding the Question

A patient with a history of hypertension, hyperlipidemia, and reactive airway disease has a Stanford Type B aortic dissection. The question asks for the most suitable long-term blood pressure medication given these conditions.

The Correct Answer: B. Calcium Channel Blocker

A **calcium channel blocker** is the most appropriate choice for long-term blood pressure control in this patient.

- **Effective for blood pressure control:** Calcium channel blockers effectively lower blood pressure.
- **Safe for reactive airway disease:** Unlike beta-blockers, which can exacerbate bronchospasm in patients with reactive airway disease, calcium channel blockers are generally safe.
- **Suitable for aortic dissection:** They can help to reduce aortic wall stress.

Why Other Options are Incorrect:

- **Beta-blocker:** While effective for blood pressure control, beta-blockers can worsen bronchospasm in patients with reactive airway disease.
- **ACE inhibitor and ARB:** These medications are generally first-line agents for hypertension but are less suitable in this patient due to the risk of inducing cough, a common side effect that can exacerbate reactive airway disease.

Additional Considerations:

- **Individualized treatment:** The choice of medication should be tailored to the patient's specific needs and comorbidities.
- **Combination therapy:** Often, blood pressure control requires a combination of medications.

- **Regular monitoring:** Blood pressure and lung function should be monitored regularly to assess the effectiveness and tolerability of the chosen medication.

Case Study: A patient with hypertension, hyperlipidemia, and reactive airway disease who has recovered from a Stanford Type B aortic dissection is started on a calcium channel blocker for blood pressure control. The patient's blood pressure is well controlled without any exacerbation of respiratory symptoms.

369. Understanding the Question

A patient with chronic kidney disease (CKD) has developed uremic pericarditis and subsequently purulent pericarditis. The question asks for the most appropriate next step in management.

The Correct Answer: D. Initiation of antibiotic therapy

Initiation of antibiotic therapy is the most crucial step in managing purulent pericarditis. This condition is a serious infection requiring immediate and aggressive antibiotic treatment to prevent complications such as sepsis and pericardial tamponade.

Why Other Options are Incorrect:

- **Repeat pericardiocentesis:** While drainage of the purulent fluid is necessary, it is not sufficient on its own. Antibiotic therapy is essential to eradicate the infection.
- **Pericardial window placement:** This procedure may be considered if antibiotic therapy fails to control the infection or if there is persistent fluid accumulation. However, it is not the initial management.
- **Pericardiectomy:** This is a major surgical procedure and is generally reserved for cases of constrictive pericarditis or recurrent pericarditis refractory to other treatments.

Additional Considerations:

- **Antibiotic selection:** The choice of antibiotic should be based on the suspected pathogen and local susceptibility patterns.
- **Drainage:** Pericardiocentesis or pericardial window placement may be necessary to drain the purulent fluid.
- **Supportive care:** Supportive care measures, including hemodynamic monitoring and respiratory support, are essential.

Case Study: A patient with CKD and purulent pericarditis is initiated on broad-spectrum antibiotics. Pericardiocentesis is performed to drain the purulent fluid and obtain cultures for specific antibiotic guidance. The patient's clinical condition is closely monitored, and additional treatments are adjusted as needed.

370. Understanding the Question

A patient with rheumatoid arthritis and septic shock has not responded to standard treatment, and there's a history of recent travel to a region endemic for fungal infections. The question asks for appropriate diagnostic tests to consider.

The Correct Answer: D. All of the above

Given the patient's clinical presentation, history of rheumatoid arthritis, and travel history, it's crucial to consider a fungal infection as a potential etiology for the persistent sepsis. Therefore, **all of the listed tests** are appropriate to investigate this possibility.

- **Fungal blood cultures:** These can directly identify the presence of fungi in the bloodstream.
- **Serum galactomannan:** This is a biomarker for invasive aspergillosis.
- **Beta-D-glucan:** This is a biomarker for invasive fungal infections, including Candida and Aspergillus.

Why Other Options are Incorrect:

Each of the listed tests provides valuable information in diagnosing invasive fungal infections, and therefore, all should be considered in this patient.

Additional Considerations:

- **Rapid diagnosis:** Early diagnosis and initiation of appropriate antifungal therapy are crucial for improving outcomes in invasive fungal infections.
- **Other diagnostic tests:** Depending on the clinical presentation, other tests such as bronchoalveolar lavage or tissue biopsy may be necessary.
- **Antifungal therapy:** Empiric antifungal therapy may be initiated while awaiting diagnostic test results if the clinical suspicion is high.

Case Study: A patient with rheumatoid arthritis and persistent sepsis after travel to an endemic region for fungal infections is found to have a positive serum galactomannan test, leading to the diagnosis of invasive aspergillosis. Early initiation of antifungal therapy resulted in improved clinical outcomes.

371. Understanding the Question

A patient with end-stage renal disease (ESRD) on hemodialysis is presenting with symptoms of altered mental status, hypotension, bradycardia, and ECG changes suggestive of hyperkalemia. The question asks for the most likely electrolyte abnormality causing these symptoms.

The Correct Answer: A. Hyperkalemia

Hyperkalemia is the most likely cause of the patient's symptoms. The classic ECG findings of peaked T waves and prolonged PR interval are characteristic of hyperkalemia. Additionally, the symptoms of altered mental status, hypotension, and bradycardia are consistent with this diagnosis.

Why Other Options are Incorrect:

- **Hypokalemia:** Would typically cause flattened T waves, not peaked T waves.
- **Hypercalcemia:** Can lead to cardiac arrhythmias, but the ECG changes would be different, and the symptoms would be more consistent with muscle weakness and confusion.
- **Hypocalcemia:** Can cause prolonged QT interval and arrhythmias, but the ECG findings and symptoms would not match the patient's presentation.

Additional Considerations:

- **Rapid treatment:** Hyperkalemia is a medical emergency requiring immediate treatment to prevent life-threatening arrhythmias.
- **Causes of hyperkalemia:** In patients with ESRD, common causes of hyperkalemia include decreased renal excretion, excessive potassium intake, and tissue breakdown.
- **Treatment options:** Treatment options for hyperkalemia include calcium gluconate for immediate stabilization, insulin and glucose to shift potassium intracellularly, and dialysis to remove excess potassium.

Case Study: A patient with ESRD on hemodialysis presents with altered mental status, hypotension, bradycardia, and peaked T waves on ECG. A diagnosis of hyperkalemia is made, and the patient is treated with calcium gluconate, insulin, glucose, and hemodialysis. The patient's symptoms improve, and potassium levels normalize.

372. Understanding the Question

A patient with HIV presents with symptoms and radiological findings suggestive of a pulmonary infection. The question asks for the most likely opportunistic infection in this context.

The Correct Answer: A. Pneumocystis pneumonia (PCP)

Pneumocystis pneumonia (PCP) is the most common opportunistic infection in patients with HIV and is highly associated with the clinical presentation and radiological findings described. Bilateral interstitial infiltrates on chest X-ray are classic findings of PCP.

Why Other Options are Incorrect:

- **Mycobacterium avium complex (MAC):** While MAC is an opportunistic infection in HIV, it typically presents with a more insidious onset, weight loss, and disseminated disease. Bilateral interstitial infiltrates are less common.

- **Cytomegalovirus (CMV) pneumonia:** CMV pneumonia is often associated with more severe immunosuppression and typically presents with a more gradual onset. Bilateral interstitial infiltrates are less common.

- **Histoplasmosis:** This is a fungal infection more common in specific geographic regions. The clinical presentation and radiological findings are less specific than those of PCP.

Additional Considerations:

- **CD4 count:** The patient's CD4 count would be crucial in determining the risk for different opportunistic infections. A lower CD4 count increases the risk for PCP.

- **Prophylaxis:** Prophylaxis against PCP is recommended for HIV-positive individuals with a CD4 count below a certain threshold.

- **Treatment:** Early diagnosis and treatment of PCP are essential to improve outcomes.

Case Study: A patient with HIV and a CD4 count of 100 presents with fever, cough, and shortness of breath. Chest X-ray shows bilateral interstitial infiltrates. Given the clinical presentation and CD4 count, PCP is strongly suspected. Induced sputum or bronchoalveolar lavage is performed to confirm the diagnosis, and treatment with trimethoprim-sulfamethoxazole is initiated.

373. Understanding the Question

A patient with COPD is experiencing a severe exacerbation despite optimal medical management and non-invasive ventilation (NIV). The question asks for the most appropriate next step in management.

The Correct Answer: D. Intubation and mechanical ventilation

Given the patient's deteriorating respiratory status despite maximal non-invasive support, **intubation and mechanical ventilation** are the most appropriate next steps. This provides optimal oxygenation and ventilation, which are critical for the patient's survival.

Why Other Options are Incorrect:

- **Tracheostomy:** While tracheostomy may be considered later in the course of management for long-term ventilation, it is not the initial step in acute respiratory failure.

- **High-frequency oscillatory ventilation (HFOV):** HFOV is a specialized form of ventilation often used in severe respiratory distress syndrome (ARDS). While it may be considered in certain circumstances, it is not the first-line treatment for COPD exacerbation.

- **Inhaled nitric oxide:** While inhaled nitric oxide can improve oxygenation in some cases, it is not a substitute for invasive ventilation when a patient is failing on NIV.

Additional Considerations:

- **Prompt intervention:** Timely intubation and mechanical ventilation are crucial to prevent further deterioration and improve outcomes.

- **Sedation and analgesia:** Appropriate sedation and analgesia are essential during the intubation process and subsequent mechanical ventilation.

- **Ventilator management:** Careful management of ventilator settings is critical to optimize oxygenation and ventilation while minimizing ventilator-induced lung injury.

Case Study: A patient with COPD and worsening respiratory failure despite NIV is intubated and placed on mechanical ventilation. The patient's oxygenation and ventilation improve, and the patient is stabilized.

374. Understanding the Question

A patient with septic shock and community-acquired pneumonia is intubated and on mechanical ventilation with a PaO_2/FiO_2 ratio of 80, indicating acute respiratory distress syndrome (ARDS). The question asks for the most common cause of refractory hypoxemia in ARDS.

The Correct Answer: C. Shunt

Shunt is the most common cause of refractory hypoxemia in ARDS. In ARDS, there is diffuse alveolar damage leading to a mismatch between ventilation and perfusion. This results in a portion of the cardiac output bypassing the oxygenated alveoli, leading to a shunt.

Why Other Options are Incorrect:

- **Pulmonary embolism:** While a pulmonary embolism can cause hypoxemia, it is less likely to be the primary cause of refractory hypoxemia in a patient with ARDS.
- **Pneumothorax:** A pneumothorax can cause hypoxemia but would usually present with sudden-onset respiratory distress and decreased breath sounds on the affected side.
- **Dead space ventilation:** Increased dead space ventilation can reduce alveolar ventilation and worsen gas exchange, but it is not the primary cause of refractory hypoxemia in ARDS.

Additional Considerations:

- **Other causes of refractory hypoxemia:** Other factors that can contribute to refractory hypoxemia in ARDS include low tidal volumes, pneumothorax, and pulmonary embolism.
- **Treatment:** Treatment of ARDS focuses on supportive care, including mechanical ventilation with low tidal volumes and positive end-expiratory pressure (PEEP), and addressing the underlying cause of the lung injury.

Case Study: A patient with ARDS is on mechanical ventilation with a low PaO2/FiO2 ratio despite increasing PEEP. A diagnosis of refractory hypoxemia is made, and the patient is managed with supportive care and close monitoring.

375. Understanding the Question

A patient with HFrEF is in cardiogenic shock despite inotropic and vasopressor support, and lactate levels remain elevated, indicating inadequate tissue perfusion. The question asks for potential interventions to improve tissue perfusion.

The Correct Answer: D. All of the above

All of the listed interventions can be considered to improve tissue perfusion in this patient. The choice of intervention depends on the specific hemodynamic profile, the underlying cause of the shock, and the patient's response to initial therapy.

- **Increase inotropic support:** This can improve cardiac output and increase blood pressure, leading to better tissue perfusion.
- **Increase vasopressor support:** This can maintain blood pressure and improve organ perfusion.

- **Inhaled pulmonary vasodilators (e.g., nitric oxide):** These can reduce pulmonary vascular resistance, improve oxygenation, and potentially increase cardiac output.

Why Other Options are Incorrect:

Each of the listed options can play a role in improving tissue perfusion, so none can be excluded as a potential intervention.

Additional Considerations:

- **Hemodynamic monitoring:** Continuous monitoring of hemodynamic parameters is crucial to guide therapy and assess response to interventions.
- **Underlying cause:** Addressing the underlying cause of cardiogenic shock, such as myocardial infarction or valvular heart disease, is essential for long-term recovery.
- **Other therapies:** Additional therapies, such as mechanical circulatory support (e.g., extracorporeal membrane oxygenation) or ultrafiltration, may be considered in refractory cases.

Case Study: A patient with HFrEF and cardiogenic shock is treated with increasing doses of inotropes and vasopressors. Despite these interventions, lactate levels remain elevated.Inhaled nitric oxide is added to the treatment regimen, leading to improved oxygenation and a decrease in lactate levels.

376. Understanding the Question

The patient has severe liver disease leading to kidney failure (hepatorenal syndrome). Terlipressin is a medication used to treat this condition. The question asks which parameter is most important to monitor to assess if the terlipressin is working.

Correct Answer: D. All of the above

Explanation:

All of the listed parameters are crucial in monitoring the effectiveness of terlipressin in a patient with hepatorenal syndrome. Let's break down why:

- **Serum creatinine:** This is a direct marker of kidney function. A decrease in serum creatinine indicates improvement in kidney function, suggesting the terlipressin is effective.
- **Urine output:** An increase in urine output is a positive sign as it reflects improved renal perfusion and glomerular filtration rate, indicating the terlipressin is working.

- **Serum sodium:** Hepatorenal syndrome is often accompanied by hyponatremia. Terlipressin can help improve sodium retention by increasing effective circulating volume. Monitoring serum sodium helps assess fluid balance and the drug's efficacy.

Why other options are incorrect: While each parameter individually provides valuable information, monitoring all three is essential for a comprehensive assessment of terlipressin's effectiveness.

Additional considerations:

- **Other monitoring parameters:** While not explicitly mentioned in the question, it's crucial to monitor blood pressure, heart rate, and for adverse effects of terlipressin like ischemic events.
- **Combination therapy:** Terlipressin is often used in combination with albumin to improve its efficacy.
- **Prognosis:** Even with successful treatment, the prognosis for patients with hepatorenal syndrome remains guarded due to the underlying liver disease.

Case Study: A 45-year-old man with cirrhosis develops rapid deterioration of kidney function. Serum creatinine rises from 1.2 to 2.5 mg/dL within a week. Urine output decreases significantly. He is diagnosed with hepatorenal syndrome and started on terlipressin and albumin. After 48 hours, his serum creatinine decreases to 1.8 mg/dL, urine output increases, and serum sodium stabilizes. These changes indicate a positive response to therapy.

By closely monitoring all the mentioned parameters, healthcare providers can assess the efficacy of terlipressin, make necessary adjustments to the treatment plan, and improve patient outcomes.

377. Understanding the Question

The patient is in critical condition with severe asthma (status asthmaticus) and is on a ventilator. The question asks which ventilator setting is best to prevent dynamic hyperinflation, a condition where air is trapped in the lungs, leading to complications.

Correct Answer: A. Low tidal volume

Explanation:

- **Low tidal volume** is the most effective setting to reduce the risk of dynamic hyperinflation in a patient with status asthmaticus. By delivering smaller amounts of air per breath, we reduce the amount of air trapped in the lungs, allowing for better expiration.

- This strategy is often combined with **permissive hypercapnia**, allowing the patient to retain some carbon dioxide to promote bronchodilation and reduce the work of breathing.

Why other options are incorrect:

- **Low respiratory rate:** While reducing respiratory rate can help, it might not be sufficient to prevent dynamic hyperinflation.
- **High inspiratory flow rate:** This setting can actually increase peak airway pressure and worsen air trapping.
- **Short expiratory time:** This would exacerbate air trapping and increase the risk of dynamic hyperinflation.

Additional considerations:

- **Other ventilator settings:** Other important settings to consider include positive end-expiratory pressure (PEEP), which can be used cautiously to improve oxygenation, and inspiratory-to-expiratory (I:E) ratio, which should be prolonged to allow more time for expiration.
- **Monitoring:** Close monitoring of lung mechanics, including peak inspiratory pressure, plateau pressure, and dynamic compliance, is crucial to assess the effectiveness of the ventilation strategy and to detect early signs of worsening lung condition.
- **Sedation and paralysis:** These may be necessary to improve patient-ventilator synchrony and reduce oxygen consumption, but should be used judiciously and monitored closely.

Case Study: A 30-year-old woman with severe asthma is intubated and placed on mechanical ventilation. Initial ventilator settings include a tidal volume of 10 ml/kg, respiratory rate of 12 breaths/min, and a high inspiratory flow rate. The patient develops increasing difficulty in exhaling, and her peak airway pressure rises. The ventilator settings are adjusted to a lower tidal volume of 6 ml/kg and a prolonged expiratory time. These changes improve lung mechanics and reduce the risk of dynamic hyperinflation.

By understanding the pathophysiology of status asthmaticus and the principles of mechanical ventilation, healthcare providers can optimize ventilator settings to improve patient outcomes and minimize complications.

378. Understanding the Question

The patient has a history of hypertension and hyperlipidemia and experienced an acute aortic dissection (a tear in the main blood vessel). The question asks about the best imaging study to assess the aorta one year later.

Correct Answer: B. Computed tomography angiography (CTA) of the chest

Explanation:

- **Computed tomography angiography (CTA)** is the most appropriate imaging modality for follow-up assessment of an aortic dissection one year after initial presentation.
- It provides excellent visualization of the aorta, its branches, and any potential aneurysmal dilatation or dissection progression.
- CTA is non-invasive, relatively quick, and offers detailed anatomical information.

Why other options are incorrect:

- **Chest X-ray:** While a chest X-ray can show aortic enlargement or calcification, it lacks the detail and specificity of CTA for assessing aortic dissection.
- **Transesophageal echocardiogram (TEE):** TEE is primarily used for evaluating the heart and proximal aorta. It is not ideal for assessing the entire thoracic and abdominal aorta.
- **Magnetic resonance imaging (MRI) of the chest:** While MRI can provide excellent image quality, it is generally less readily available than CTA and can be time-consuming. Additionally, patients with certain implants or claustrophobia may not be suitable candidates for MRI.

Additional considerations:

- **Follow-up imaging:** The frequency of follow-up imaging depends on the extent of the initial dissection, the presence of risk factors (e.g., hypertension, connective tissue disorders), and the patient's overall clinical condition.
- **Aortic aneurysm:** Patients with aortic dissection are at increased risk of developing an aortic aneurysm, which is another reason for regular follow-up imaging.
- **Treatment:** If the CTA demonstrates progression of the aortic dissection or development of an aneurysm, surgical or endovascular intervention may be considered.

Case Study: A 60-year-old man with a history of hypertension and a repaired aortic dissection undergoes a CTA one year after the initial event. The CTA demonstrates no evidence of dissection propagation or aortic aneurysm formation. He is continued on antihypertensive medication and scheduled for another CTA in two years.

By using CTA for follow-up imaging, healthcare providers can monitor the aorta for changes and intervene as needed to prevent complications.

379. Understanding the Question

The patient has chronic kidney disease (CKD) and has developed inflammation of the sac around the heart (uremic pericarditis). The question asks about the most common ECG finding in this condition.

Correct Answer: A. ST-segment elevation

Explanation:

- **ST-segment elevation** is the most common ECG finding in uremic pericarditis. This is often diffuse and concave upward, different from the typical ST-elevation seen in acute coronary syndromes.

- It's important to differentiate uremic pericarditis from acute coronary syndrome (heart attack), as both can present with ST-segment elevation.

Why other options are incorrect:

- **PR depression:** While PR depression can occur in pericarditis, it's not as specific or common as ST-segment elevation.

- **Electrical alternans:** This ECG finding is associated with cardiac tamponade, a severe complication of pericarditis where the heart is compressed by fluid.

- **Diffuse ST-segment depression and T-wave flattening:** This pattern is more suggestive of ischemic changes rather than pericarditis.

Additional considerations:

- **Other ECG findings:** In addition to ST-segment elevation, other ECG changes in uremic pericarditis may include PR depression, T-wave inversions, and low QRS voltage.

- **Clinical presentation:** Patients with uremic pericarditis may present with chest pain, dyspnea, and tachycardia.

- **Treatment:** Management includes addressing the underlying CKD, pericarditic effusion drainage (if necessary), and dialysis.

Case Study: A 72-year-old woman with CKD presents with chest pain. Her ECG shows diffuse ST-segment elevation. Pericardial effusion is confirmed on echocardiogram. She undergoes hemodialysis and improves symptomatically.

Understanding the ECG findings of uremic pericarditis is crucial for early diagnosis and appropriate management to prevent complications like pericardial tamponade.

380. Understanding the Question

A patient with rheumatoid arthritis developed septic shock secondary to pneumonia. Despite antibiotic therapy and vasopressor support, her condition is deteriorating. The question asks for the appropriate next steps if a non-infectious cause is suspected.

Correct Answer: D. All of the above

Explanation:

Given the patient's persistent septic shock without a clear infectious etiology, considering non-infectious causes is crucial. All of the options presented are relevant and should be explored:

- **Discontinuation of antibiotics:** If the patient is not responding to antibiotics and there's a growing suspicion of a non-infectious cause, it's reasonable to consider stopping the antibiotic therapy to avoid unnecessary exposure.
- **Initiation of immunosuppressive therapy:** Given the patient's underlying rheumatoid arthritis, an autoimmune process could be contributing to her condition. Immunosuppressive therapy might be beneficial in certain cases, but it's essential to weigh the risks and benefits carefully.
- **Evaluation for underlying malignancy:** Some malignancies can present with symptoms mimicking infection. A comprehensive evaluation to rule out or diagnose cancer is warranted.

Why other options are incorrect:

- Options A, B, and C are all valid considerations in this scenario, so eliminating any one would be incorrect.

Additional considerations:

- **Source control:** Ensuring adequate source control for the suspected pneumonia is essential, even if a non-infectious cause is suspected.
- **Diagnostic evaluation:** Further diagnostic tests, such as echocardiography, CT scans, or biopsies, might be necessary to identify the underlying cause.
- **Supportive care:** Maintaining adequate hemodynamic support, organ perfusion, and infection control measures is crucial throughout the evaluation and treatment process.

Case Study: A 52-year-old woman with rheumatoid arthritis develops septic shock due to pneumonia. Despite broad-spectrum antibiotics and vasopressor support, her condition worsens. Blood cultures remain negative. An echocardiogram reveals a large pericardial effusion, suggesting a possible autoimmune pericarditis. The patient is started on immunosuppressive therapy, and the pericardial effusion gradually resolves.

This case highlights the importance of considering non-infectious causes in patients with persistent septic shock, even in the presence of an apparent infection.

381. Understanding the Question

A patient with risk factors for heart disease is presenting with classic symptoms of a heart attack (chest pain radiating to the arm and jaw). The ECG shows ST-segment elevation in specific leads. The question is asking which coronary artery is most likely blocked.

Correct Answer: C. Right coronary artery (RCA)

Explanation:

- **ST-segment elevation in leads II, III, and aVF** is typically indicative of an **inferior wall myocardial infarction**.
- The inferior wall of the heart is primarily supplied by the **right coronary artery (RCA)**.

Why other options are incorrect:

- **Left anterior descending artery (LAD):** This artery primarily supplies the anterior wall of the heart. ECG changes would be seen in the chest leads (V1-V4) in this case.
- **Left circumflex artery (LCx):** This artery primarily supplies the lateral wall of the heart. ECG changes would be seen in the lateral leads (I, aVL, V5, V6) in this case.
- **Left main coronary artery (LMCA):** Occlusion of the LMCA would result in a massive heart attack with widespread ST-segment elevation and often immediate hemodynamic instability.

Additional Considerations:

- This is a classic presentation of an inferior wall myocardial infarction, a common type of heart attack.
- Prompt diagnosis and treatment are crucial for improving outcomes.

- Other diagnostic tests like cardiac enzymes (troponin) and echocardiogram can help confirm the diagnosis.

Case Study: A 68-year-old man presents with severe chest pain radiating to his left arm. His ECG shows ST-segment elevation in leads II, III, and aVF. He is immediately taken to the catheterization lab where an RCA occlusion is confirmed and successfully treated with a stent.

Understanding the relationship between ECG findings and coronary artery anatomy is crucial for rapid diagnosis and appropriate management of acute coronary syndromes.

382. Understanding the Question

A patient with systemic lupus erythematosus (SLE) is presenting with severe symptoms including altered mental status, hypotension, kidney failure, and fever. The question is asking about the most appropriate initial intervention.

Correct Answer: C. Fluid resuscitation with crystalloids

Explanation:

- The patient is presenting with signs of **septic shock**, including hypotension, altered mental status, and elevated creatinine.
- The initial focus should be on **resuscitating the patient** by expanding the intravascular volume.
- **Fluid resuscitation with crystalloids** is the cornerstone of initial management for septic shock.

Why other options are incorrect:

- **Broad-spectrum antibiotics:** While infection is a possibility, it is not the immediate life-threatening issue. Fluid resuscitation takes priority. Antibiotics can be initiated concurrently after initial fluid boluses.
- **Intravenous corticosteroids:** Corticosteroids are a mainstay of SLE treatment, but they are not the first-line therapy in this acute septic shock scenario.
- **Dialysis:** While the patient has kidney injury, dialysis is not indicated at this point. Fluid resuscitation should be attempted first to improve renal perfusion. Dialysis can be considered if there is no improvement in renal function after fluid resuscitation.

Additional Considerations:

- Rapid assessment and management of septic shock are crucial to improve patient outcomes.
- Other supportive measures, such as vasopressors, may be required if fluid resuscitation is not sufficient to maintain adequate blood pressure.
- Early identification and treatment of the underlying cause of sepsis are essential.

Case Study: A 45-year-old woman with SLE presents with fever, altered mental status, and hypotension. Initial labs show elevated creatinine and lactate. She is started on rapid fluid resuscitation with crystalloids. Blood cultures are obtained, and broad-spectrum antibiotics are initiated. After fluid resuscitation, her blood pressure improves, and mental status becomes clearer.

Prompt fluid resuscitation is crucial in improving survival and organ function in patients with septic shock.

383. Understanding the Question

A patient with chronic obstructive pulmonary disease (COPD) is critically ill and on a ventilator. The question asks about the best ventilator strategy to prevent ventilator-induced lung injury (VILI).

Correct Answer: D. Low Vt ventilation

Explanation:

- **Low tidal volume (Vt) ventilation** is the cornerstone of lung-protective ventilation strategies to prevent VILI. By delivering smaller amounts of air per breath, we reduce the risk of overdistending the alveoli, which is a primary cause of VILI.

Why other options are incorrect:

- **High tidal volume ventilation (Vt):** This is directly associated with increased risk of VILI and should be avoided.
- **High respiratory rate (RR):** While respiratory rate can be adjusted to maintain adequate ventilation, excessively high rates can increase tidal volume and contribute to VILI.
- **High positive end-expiratory pressure (PEEP):** While PEEP is important to prevent alveolar collapse, excessively high levels can also lead to VILI.

Additional Considerations:

- Lung-protective ventilation strategies also include other factors like plateau pressure monitoring, limiting peak inspiratory pressure, and using appropriate PEEP levels.
- The specific ventilator settings should be tailored to the individual patient based on their clinical condition and lung mechanics.
- Early mobilization and sedation management are also crucial in preventing VILI.

Case Study: A 72-year-old man with COPD is intubated for acute respiratory failure. The ventilator is set to a low tidal volume of 6 ml/kg predicted body weight, with appropriate PEEP and respiratory rate. Regular monitoring of lung mechanics and blood gases is performed.

By implementing lung-protective ventilation strategies, healthcare providers can significantly reduce the risk of VILI and improve patient outcomes.

384. **Understanding the Question**

A young woman with no significant medical history is in septic shock despite initial treatment. The question asks for the most appropriate next step in management.

Correct Answer: C. Administer hydrocortisone

Explanation:
- The patient is exhibiting signs of refractory septic shock, meaning she is not responding adequately to initial fluid resuscitation and vasopressor therapy.
- **Adrenal insufficiency** is a common complication of severe sepsis and septic shock.
- **Hydrocortisone** is recommended as part of the Surviving Sepsis Campaign guidelines for patients with septic shock who remain hypotensive despite fluid resuscitation and vasopressors.

Why other options are incorrect:
- **Increase norepinephrine dose:** While increasing the dose of norepinephrine might be considered, it's often not the most effective next step in refractory septic shock.
- **Start vasopressin infusion:** Vasopressin is a second-line vasopressor and is typically used after failing to achieve adequate blood pressure with norepinephrine.

- **Start epinephrine infusion:** Epinephrine is a high-dose vasopressor and should be reserved for extreme cases of refractory shock when other agents have failed.

Additional Considerations:

- It's essential to continue reassessing the patient's fluid status and optimizing vasopressor therapy while initiating hydrocortisone.
- Other potential causes of refractory shock, such as adrenal hemorrhage or sepsis-induced cardiomyopathy, should be considered.
- Early goal-directed therapy, including lactate clearance and blood culture results, is crucial in managing septic shock.

Case Study: A 32-year-old woman with pyelonephritis develops septic shock despite fluid resuscitation and norepinephrine. She remains hypotensive with cool extremities. Hydrocortisone is initiated, and her blood pressure gradually improves. Blood cultures later confirm E. coli as the causative organism.

By recognizing the potential for adrenal insufficiency in refractory septic shock and initiating hydrocortisone early, healthcare providers can improve patient outcomes.

385. Understanding the Question

A patient with severe heart failure is in cardiogenic shock despite maximal medical therapy. The question asks about contraindications for Intra-Aortic Balloon Pump (IABP) placement.

Correct Answer: C. Severe aortic atherosclerosis

Explanation:

- **Severe aortic atherosclerosis** is a contraindication for IABP placement. The balloon in the IABP can dislodge atherosclerotic plaque, leading to embolization and potentially catastrophic consequences.

Why other options are incorrect:

- **Aortic regurgitation:** While aortic regurgitation can be a challenge in patients with IABP, it's generally not an absolute contraindication. The IABP can actually improve coronary perfusion in some cases of aortic regurgitation.
- **Peripheral arterial disease (PAD):** While PAD can increase the risk of complications during IABP insertion, it's not an absolute contraindication. Careful patient selection and technique can mitigate these risks.

Additional Considerations:

- IABP is a temporary support device used to improve coronary blood flow and reduce afterload in patients with cardiogenic shock.
- Other contraindications for IABP include aortic dissection, severe peripheral vascular disease, and irreversible end-organ damage.
- Careful patient selection and risk-benefit assessment are crucial before proceeding with IABP placement.

Case Study: A 68-year-old man with HFrEF develops cardiogenic shock after an acute MI. Despite maximal medical therapy, his cardiac index remains low. An IABP is considered, but a CT angiogram reveals severe aortic atherosclerosis. The decision is made to proceed with an extracorporeal membrane oxygenation (ECMO) due to the high risk of embolization with IABP.

Understanding the contraindications for IABP is essential for appropriate patient selection and to prevent complications.

386. Understanding the Question

A patient with severe liver disease (alcoholic hepatitis) has developed kidney failure (hepatorenal syndrome). The question asks about the medication most likely to improve short-term survival.

Correct Answer: D. Albumin

Explanation:
- **Albumin** has been shown to improve short-term survival in patients with hepatorenal syndrome. It works by increasing intravascular volume and oncotic pressure, which helps to maintain renal perfusion.

Why other options are incorrect:
- **Terlipressin:** While terlipressin can improve renal function in hepatorenal syndrome, it hasn't been shown to improve overall survival.
- **Midodrine:** This medication is primarily used for symptomatic management of orthostatic hypotension, not for improving renal function or survival in hepatorenal syndrome.
- **Octreotide:** This medication is used to manage complications of liver disease, such as variceal bleeding, but it doesn't have a direct impact on renal function or survival in hepatorenal syndrome.

Additional Considerations:
- Albumin is often used in combination with terlipressin for the management of hepatorenal syndrome.

- Liver transplantation is the definitive treatment for hepatorenal syndrome, but it's not always feasible in the short term.
- Supportive care, including dialysis, is essential for managing complications of liver and kidney failure.

Case Study: A 42-year-old man with alcoholic hepatitis develops hepatorenal syndrome. He is started on albumin and terlipressin. His renal function improves, and his overall condition stabilizes.

Albumin is an essential component of the management of hepatorenal syndrome and can significantly improve patient outcomes.

387. Understanding the Question

A patient with severe asthma (status asthmaticus) is on a ventilator and receiving high-dose inhaled beta-agonists. The question asks about a potential complication of this treatment.

Correct Answer: A. Hypokalemia

Explanation:

- **Hypokalemia** (low potassium levels) is a common side effect of high-dose beta-agonist therapy. Beta-agonists stimulate the beta-2 receptors, which can lead to intracellular potassium shifting and subsequent hypokalemia.
- This is especially important to monitor in critically ill patients like those with status asthmaticus, as hypokalemia can exacerbate arrhythmias and worsen respiratory muscle function.

Why other options are incorrect:

- **Hyperkalemia:** This is not a typical side effect of beta-agonist therapy.
- **Hypoglycemia and hyperglycemia:** These are more commonly associated with insulin therapy or other metabolic conditions, not beta-agonist use.

Additional Considerations:

- Regular monitoring of potassium levels is essential in patients receiving high-dose beta-agonists.
- Potassium supplementation may be necessary in some cases.
- Other potential side effects of beta-agonist therapy include tachycardia, tremor, and anxiety.

Case Study: A 28-year-old woman with status asthmaticus is treated with high-dose albuterol. After several hours, her potassium level drops to 2.8 mEq/L. She is started on potassium supplementation and her potassium level gradually normalizes.

Understanding the potential side effects of beta-agonist therapy is crucial for preventing complications and optimizing patient care.

388. Understanding the Question

The patient has a Type B aortic dissection and is being managed medically. The question asks for the most common long-term complication of this condition.

Correct Answer: A. Aortic aneurysm formation

Explanation:

- **Aortic aneurysm formation** is the most common long-term complication of Type B aortic dissection. The weakened aortic wall due to the dissection process can lead to dilation and formation of an aneurysm over time.

Why other options are incorrect:

- **Aortic rupture:** While a catastrophic complication, it is less common than aneurysm formation in the long term.
- **Stroke:** This is more commonly associated with Type A aortic dissection involving the ascending aorta, where there's a higher risk of embolization to the brain.
- **Renal failure:** While renal artery involvement can occur in aortic dissection, it is not the most common long-term complication.

Additional Considerations:

- Regular follow-up imaging (CT angiography) is crucial to monitor for aortic aneurysm formation.
- Blood pressure control is essential to prevent progression of the aneurysm.
- Surgical intervention may be considered if the aneurysm grows to a critical size or becomes symptomatic.

Case Study: A 58-year-old man with a history of Type B aortic dissection is followed with regular CT angiograms. Five years after the initial event, he is found to have an enlarging aortic aneurysm. Surgical intervention is planned to prevent rupture.

Understanding the long-term complications of aortic dissection is essential for appropriate follow-up and management.

389. Understanding the Question

A patient with chronic kidney disease (CKD) has developed uremic pericarditis with persistent or recurrent cardiac tamponade. The question asks for the most definitive treatment.

Correct Answer: D. Pericardiectomy

Explanation:

- **Pericardiectomy** is the definitive treatment for persistent or recurrent cardiac tamponade due to uremic pericarditis. It involves surgically removing the pericardium to prevent fluid accumulation and recurrence of tamponade.

Why other options are incorrect:

- **Hemodialysis:** While essential for managing CKD and uremic toxins, it alone is not sufficient to resolve persistent or recurrent cardiac tamponade.
- **Pericardiocentesis:** This is a temporary measure to relieve cardiac tamponade by draining fluid from the pericardial sac. It is not a definitive treatment and often needs to be repeated.
- **Pericardial window:** This procedure creates a window in the pericardium to allow fluid drainage. While it can be effective in some cases, it may not prevent recurrent tamponade.

Additional Considerations:

- Pericardiectomy is a major surgical procedure with associated risks, and it should be considered for patients with refractory or recurrent cardiac tamponade despite other interventions.
- Other management strategies for uremic pericarditis include dialysis, corticosteroids, and supportive care.

Case Study: A 72-year-old woman with CKD develops uremic pericarditis and undergoes pericardiocentesis for cardiac tamponade. Despite repeated pericardiocenteses, she experiences recurrent tamponade. A pericardiectomy is performed, and she recovers without further complications.

Pericardiectomy is the definitive treatment for persistent or recurrent cardiac tamponade due to uremic pericarditis, improving long-term outcomes for these patients.

390. Understanding the Question

A patient with rheumatoid arthritis and septic shock of unknown origin has a history of recent travel to the southwestern United States. The question asks for the most likely diagnosis given this information.

Correct Answer: B. Coccidioidomycosis

Explanation:

- **Coccidioidomycosis** is a fungal infection caused by the fungus Coccidioides, which is endemic to the southwestern United States, including California, Arizona, New Mexico, and Texas.
- Given the patient's recent travel to this region and persistent symptoms despite antibiotic therapy, coccidioidomycosis is the most likely diagnosis.

Why other options are incorrect:

- **Histoplasmosis:** While a fungal infection, it is more commonly associated with the Ohio and Mississippi River valleys.
- **Blastomycosis:** This fungal infection is primarily found in the central and eastern United States.
- **Aspergillosis:** This fungal infection is an opportunistic infection that is more common in immunocompromised patients and is not typically associated with geographic location.

Additional Considerations:

- Coccidioidomycosis can cause a variety of symptoms, including fever, cough, chest pain, and fatigue.
- In severe cases, it can lead to disseminated disease and involve multiple organs.
- Diagnosis can be confirmed through blood tests, culture, or imaging studies.
- Treatment typically involves antifungal medications.

Case Study: A 52-year-old woman with rheumatoid arthritis presents with septic shock after a recent trip to Arizona. Blood cultures are negative, and she does not respond to antibiotics. A chest X-ray shows pulmonary infiltrates. Coccidioidomycosis is suspected and confirmed with a blood test. She is started on antifungal therapy and improves.

Understanding the geographic distribution of fungal infections is crucial for accurate diagnosis and appropriate management of patients with suspected infectious diseases.

391. Understanding the Question

A patient with atrial fibrillation and rapid ventricular response (RVR) is hemodynamically unstable. Given her comorbidities, the question asks for the most appropriate next step in management.

Correct Answer: A. Perform electrical cardioversion
Explanation:
• The patient is **hemodynamically unstable** due to rapid ventricular response in atrial fibrillation. This requires immediate intervention to restore normal heart rhythm and improve blood pressure.
• **Electrical cardioversion** is the most effective and rapid method to achieve this in a hemodynamically unstable patient.
Why other options are incorrect:
• **Initiate amiodarone for rhythm control:** While amiodarone can be used for rhythm control in atrial fibrillation, it is not the first-line treatment for hemodynamic instability.
• **Assess and correct underlying causes of atrial fibrillation:** This is important for long-term management but does not address the immediate hemodynamic compromise.
• **Start intravenous heparin infusion:** While anticoagulation is important to prevent stroke in atrial fibrillation, it does not address the immediate need for rapid heart rate control.
Additional Considerations:
• Before performing cardioversion, it's essential to assess the duration of atrial fibrillation. If it's been less than 48 hours, anticoagulation should be considered to reduce the risk of embolization.
• Post-cardioversion, the patient will require anticoagulation to prevent stroke recurrence.
• Underlying causes of atrial fibrillation should be investigated and addressed to prevent future episodes.
Case Study: A 65-year-old woman with atrial fibrillation and RVR presents with hypotension and altered mental status. Immediate synchronized cardioversion is performed, and her blood pressure improves. She is subsequently started on anticoagulation and evaluated for underlying causes of atrial fibrillation.
Rapid intervention with electrical cardioversion is crucial in managing hemodynamically unstable patients with atrial fibrillation.

392. **Understanding the Question**
A patient with a history of infective endocarditis has undergone successful surgical treatment but is now presenting with recurrent symptoms suggestive of

infection. The question asks for the most likely diagnostic test to identify the source of the infection after a negative transesophageal echocardiogram (TEE).

Correct Answer: A. 18F-FDG PET/CT scan

Explanation:

- An **18F-FDG PET/CT scan** is the most likely diagnostic test to identify the source of a recurrent infection in this patient.
- FDG (fluorodeoxyglucose) is a type of sugar that is taken up by active metabolic tissues, including infected areas. The PET scan can visualize these areas of increased metabolic activity, while the CT scan provides anatomical information.
- This combination makes it a powerful tool for detecting occult infections.

Why other options are incorrect:

- **Gallium scan:** While gallium scans can be used to detect inflammation, they are less specific than PET/CT scans and may produce false-positive results.
- **Indium-111-labeled white blood cell scan:** This scan can be used to identify areas of infection but is less sensitive and specific than PET/CT scans.
- **Computed tomography (CT) scan of the chest:** A CT scan can identify structural abnormalities but is not as effective as PET/CT in detecting active infections.

Additional Considerations:

- Other diagnostic tests, such as blood cultures, bone marrow biopsy, and lumbar puncture, may be necessary depending on the clinical presentation.
- Early identification and treatment of the underlying infection are crucial to prevent complications.

Case Study: A 48-year-old man with a history of infective endocarditis undergoes surgical valve replacement and debridement. Six weeks later, he develops recurrent fever and fatigue. Blood cultures are negative, and a TEE is unremarkable. An 18F-FDG PET/CT scan reveals a focal area of increased uptake in the right kidney, suggestive of a renal abscess.

An 18F-FDG PET/CT scan is a valuable tool for diagnosing occult infections in complex cases like this.

393. **Understanding the Question**

A patient with COPD, acute respiratory failure, and Pseudomonas aeruginosa pneumonia is on continuous renal replacement therapy (CRRT) due to acute kidney injury (AKI). The question asks for the most appropriate antibiotic choice for this patient.

Correct Answer: C. Ceftazidime/avibactam with dose adjustment based on CRRT clearance

Explanation:

- **Ceftazidime/avibactam** is an excellent choice for treating Pseudomonas aeruginosa pneumonia, especially in patients with limited antibiotic options.
- The combination of ceftazidime and avibactam provides coverage against many beta-lactamase-producing strains of Pseudomonas aeruginosa.
- Given the patient's renal impairment, **dose adjustment based on CRRT clearance** is crucial to optimize therapy and minimize toxicity.

Why other options are incorrect:

- **Cefepime:** While cefepime is active against Pseudomonas aeruginosa, its activity against certain resistant strains is limited. Additionally, extended interval dosing may not be optimal in severe infections.
- **Meropenem:** Although effective against Pseudomonas aeruginosa, meropenem has a higher risk of nephrotoxicity, which is a concern in a patient with AKI.
- **Imipenem/cilastatin:** This combination also carries a risk of nephrotoxicity and may not be the best choice in a patient with AKI.

Additional Considerations:

- The choice of antibiotic should always be guided by local susceptibility patterns.
- Close monitoring of renal function and antibiotic levels is essential in patients on CRRT.
- Combination therapy with other antibiotics may be considered in severe cases or if there is evidence of resistance.

Case Study: A 72-year-old man with COPD develops Pseudomonas aeruginosa pneumonia and requires CRRT for AKI. Ceftazidime/avibactam is initiated with dose adjustment based on CRRT clearance. The patient shows clinical improvement, and the infection resolves successfully.

Choosing the right antibiotic with appropriate dosing is crucial for optimizing treatment outcomes in patients with complex infections and renal impairment.

394. Understanding the Question

A patient with septic shock secondary to a pelvic abscess is hypotensive despite fluid resuscitation and norepinephrine. The question asks for the most appropriate intervention to improve cardiac output.

Correct Answer: A. Dobutamine infusion

Explanation:

- **Dobutamine** is a beta-adrenergic agonist with primarily inotropic effects, meaning it increases the force of heart muscle contractions.
- Given that the patient is hypotensive despite adequate fluid resuscitation and vasopressor support, it is likely that cardiac output is compromised.
- Dobutamine can help improve cardiac output by increasing heart contractility.

Why other options are incorrect:

- **Increase in norepinephrine dose:** Increasing the dose of norepinephrine would primarily increase peripheral vasoconstriction, which may worsen tissue perfusion.
- **Vasopressin infusion:** Vasopressin is a potent vasoconstrictor and would likely worsen tissue perfusion in a patient with already compromised cardiac output.
- **Epinephrine infusion:** Epinephrine has both alpha and beta-adrenergic effects, but its primary effect is vasoconstriction, which is not ideal in this scenario.

Additional Considerations:

- It's important to monitor cardiac output and other hemodynamic parameters closely during dobutamine infusion.
- Dobutamine can increase heart rate and myocardial oxygen demand, so it should be used cautiously in patients with ischemic heart disease.
- Other factors affecting cardiac output, such as preload and afterload, should also be considered.

Case Study: A 32-year-old woman with septic shock secondary to a pelvic abscess remains hypotensive despite fluid resuscitation and norepinephrine. A dobutamine infusion is initiated, and her blood pressure and cardiac index improve.

Dobutamine can be a valuable tool in managing patients with septic shock and low cardiac output.

395. Understanding the Question

A patient with heart failure with preserved ejection fraction (HFpEF) is refractory to high-dose loop diuretics and metolazone. The question asks for a suitable adjunctive diuretic for this patient with renal insufficiency.

Correct Answer: B. Acetazolamide

Explanation:

- **Acetazolamide** is a carbonic anhydrase inhibitor that acts as a diuretic by reducing bicarbonate reabsorption in the proximal tubule.
- It can be a useful adjunct to loop diuretics in patients with refractory edema, including those with renal insufficiency.

Why other options are incorrect:

- **Chlorothiazide:** While another diuretic, it is less potent than loop diuretics and is less likely to be effective in this setting of refractory edema.
- **Low-dose dopamine:** Primarily used for renal protection, it has limited diuretic effects and is not the best choice for this patient.
- **Tolvaptan or conivaptan:** These agents are vasopressin receptor antagonists primarily used in patients with acute decompensated heart failure with hyponatremia. They are not indicated in this patient with renal insufficiency and refractory edema.

Additional Considerations:

- Acetazolamide can cause metabolic acidosis, which should be monitored.
- Other adjunctive therapies for refractory edema include ultrafiltration and dialysis.
- The underlying cause of the patient's fluid retention should be investigated, as it may require specific treatment.

Case Study: A 68-year-old woman with HFpEF is refractory to high-dose loop diuretics and metolazone. Acetazolamide is added to the regimen, resulting in increased diuresis and improvement in symptoms.

Acetazolamide can be a valuable tool in managing refractory edema in patients with heart failure and renal insufficiency.

396. Understanding the Question

A patient with alcoholic hepatitis and acute liver failure has developed hepatorenal syndrome and is being treated with terlipressin. The question asks about the optimal duration of terlipressin therapy.

Correct Answer: D. Until renal function improves

Explanation:

- The duration of terlipressin therapy in hepatorenal syndrome is not fixed and depends on the patient's clinical response.
- The goal of treatment is to improve renal function, and **therapy should be continued until there is a sustained improvement in renal parameters**.
- This often requires several days of treatment, and the exact duration varies from patient to patient.

Why other options are incorrect:

- Options A, B, and C suggest fixed durations for terlipressin therapy, which is not optimal as patient responses can vary significantly.

Additional Considerations:

- Terlipressin should be used in combination with albumin for optimal efficacy.
- Close monitoring of renal function, blood pressure, and other vital parameters is essential during treatment.
- Liver transplantation is the definitive treatment for hepatorenal syndrome, but it's not always feasible in the short term.

Case Study: A 45-year-old man with alcoholic hepatitis develops hepatorenal syndrome. He is started on terlipressin and albumin. His renal function gradually improves over a week, and the terlipressin is continued until there is a sustained increase in urine output and improvement in creatinine levels.

The duration of terlipressin therapy should be individualized based on the patient's response and clinical course.

397. Understanding the Question

A patient with status asthmaticus is intubated and fails a spontaneous breathing trial (SBT). The question asks for a suitable adjunctive therapy to facilitate extubation.

Correct Answer: A. Noninvasive ventilation (NIV)

Explanation:

- **Noninvasive ventilation (NIV)** is a valuable tool to support respiratory function in patients with acute respiratory failure, including those with exacerbations of chronic respiratory diseases like asthma.
- It can help to improve oxygenation and reduce the work of breathing, thereby increasing the likelihood of successful extubation.

Why other options are incorrect:

- **Heliox:** While heliox can improve gas exchange in certain conditions, it is not typically used as a primary therapy for extubation facilitation.
- **Methylxanthines:** These medications have limited efficacy in acute respiratory failure and are not recommended for extubation support.
- **Inhaled anesthetics:** These agents are used for sedation during surgery or procedures and are not appropriate for extubation facilitation.

Additional Considerations:

- NIV should be considered in carefully selected patients who meet specific criteria, such as adequate mental status, ability to protect the airway, and stable hemodynamics.
- Other factors influencing extubation success include optimal medical management, physiotherapy, and patient-centered care.

Case Study: A 28-year-old woman with severe asthma is intubated for status asthmaticus. After a failed SBT, she is transitioned to noninvasive ventilation. Her respiratory status improves, and she is successfully extubated two days later.

Noninvasive ventilation can be a valuable tool in facilitating extubation in patients with acute respiratory failure, reducing the need for prolonged invasive ventilation.

398. Correct Answer: B. Computed tomography angiography (CTA) of the chest
Explanation:

- **Computed tomography angiography (CTA)** remains the gold standard for follow-up imaging of aortic dissections.
- It provides excellent visualization of the aorta, allowing for assessment of aortic diameter, aneurysm formation, and any evidence of dissection progression.

Why other options are incorrect:

- **Chest X-ray:** While a chest X-ray can show gross aortic enlargement, it lacks the detail and specificity of CTA for evaluating aortic dissection and its complications.
- **Transesophageal echocardiogram (TEE):** Primarily used for evaluating the heart and proximal aorta, TEE is not optimal for assessing the entire thoracic and abdominal aorta.
- **Magnetic resonance imaging (MRI) of the chest:** While MRI can provide excellent image quality, it is generally less readily available than CTA and can be time-consuming. Additionally, patients with certain implants or claustrophobia may not be suitable candidates for MRI.

Additional Considerations:
- The frequency of follow-up CTAs depends on the patient's risk factors, the extent of the initial dissection, and the presence of complications.
- Early detection of aortic aneurysm formation is crucial to prevent rupture.
- Other imaging modalities, such as echocardiography, may be used to assess cardiac function and complications related to the aortic dissection.

Case Study: A 57-year-old man with a history of Type B aortic dissection undergoes a follow-up CTA five years after the initial event. The CTA demonstrates no evidence of aortic aneurysm formation or dissection progression. He is scheduled for another CTA in two years.

Regular follow-up with CTA is essential for long-term management of patients with aortic dissection.

399.Correct Answer: D. Pericardial fluid creatinine

Explanation:
- **Pericardial fluid creatinine** is the most helpful test to differentiate uremic pericarditis from other causes.
- In patients with CKD and uremic pericarditis, the pericardial fluid creatinine level will be significantly elevated due to the high creatinine concentration in the blood.
- This finding is highly suggestive of uremic pericarditis.

Why other options are incorrect:
- **Pericardial fluid culture:** This test is useful for identifying infectious pericarditis but is unlikely to be positive in uremic pericarditis.

- **Pericardial fluid cytology:** This test can help identify malignant or inflammatory cells but is not specific for uremic pericarditis.
- **Pericardial fluid glucose:** While glucose levels can be helpful in certain conditions, they are not specific for differentiating uremic pericarditis.

Additional Considerations:

- Other tests, such as pericardial fluid protein and lactate dehydrogenase (LDH) levels, can also be helpful in evaluating pericardial fluid but are not as specific as creatinine for uremic pericarditis.
- The diagnosis of uremic pericarditis is often based on clinical presentation, laboratory findings, and imaging studies.

Case Study: A 75-year-old woman with CKD and pericarditis undergoes pericardiocentesis. The pericardial fluid is bloody, and the creatinine level is found to be significantly elevated, confirming the diagnosis of uremic pericarditis.

Measuring pericardial fluid creatinine is a valuable tool in the diagnostic workup of pericarditis.

400. Correct Answer: A. Macrophage Activation Syndrome (MAS)

Macrophage Activation Syndrome (MAS) is a hyperinflammatory condition that can occur in patients with autoimmune diseases, most commonly systemic lupus erythematosus (SLE) but also in rheumatoid arthritis. It's characterized by high ferritin levels, cytopenias, and organ dysfunction. The patient's persistent shock despite antibiotic therapy and elevated ferritin strongly suggest MAS.

Why Other Options Are Incorrect:

- **B. Drug-induced lupus:** While drug-induced lupus can present with fever and fatigue, it typically doesn't cause shock or have such dramatically elevated ferritin levels.
- **C. Adult-onset Still's disease:** This condition can mimic an infectious process and cause high ferritin, but it usually presents with a characteristic rash, arthritis, and elevated white blood cell count, which are not described in the scenario.
- **D. All of the above:** Given the specific clinical picture and the high ferritin level, MAS is the most likely diagnosis.

Additional Considerations:

- **Prompt recognition and treatment** of MAS are crucial as it can rapidly progress to multi-organ failure and death.
- **Diagnostic criteria** for MAS include fever, cytopenias, elevated ferritin, elevated triglycerides, hyperferritinemia, elevated transaminases, and evidence of macrophage activation.
- **Treatment** involves high-dose corticosteroids and often cyclosporine or other immunosuppressive agents.

This case highlights the importance of considering non-infectious causes in patients with persistent sepsis-like illness, especially those with underlying autoimmune conditions. Early recognition and treatment of MAS are essential for improving patient outcomes.

401. Correct Answer: C. Perform coronary angiography with possible percutaneous coronary intervention (PCI)

The patient is presenting with a high likelihood of acute coronary syndrome (ACS). Her risk factors (hypertension, coronary artery disease), hemodynamic instability (hypotension), and ECG changes are all consistent with ACS. In this scenario, **immediate reperfusion therapy** is the priority. Coronary angiography with potential PCI is the gold standard for diagnosing and treating ACS.

Why Other Options Are Incorrect:
- **A. Perform emergent electrical cardioversion:** While rapid ventricular response (RVR) in atrial fibrillation can be hemodynamically unstable, in the presence of suspected ACS, restoring sinus rhythm is not the immediate priority. Cardioversion carries the risk of dislodging a coronary thrombus, worsening myocardial ischemia.
- **B. Initiate amiodarone for rhythm control:** While amiodarone is a useful antiarrhythmic, it is not indicated as first-line therapy in this patient. The focus should be on reperfusion rather than rhythm control.
- **D. Start intravenous heparin infusion:** While heparin is often used in the management of ACS to prevent thrombus growth, it is not the most immediate intervention. Reperfusion of the blocked coronary artery is the priority.

Additional Considerations:
- **Time is muscle:** Early reperfusion is crucial in limiting myocardial damage in ACS.

- **Other diagnostic tests** (e.g., troponin, BNP) can support the diagnosis of ACS.
- **Adjunctive therapies** (e.g., aspirin, clopidogrel, beta-blockers) should be initiated promptly after reperfusion.

This case highlights the importance of recognizing and rapidly managing acute coronary syndrome in patients with atrial fibrillation. Timely reperfusion is essential for improving outcomes.

402.

Correct Answer: A. Empiric antibiotic therapy for prosthetic valve endocarditis

Recurrent fever and systemic symptoms after successful surgical treatment for infective endocarditis are highly suggestive of prosthetic valve endocarditis (PVE). Despite negative blood cultures, PVE can be challenging to diagnose, and the patient's risk factors (IV drug use, previous endocarditis) make this diagnosis highly likely.

Why Other Options Are Incorrect:
- **B. Repeat surgical intervention:** Given that the patient underwent recent surgery and there's no clear indication of a recurrent abscess or mechanical complication, repeat surgery is not warranted at this time.
- **C. Continue observation and supportive care:** Continuing observation is not appropriate given the patient's clinical presentation and the high suspicion of PVE. Delaying treatment can lead to severe complications.
- **D. Initiate antifungal therapy:** There is no clinical evidence to suggest a fungal infection. The patient's symptoms and history are more consistent with bacterial endocarditis.

Additional Considerations:
- **Empiric antibiotic therapy** should cover organisms typically associated with PVE, such as staphylococci, enterococci, and gram-negative bacilli.
- **Transesophageal echocardiogram (TEE)** is often used to diagnose PVE as it can visualize vegetation on the prosthetic valve.
- **Duration of antibiotic therapy** for PVE is typically prolonged (4-6 weeks).

This case emphasizes the importance of maintaining a high index of suspicion for PVE in patients with previous endocarditis, especially those with persistent symptoms despite initial treatment. Early initiation of appropriate antibiotic therapy is crucial for improving outcomes.

403. Correct Answer: D. Aztreonam

Aztreonam is the most appropriate antibiotic in this case. It is a monobactam antibiotic with excellent activity against Pseudomonas aeruginosa and other gram-negative organisms. Importantly, it does not have cross-allergenicity with penicillins or cephalosporins, making it a safe choice for this patient.

Why Other Options Are Incorrect:
• **A. Cefepime:** This is a cephalosporin and would be contraindicated due to the patient's allergy.
• **B. Meropenem:** This is a carbapenem and while effective against Pseudomonas aeruginosa, it is a broader-spectrum antibiotic than necessary in this case. Additionally, carbapenems are often reserved for more resistant organisms due to concerns about increasing antimicrobial resistance.
• **C. Ceftazidime/avibactam:** This is a combination antibiotic with activity against carbapenemase-producing organisms. While effective against Pseudomonas aeruginosa, it is unnecessary in this case and carries the risk of contributing to antimicrobial resistance.

Additional Considerations:
• It's essential to consider the patient's overall clinical status, including renal function, when selecting an antibiotic.
• If the patient develops resistance to aztreonam, other options may include aminoglycosides (e.g., gentamicin, tobramycin) or fluoroquinolones (e.g., ciprofloxacin, levofloxacin).
• Combination therapy is often used for severe Pseudomonas aeruginosa infections, but the specific choice of antibiotics depends on the patient's clinical condition and local antibiogram data.

This case highlights the importance of careful antibiotic selection based on the patient's specific clinical characteristics, including allergies and the infecting organism.

404. Correct Answer: C. ScvO2 > 70%

ScvO2 (central venous oxygen saturation) is a measure of oxygen content in mixed venous blood, reflecting the balance between oxygen delivery and consumption. A target ScvO2 of **>70%** is generally recommended in patients with septic shock who are not responding to initial resuscitation. This goal is based on evidence from the Surviving Sepsis Campaign guidelines, which emphasize the importance of early goal-directed therapy in improving outcomes.

Why Other Options Are Incorrect:

- **A. ScvO2 > 50%:** This is too low and indicates inadequate oxygen delivery.
- **B. ScvO2 > 60%:** While better than 50%, it is still suboptimal and may not be sufficient to meet tissue oxygen demands in septic shock.
- **D. ScvO2 > 80%:** While a high ScvO2 might seem desirable, excessive oxygen delivery without adequate oxygen consumption can lead to hyperoxia and potential harm. The goal is to optimize oxygen delivery and consumption, not simply maximize ScvO2.

Additional Considerations:

- ScvO2 is a dynamic parameter and should be interpreted in conjunction with other hemodynamic variables (e.g., blood pressure, heart rate, cardiac output).
- Achieving a ScvO2 > 70% may require aggressive fluid resuscitation, vasopressor support, and potentially blood transfusion.
- It's essential to monitor for signs of fluid overload and other complications during resuscitation.

This case highlights the importance of using ScvO2 as a guide for goal-directed therapy in septic shock. Achieving an adequate ScvO2 is crucial for optimizing tissue oxygenation and improving patient outcomes.

405. Correct Answer: B. Nesiritide

Nesiritide is a recombinant form of B-type natriuretic peptide (BNP). It acts as a potent vasodilator, reducing preload and afterload. This leads to increased renal blood flow and diuresis. It can be a valuable option for patients with acute decompensated heart failure who are refractory to standard diuretic therapy, especially those with renal insufficiency.

Why Other Options Are Incorrect:

- **A. Low-dose dopamine:** While dopamine can increase renal blood flow, its overall effect on diuresis is inconsistent and often limited. It is generally not considered a first-line agent for managing fluid overload in heart failure.
- **C. Milrinone:** Milrinone is a phosphodiesterase inhibitor that increases cardiac output. While it may improve hemodynamics, its primary effect is inotropic, and it doesn't have a specific diuretic action.

- **D. Continuous renal replacement therapy (CRRT):** CRRT is an effective way to remove fluid and solutes in patients with acute kidney injury. However, it is an invasive procedure and should be considered when diuretic therapy has failed and the patient is developing or has developed acute kidney injury. In this case, nesiritide would be a more appropriate initial step.

Additional Considerations:

- The use of nesiritide should be monitored closely due to the risk of hypotension.
- Other adjunctive therapies, such as ultrafiltration, can be considered in refractory cases.
- The underlying cause of the patient's fluid overload should be addressed, such as treating underlying infections or exacerbations of comorbidities.

This case highlights the challenges of managing fluid overload in patients with HFpEF. Nesiritide can be a valuable tool in the management of these patients when diuretic therapy is inadequate.

406. Correct Answer: A. Liver transplantation

Liver transplantation is the definitive treatment for hepatorenal syndrome. It addresses the underlying liver disease, which is the primary cause of HRS. By restoring liver function, it can reverse the renal dysfunction and improve overall survival.

Why Other Options Are Incorrect:

- **B. Terlipressin:** While terlipressin can improve renal function in some patients with HRS, it is a temporary measure and does not address the underlying liver disease.
- **C. Midodrine and octreotide:** These medications are often used in the management of HRS to improve hemodynamics, but they do not alter the underlying liver disease and their impact on survival is limited.
- **D. Albumin:** Albumin is a component of the standard treatment for HRS, but it is used to support hemodynamic stability and does not directly improve survival.

Additional Considerations:

- Early recognition and treatment of HRS are crucial for improving outcomes.
- Liver transplantation is a complex procedure with significant risks, and patient selection is essential.

- Supportive care, including dialysis, may be required while awaiting liver transplantation.

This case highlights the importance of recognizing HRS as a complication of advanced liver disease and the role of liver transplantation in improving survival.

407. Correct Answer: C. Magnesium sulfate

Magnesium sulfate has been shown to have bronchodilator and anti-inflammatory effects. In severe asthma, it can help to reduce airway hyperresponsiveness and improve lung function. It's considered a safe and effective adjunctive therapy in refractory status asthmaticus.

Why Other Options Are Incorrect:

- **A. Ketamine infusion:** While ketamine has bronchodilator properties, it is primarily used as an anesthetic and analgesic. Its role in treating severe asthma is limited.

- **B. Inhaled helium-oxygen mixture (heliox):** Heliox can reduce airway resistance and improve gas exchange, but its primary benefit is in reducing the work of breathing. It does not directly address airway inflammation or hyperresponsiveness.

- **D. Bronchial thermoplasty:** This is a long-term treatment for severe asthma that involves reducing smooth muscle mass in the airways. It is not appropriate for acute exacerbations like status asthmaticus.

Additional Considerations:

- Magnesium sulfate should be administered cautiously in patients with renal impairment.

- Other potential adjunctive therapies for severe asthma include inhaled nitric oxide and extracorporeal membrane oxygenation (ECMO).

- The decision to use adjunctive therapies should be based on the severity of the asthma, the patient's response to standard treatments, and the availability of resources.

This case highlights the importance of considering adjunctive therapies in refractory status asthmaticus. Magnesium sulfate is a valuable option for reducing airway hyperresponsiveness and inflammation in these patients.

408. Correct Answer: B. Computed tomography angiography (CTA) of the chest

CTA of the chest is the most appropriate imaging modality for assessing the progression or stabilization of a Stanford Type B aortic dissection. It provides detailed anatomical information about the aorta, including the extent of the dissection, the presence of any complications (e.g., aortic rupture, malperfusion), and the overall size of the aorta. This information is crucial for determining the need for surgical or endovascular intervention.

Why Other Options Are Incorrect:
- **A. Chest X-ray:** While a chest X-ray can show mediastinal widening, it is not specific for aortic dissection and cannot provide enough detail to assess the dissection's progression.
- **C. Transesophageal echocardiogram (TEE):** TEE is primarily used for evaluating the aortic arch and ascending aorta. It is less suitable for assessing the descending thoracic aorta, which is the primary focus in Stanford Type B dissections.
- **D. Magnetic resonance imaging (MRI) of the chest:** While MRI can provide excellent image quality, it is time-consuming and requires patient cooperation, making it less practical for acute management of aortic dissection.

Additional Considerations:
- CTA can be repeated serially to monitor the dissection's progression.
- Other imaging modalities, such as echocardiography, may be used to assess cardiac function and complications.
- Close clinical monitoring is essential for early detection of complications that may require urgent intervention.

This case highlights the importance of imaging in the management of aortic dissection. CTA is a valuable tool for assessing disease progression and guiding treatment decisions.

409. Correct Answer: C. Pericardial fluid with high urea and creatinine levels

Pericardial fluid with high urea and creatinine levels is the most specific laboratory finding for uremic pericarditis. This indicates that the pericardial fluid is derived from the uremic milieu, which is characteristic of this condition.

Why Other Options Are Incorrect:

- **A. Elevated C-reactive protein (CRP):** While CRP is often elevated in pericarditis, it is a nonspecific marker of inflammation and can be elevated in various conditions, including infections and autoimmune diseases.
- **B. Elevated erythrocyte sedimentation rate (ESR):** Similar to CRP, ESR is a nonspecific marker of inflammation and is not specific for uremic pericarditis.
- **D. Pericardial fluid with positive bacterial culture:** This would indicate infectious pericarditis, not uremic pericarditis.

Additional Considerations:

- Other diagnostic tools, such as echocardiography, can help confirm the diagnosis of pericarditis and assess its severity.
- The management of uremic pericarditis primarily involves improving kidney function through dialysis.
- Pericardial effusion can be a complication of uremic pericarditis and may require pericardiocentesis.

This case highlights the importance of considering the underlying kidney disease when evaluating a patient with pericarditis. The presence of high urea and creatinine levels in pericardial fluid is a strong indicator of uremic pericarditis.

410. Correct Answer: A. Hemophagocytic Lymphohistiocytosis (HLH)

Hemophagocytic Lymphohistiocytosis (HLH) is a hyperinflammatory syndrome characterized by excessive immune activation, leading to a cytokine storm. It often presents with fever, cytopenias, organ dysfunction, and elevated ferritin. Given the patient's refractory septic shock, elevated ferritin, and underlying autoimmune disease (rheumatoid arthritis), HLH is a strong consideration.

Why Other Options Are Incorrect:

- **B. Systemic mastocytosis:** While associated with elevated ferritin, systemic mastocytosis typically presents with skin findings, gastrointestinal symptoms, and flushing. It is less likely to explain the patient's severe sepsis-like presentation.
- **C. Castleman disease:** This is a rare lymphoproliferative disorder that can cause hyperferritinemia, but it is less likely to present with such severe systemic symptoms as seen in this patient.
- **D. All of the above:** Given the specific clinical presentation and the high ferritin level, HLH is the most likely diagnosis.

Additional Considerations:

- HLH can be triggered by infections, autoimmune diseases, or malignancies.
- Early diagnosis and treatment are crucial for improving outcomes.
- Treatment typically involves immunosuppressive therapy, including corticosteroids and cyclosporine.

This case highlights the importance of considering non-infectious causes in patients with persistent sepsis-like illness, especially those with underlying autoimmune conditions. Early recognition of HLH is essential for initiating appropriate therapy.

411. **Correct Answer: C. Perform coronary angiography with possible percutaneous coronary intervention (PCI)**
The patient is presenting with a high likelihood of acute coronary syndrome (ACS). Her risk factors (hypertension, coronary artery disease), hemodynamic instability (hypotension), and ECG changes are all consistent with ACS. In this scenario, **immediate reperfusion therapy** is the priority. Coronary angiography with potential PCI is the gold standard for diagnosing and treating ACS.

Why Other Options Are Incorrect:

- **A. Perform emergent electrical cardioversion:** While rapid ventricular response (RVR) in atrial fibrillation can be hemodynamically unstable, in the presence of suspected ACS, restoring sinus rhythm is not the immediate priority. Cardioversion carries the risk of dislodging a coronary thrombus, worsening myocardial ischemia.
- **B. Initiate amiodarone for rhythm control:** While amiodarone is a useful antiarrhythmic, it is not indicated as first-line therapy in this patient. The focus should be on reperfusion rather than rhythm control.
- **D. Perform transesophageal echocardiogram (TEE) to assess for left atrial appendage thrombus before cardioversion:** While assessing for left atrial appendage thrombus is important in patients with atrial fibrillation, it is not the immediate priority in this patient with suspected ACS. Reperfusion therapy takes precedence.

Additional Considerations:

- **Time is muscle:** Early reperfusion is crucial in limiting myocardial damage in ACS.

- **Other diagnostic tests** (e.g., troponin, BNP) can support the diagnosis of ACS.
- **Adjunctive therapies** (e.g., aspirin, clopidogrel, beta-blockers) should be initiated promptly after reperfusion.

This case highlights the importance of recognizing and rapidly managing acute coronary syndrome in patients with atrial fibrillation. Timely reperfusion is essential for improving outcomes.

412. Correct Answer: B. 18F-FDG PET/CT scan

An **18F-FDG PET/CT scan** is the most appropriate next step in this patient. It is a highly sensitive imaging modality that can detect areas of increased metabolic activity, which is often seen in active infections. It can help identify potential sources of infection, such as residual abscesses, prosthetic valve infection, or distant foci of infection.

Why Other Options Are Incorrect:

- **A. Repeat TEE:** A TEE has already been performed and was negative. Repeating it is unlikely to provide new information.
- **C. Gallium scan:** While gallium scans can detect areas of inflammation, they are less specific than PET/CT scans and have lower diagnostic accuracy.
- **D. Indium-111-labeled white blood cell scan:** This scan can be used to detect areas of infection, but it is less sensitive and specific than PET/CT scans, and it requires several hours for image acquisition.

Additional Considerations:

- If the PET/CT scan is positive, further diagnostic and therapeutic steps will be guided by the specific findings.
- Other diagnostic modalities, such as MRI or CT scans of specific regions, may be considered based on the PET/CT findings.
- The management of persistent infection after cardiac surgery is complex and often requires a multidisciplinary approach.

This case highlights the importance of using advanced imaging techniques to investigate persistent infections in complex cases. PET/CT scans can provide valuable information for guiding further management.

413. Correct Answer: B. Meropenem with dose adjustment based on CRRT clearance

Meropenem is a broad-spectrum carbapenem with excellent activity against Pseudomonas aeruginosa. It is a suitable choice for this patient despite the penicillin allergy as carbapenems have a different structure. Given the patient's renal impairment and CRRT, the dose of meropenem should be adjusted based on the patient's CRRT clearance to prevent toxicity.

Why Other Options Are Incorrect:

• **A. Cefepime with extended interval dosing:** While cefepime can be used for Pseudomonas aeruginosa, it is less active than carbapenems. Additionally, the patient has a penicillin allergy, making cephalosporins contraindicated.

• **C. Ceftazidime/avibactam with dose adjustment based on CRRT clearance:** This combination is effective against carbapenemase-producing organisms but is not necessary for this patient. It is also a broader-spectrum antibiotic than needed, increasing the risk of antimicrobial resistance.

• **D. Levofloxacin:** Fluoroquinolones like levofloxacin have variable activity against Pseudomonas aeruginosa and are not the first-line choice for severe infections like pneumonia. Additionally, fluoroquinolones carry the risk of adverse effects, including tendinitis and tendon rupture, which may be increased in patients with renal impairment.

Additional Considerations:

• Close monitoring of renal function is essential when using meropenem in patients with renal impairment.

• Combination therapy with an aminoglycoside (e.g., gentamicin, tobramycin) can be considered for severe infections.

• The duration of antibiotic therapy should be based on the patient's clinical response and culture results.

This case highlights the importance of careful antibiotic selection based on the patient's specific clinical characteristics, including allergies, renal function, and the infecting organism.

414. Correct Answer: C. SvO2 > 70%

SvO2 (mixed venous oxygen saturation) is a measure of oxygen content in mixed venous blood, reflecting the balance between oxygen delivery and consumption. A target SvO2 of **>70%** is generally recommended in patients with septic shock who are not responding to initial resuscitation. This goal is based on evidence from the Surviving Sepsis Campaign guidelines, which emphasize the importance of early goal-directed therapy in improving outcomes.

Why Other Options Are Incorrect:

- **A. SvO2 > 50%:** This is too low and indicates inadequate oxygen delivery.
- **B. SvO2 > 60%:** While better than 50%, it is still suboptimal and may not be sufficient to meet tissue oxygen demands in septic shock.
- **D. SvO2 > 80%:** While a high SvO2 might seem desirable, excessive oxygen delivery without adequate oxygen consumption can lead to hyperoxia and potential harm. The goal is to optimize oxygen delivery and consumption, not simply maximize SvO2.

Additional Considerations:

- SvO2 is a dynamic parameter and should be interpreted in conjunction with other hemodynamic variables (e.g., blood pressure, heart rate, cardiac output).
- Achieving a SvO2 > 70% may require aggressive fluid resuscitation, vasopressor support, and potentially blood transfusion.
- It's essential to monitor for signs of fluid overload and other complications during resuscitation.

This case highlights the importance of using SvO2 as a guide for goal-directed therapy in septic shock. Achieving an adequate SvO2 is crucial for optimizing tissue oxygenation and improving patient outcomes.

415. Correct Answer: B. Acetazolamide

Acetazolamide is a carbonic anhydrase inhibitor that promotes diuresis by inhibiting sodium reabsorption in the proximal tubule. It is often used as an adjunctive diuretic in patients with refractory edema, especially those with renal insufficiency. Additionally, it has a potassium-sparing effect, which is beneficial for this patient with hyperkalemia.

Why Other Options Are Incorrect:

- **A. Chlorothiazide:** While a thiazide diuretic, chlorothiazide can exacerbate hyperkalemia, making it unsuitable for this patient.
- **C. Low-dose dopamine:** While dopamine can increase renal blood flow, its effect on diuresis is inconsistent and limited. It is not a primary treatment for fluid overload.

- **D. Milrinone:** A phosphodiesterase inhibitor, milrinone, primarily increases cardiac output and has no direct diuretic effect.

Additional Considerations:

- Acetazolamide can cause metabolic acidosis, which should be monitored.
- Other adjunctive therapies, such as ultrafiltration, can be considered in refractory cases.
- The underlying cause of the patient's fluid overload should be addressed, such as treating underlying infections or exacerbations of comorbidities.

This case highlights the importance of careful diuretic selection in patients with complex conditions like HFpEF, renal insufficiency, and hyperkalemia. Acetazolamide can be a valuable option in these challenging cases.

416. Correct Answer: A. Hyponatremia

Hyponatremia is the most common electrolyte abnormality seen in patients with hepatorenal syndrome (HRS). It is primarily due to the impaired ability of the liver to synthesize and release vasopressin (antidiuretic hormone), leading to increased free water retention and dilutional hyponatremia.

Why Other Options Are Incorrect:

- **B. Hypernatremia:** This is less common in HRS and would typically indicate severe fluid loss or inadequate water intake.
- **C. Hypokalemia:** While electrolyte disturbances can occur in liver disease, hypokalemia is not specifically associated with HRS.
- **D. Hyperkalemia:** Hyperkalemia is more commonly associated with acute kidney injury, which can occur as a complication of HRS, but it is not the most common electrolyte abnormality in HRS itself.

Additional Considerations:

- Hyponatremia in HRS can be severe and can lead to neurological complications.
- Treatment of hyponatremia in HRS focuses on fluid restriction and careful sodium replacement.
- Other electrolyte abnormalities, such as hypokalemia and hypomagnesemia, can also occur in patients with HRS and should be monitored.

This case highlights the importance of careful electrolyte monitoring in patients with HRS. Hyponatremia is a common and potentially serious complication that requires appropriate management.

417. Correct Answer: C. Magnesium sulfate

Magnesium sulfate is the most appropriate choice in this scenario. It has both bronchodilator and anti-inflammatory effects, and can be particularly beneficial in patients with eosinophilic asthma. It's a safe and effective adjunctive therapy for refractory status asthmaticus.

Why Other Options Are Incorrect:

- **A. Ketamine infusion:** While ketamine has bronchodilator properties, it is primarily used as an anesthetic and analgesic. Its role in treating severe asthma is limited.

- **B. Inhaled helium-oxygen mixture (heliox):** Heliox can reduce airway resistance and improve gas exchange, but its primary benefit is in reducing the work of breathing. It does not directly address airway inflammation or hyperresponsiveness.

- **D. Bronchial thermoplasty:** This is a long-term treatment for severe asthma that involves reducing smooth muscle mass in the airways. It is not appropriate for acute exacerbations like status asthmaticus.

Additional Considerations:

- Magnesium sulfate should be administered cautiously in patients with renal impairment.

- Other potential adjunctive therapies for severe asthma include inhaled nitric oxide and extracorporeal membrane oxygenation (ECMO).

- The decision to use adjunctive therapies should be based on the severity of the asthma, the patient's response to standard treatments, and the availability of resources.

This case highlights the importance of considering adjunctive therapies in refractory status asthmaticus, especially in patients with eosinophilic asthma. Magnesium sulfate is a valuable option for reducing airway hyperresponsiveness and inflammation in these patients.

418. Correct Answer: B. Computed tomography angiography (CTA) of the chest

CTA of the chest remains the most appropriate imaging modality for long-term follow-up of a Stanford Type B aortic dissection. It provides detailed anatomical information about the aorta, allowing for assessment of aortic dilation, dissection progression, and the development of any complications such as aneurysm formation or rupture.

Why Other Options Are Incorrect:

• **A. Chest X-ray:** While a chest X-ray can show mediastinal widening, it is not specific for aortic dissection and cannot provide enough detail for long-term follow-up.

• **C. Transesophageal echocardiogram (TEE):** TEE is primarily used for evaluating the aortic arch and ascending aorta. It is less suitable for assessing the descending thoracic aorta, which is the primary focus in Stanford Type B dissections.

• **D. Magnetic resonance imaging (MRI) of the chest:** While MRI can provide excellent image quality, it is time-consuming and requires patient cooperation, making it less practical for routine follow-up.

Additional Considerations:

• CTA can be repeated annually or as clinically indicated to monitor the dissection's progression.

• Other imaging modalities, such as echocardiography, may be used to assess cardiac function and complications.

• Close clinical monitoring is essential for early detection of complications that may require urgent intervention.

This case highlights the importance of ongoing surveillance in patients with aortic dissection. CTA is a valuable tool for assessing the long-term course of the disease and guiding treatment decisions.

419. Correct Answer: A. Pericardial effusion

Pericardial effusion is the most common complication of uremic pericarditis. As inflammation increases around the heart, fluid accumulates in the pericardial space.

Why Other Options Are Incorrect:

• **B. Cardiac tamponade:** While a serious complication, cardiac tamponade is less common than pericardial effusion. It occurs when the pericardial effusion becomes so large that it compresses the heart, impairing its ability to pump blood effectively.

• **C. Constrictive pericarditis:** This is a chronic condition where the pericardium becomes thickened and scarred, restricting the heart's ability to fill with blood. It is a rare complication of uremic pericarditis.

- **D. Pericardial calcification:** This is a long-term complication that can occur after repeated episodes of pericarditis, but it is not the most common initial complication.

Additional Considerations:

- Early recognition and management of uremic pericarditis are crucial to prevent complications.
- Pericardial effusion can be monitored with echocardiography.
- If the pericardial effusion becomes symptomatic or large, pericardiocentesis may be required.

This case highlights the importance of recognizing the potential complications of uremic pericarditis and monitoring patients closely for the development of pericardial effusion.

420. Correct Answer: A. Macrophage Activation Syndrome (MAS)

Macrophage Activation Syndrome (MAS) is the most likely diagnosis based on the given clinical picture. The combination of fever, cytopenias, hepatosplenomegaly, and hyperferritinemia in a patient with an underlying autoimmune disease is highly suggestive of MAS.

Why Other Options Are Incorrect:

- **B. Drug-induced lupus:** While drug-induced lupus can present with fever and cytopenias, it typically doesn't cause such severe organ dysfunction or hepatosplenomegaly.
- **C. Adult-onset Still's disease:** This condition can mimic an infectious process and cause high ferritin, but it usually presents with a characteristic rash and arthritis, which are not described in the scenario.
- **D. Systemic vasculitis:** Vasculitis can cause fever, cytopenias, and organ dysfunction, but it typically involves specific organ systems (e.g., kidneys, lungs) and often has characteristic patterns of inflammation on imaging studies.

Additional Considerations:

- Prompt recognition and treatment of MAS are crucial as it can rapidly progress to multi-organ failure and death.
- Diagnostic criteria for MAS include fever, cytopenias, elevated ferritin, elevated triglycerides, hyperferritinemia, elevated transaminases, and evidence of macrophage activation.

- Treatment involves high-dose corticosteroids and often cyclosporine or other immunosuppressive agents.

This case highlights the importance of considering non-infectious causes in patients with persistent sepsis-like illness, especially those with underlying autoimmune conditions. Early recognition and treatment of MAS are essential for improving patient outcomes.

421.Correct Answer:

C. Perform coronary angiography with possible percutaneous coronary intervention (PCI)

Explanation:

The patient presents with a classic picture of acute coronary syndrome (ACS) - new-onset chest pain and ECG changes. Given his hemodynamic instability (hypotension) secondary to rapid ventricular response, the priority is to rapidly assess and treat the underlying coronary occlusion. Coronary angiography with potential PCI is the gold standard for diagnosing and treating ACS.

Why other options are incorrect:

- **A. Perform emergent electrical cardioversion:** While rapid ventricular rate control is crucial, in the setting of acute myocardial ischemia, restoring coronary blood flow takes precedence. Cardioversion can be considered after stabilization of the patient.

- **B. Initiate amiodarone for rhythm control:** Amiodarone is a rhythm control medication, but it is not the first-line treatment for hemodynamically unstable patients with ACS. Rate control with beta-blockers or calcium channel blockers is often initiated first.

- **D. Perform transesophageal echocardiogram (TEE) to assess for left atrial appendage thrombus before cardioversion:** While TEE is important to rule out left atrial thrombus before cardioversion in patients with atrial fibrillation, it is not the immediate priority in this case. The patient's hemodynamic instability and suspected ACS require immediate attention.

Additional Considerations:

- The patient's CHA2DS2-VASc score of 0 indicates a low risk of stroke, which is relevant when considering anticoagulation.

- Other interventions, such as vasopressors and inotropic support, may be necessary to manage the patient's hemodynamic instability.

- Continuous cardiac monitoring is essential to assess for changes in rhythm and ST-segment elevations.

This case highlights the importance of rapid assessment and decision-making in critically ill patients. Understanding the priorities in managing acute coronary syndrome and atrial fibrillation is crucial for optimal patient outcomes.

422. Correct Answer:

B. 18F-FDG PET/CT scan

Explanation:

Given the persistent symptoms suggestive of infection, the negative blood cultures, and the inconclusive TEE, a more sensitive imaging modality is needed. A PET/CT scan with 18F-FDG (fluorodeoxyglucose) is an excellent choice for this scenario. It can detect inflammatory activity, including that associated with PVE, even in the absence of positive blood cultures.

Why other options are incorrect:

- **A. Repeat TEE:** While TEE can be helpful in diagnosing PVE, it has limitations, especially in the absence of vegetation or abscess. A repeat TEE is unlikely to provide new information in this case.

- **C. Gallium scan:** Gallium scans were previously used for infection detection, but they have been largely replaced by PET/CT scans due to their lower sensitivity and specificity.

- **D. Empirical antibiotic therapy for PVE:** Initiating antibiotic therapy without a definitive diagnosis is not recommended. It can lead to the development of antibiotic resistance and mask the underlying infection.

Additional Considerations:

- Other imaging modalities, such as cardiac MRI, may also be considered in specific cases.

- If the PET/CT scan is positive, further diagnostic steps, such as transvenous echocardiography or endocardial biopsy, may be necessary.

- Management of PVE is complex and involves a multidisciplinary approach, including infectious disease specialists and cardiac surgeons.

By understanding the strengths and limitations of different diagnostic modalities, you can effectively evaluate patients with suspected PVE and guide appropriate management strategies.

423. Correct Answer:

C. Ceftazidime/avibactam with dose adjustment based on CRRT clearance and vancomycin

Explanation:

The patient has severe pneumonia caused by Pseudomonas aeruginosa, a multidrug-resistant organism. The antibiotic choice must be effective against this pathogen, considering the patient's renal impairment (requiring dose adjustment), penicillin allergy, and MRSA colonization.

- **Ceftazidime/avibactam** is an excellent choice because it has a broad spectrum of activity, including Pseudomonas aeruginosa, and it is not affected by common resistance mechanisms. The avibactam component overcomes carbapenemases.

- **Dose adjustment** is necessary due to the patient's renal impairment and CRRT.

- **Vancomycin** is added to cover MRSA, although it is important to monitor for red man syndrome and nephrotoxicity.

Why other options are incorrect:

- **A. Cefepime with extended interval dosing and vancomycin:** While cefepime can be effective against Pseudomonas aeruginosa, it is susceptible to various resistance mechanisms, and extended interval dosing may not be optimal in severe infections.

- **B. Meropenem with dose adjustment based on CRRT clearance and vancomycin:** Meropenem is another carbapenem option, but it is susceptible to carbapenemases, which are increasingly prevalent.

- **D. Levofloxacin and vancomycin:** Fluoroquinolones like levofloxacin should be reserved for cases where other options are not available due to the increasing risk of resistance. Moreover, they have limited activity against Pseudomonas aeruginosa compared to other options.

Additional Considerations:

- Close monitoring of renal function is crucial due to the use of both ceftazidime/avibactam and vancomycin.

- Combination therapy is often necessary for severe Pseudomonas aeruginosa infections.

- The duration of antibiotic therapy should be guided by clinical response and microbiological data.

This case highlights the importance of careful antibiotic selection in complex patients. Consideration of the pathogen's susceptibility, patient factors, and potential drug interactions is essential for optimal outcomes.

424. Correct Answer:

B. Lactate clearance > 20%

Explanation:

Lactate clearance is a valuable marker of tissue perfusion and oxygenation in patients with septic shock. A lactate clearance of greater than 10% is generally considered a positive response to resuscitation. However, in patients who are not responding to initial resuscitation, a more aggressive lactate clearance goal of **>20%** is often recommended. This indicates improved tissue perfusion and oxygenation.

Why other options are incorrect:

• **A. Lactate clearance > 10%:** While this is a positive response to resuscitation, it is not aggressive enough for patients who are not responding to initial measures.

• **C. Lactate clearance > 30% and D. Lactate clearance > 40%:** While achieving these high levels of lactate clearance is ideal, they may be unrealistic in many patients with severe septic shock. The focus should be on achieving a significant and sustained improvement in lactate clearance.

Additional Considerations:

• It is important to remember that lactate clearance is just one marker of tissue perfusion and should be interpreted in conjunction with other clinical parameters, such as blood pressure, heart rate, urine output, and mental status.

• Other resuscitation goals include maintaining adequate mean arterial pressure, optimizing fluid resuscitation, and administering appropriate antibiotics and vasopressors.

By targeting a lactate clearance of >20% in patients with septic shock who are not responding to initial resuscitation, clinicians can improve the likelihood of successful resuscitation and reduce the risk of complications.

425. Correct Answer:

B. Acetazolamide

Explanation:

Acetazolamide is a carbonic anhydrase inhibitor that can be used as adjunctive therapy for refractory edema. It works by inhibiting proximal tubular bicarbonate reabsorption, leading to increased sodium and water excretion. It is particularly useful in patients with renal insufficiency as it has a different mechanism of action compared to loop diuretics.

Why other options are incorrect:

- **A. Chlorothiazide:** This is a thiazide diuretic, and its efficacy is likely to be limited in a patient with refractory edema.
- **C. Low-dose dopamine:** While dopamine can improve renal blood flow, it has not been shown to be effective in increasing diuresis in patients with acute decompensated heart failure.
- **D. Hypertonic saline with furosemide:** This combination is used in the management of severe hyponatremia, but it is not indicated for refractory edema in this patient with hyperkalemia.

Additional Considerations:

- Acetazolamide can cause metabolic acidosis and hypokalemia, which should be monitored closely.
- Other potential adjunctive therapies for refractory edema include ultrafiltration and nesiritide.
- The underlying cause of refractory edema should be investigated, as it may be due to a non-diuretic-responsive factor such as renal artery stenosis or constrictive pericarditis.

By understanding the different classes of diuretics and their mechanisms of action, you can effectively manage patients with refractory edema and optimize their outcomes.

426.Correct Answer:

A. MELD score

Explanation:

The **MELD (Model for End-Stage Liver Disease) score** is the primary determinant for prioritization of patients on the liver transplant waiting list. It incorporates factors such as bilirubin, creatinine, INR, and sodium levels, which accurately reflect the severity of liver disease and the patient's prognosis. In the context of type 1 HRS, which is a severe complication of liver disease, the MELD score will typically be elevated, further emphasizing the need for liver transplantation.

Why other options are incorrect:

• **B. Child-Pugh score:** While the Child-Pugh score is a useful tool for assessing liver disease severity, it is less predictive of short-term mortality compared to the MELD score, especially in the context of HRS.

• **C. Presence of ascites:** Ascites is a common complication of liver disease but is not as strong a predictor of mortality as the MELD score, especially in the setting of HRS.

• **D. Age:** While age can be a factor in transplant decision-making, it is not the primary determinant. The MELD score is a more objective and accurate measure of disease severity.

Additional Considerations:

• Other factors, such as the patient's overall health status, social support, and compliance with post-transplant care, may also be considered in the transplantation decision-making process.

• Early referral for liver transplantation is crucial in patients with type 1 HRS, as the condition carries a high mortality rate.

By understanding the role of the MELD score in assessing the severity of liver disease and prioritizing patients for transplantation, you can optimize patient care and improve outcomes.

427. Correct Answer:

C. Leukotriene modifiers (e.g., montelukast)

Explanation:

Leukotrienes are potent inflammatory mediators involved in asthma pathogenesis. In patients with eosinophilic asthma, leukotriene modifiers can be effective in reducing airway inflammation and hyperresponsiveness. Montelukast is a commonly used oral leukotriene receptor antagonist.

Why other options are incorrect:

• **A. Ketamine infusion:** Ketamine has been studied in the management of refractory asthma, but its role is not well-established, and it is not a first-line therapy.

- **B. Inhaled helium-oxygen mixture (heliox):** Heliox can improve gas exchange in patients with severe airflow obstruction, but it does not directly address airway inflammation or hyperresponsiveness.
- **D. Bronchial thermoplasty:** This is a procedural intervention for chronic severe asthma that is not indicated in acute exacerbations.

Additional Considerations:
- Other potential adjunctive therapies for refractory asthma include omalizumab (anti-IgE antibody) and inhaled corticosteroids.
- It is essential to optimize conventional therapy, including high-dose inhaled beta-agonists, corticosteroids, and bronchodilators, before considering additional agents.
- Early identification and treatment of underlying triggers, such as infections, are crucial in managing asthma exacerbations.

By understanding the role of different inflammatory mediators in asthma and the available therapeutic options, you can effectively manage patients with refractory asthma and improve their outcomes.

428. Correct Answer:

A. Blood pressure

Explanation:

Blood pressure is the most critical factor to monitor in patients with Stanford Type B aortic dissection. Elevated blood pressure increases the shear stress on the aortic wall, which can lead to increased dissection propagation and the risk of rupture. Aggressive blood pressure control is essential to reduce this risk.

Why other options are incorrect:
- **B. Heart rate:** While heart rate can influence blood pressure, it is not as direct a factor in aortic dissection progression as blood pressure itself.
- **C. Aortic diameter:** While aortic diameter is important to monitor for potential enlargement and rupture, it is not as immediate a predictor of imminent rupture as blood pressure. Serial imaging studies would be used to assess aortic diameter changes.
- **D. Pain intensity:** Pain is a symptom of aortic dissection but does not directly correlate with the risk of rupture.

Additional Considerations:
- Other factors to monitor include heart rate, rhythm, and pain characteristics.

- Serial imaging studies, such as CT or MRI, may be used to assess aortic dissection progression.
- Patients with Stanford Type B aortic dissection should be managed in a monitored setting with close hemodynamic monitoring.

By understanding the critical role of blood pressure control in managing Stanford Type B aortic dissection, you can effectively reduce the risk of complications and improve patient outcomes.

429. Correct Answer:

D. Initiation of antibiotic therapy

Explanation:

Purulent pericarditis is a medical emergency that requires immediate and aggressive treatment. The presence of purulent fluid in the pericardium indicates a bacterial infection, which can rapidly progress to cardiac tamponade and septic shock. Therefore, the **initiation of appropriate antibiotic therapy** is the most critical step in management.

Why other options are incorrect:

- **A. Repeat pericardiocentesis:** While pericardiocentesis is a valuable diagnostic tool, it is not the primary treatment for purulent pericarditis. Repeated pericardiocentesis may not effectively address the underlying infection and can worsen hemodynamic instability.
- **B. Pericardial window placement:** Pericardial window placement is indicated for recurrent pericarditis or persistent pericardial effusion despite medical management. It is not the initial treatment for purulent pericarditis and hemodynamic instability.
- **C. Pericardiectomy:** Pericardiectomy is a surgical procedure reserved for refractory or recurrent pericarditis that does not respond to medical or percutaneous interventions. It is not indicated in the acute setting of purulent pericarditis and hemodynamic instability.

Additional Considerations:

- Broad-spectrum antibiotics should be initiated promptly based on the patient's clinical condition and local epidemiology.
- Hemodynamic support, including vasopressors and inotropes, may be necessary to manage the patient's instability.

- Pericardiocentesis may need to be repeated for diagnostic or therapeutic purposes, but antibiotic therapy is the cornerstone of management.

Early recognition and aggressive management of purulent pericarditis are crucial for improving patient outcomes.

430.

Correct Answer:

A. Macrophage Activation Syndrome (MAS)

Explanation:

Macrophage Activation Syndrome (MAS) is a severe and often life-threatening complication of autoimmune diseases, including rheumatoid arthritis. It is characterized by a hyperinflammatory state with features such as fever, cytopenias, hepatosplenomegaly, and elevated ferritin. The finding of hemophagocytosis on bone marrow biopsy is diagnostic of MAS.

Why other options are incorrect:

- **B. Drug-induced lupus:** While drug-induced lupus can present with fever and cytopenias, it typically does not cause the severe organ dysfunction and hemophagocytosis seen in MAS.

- **C. Adult-onset Still's disease:** This is a rare inflammatory condition that can mimic sepsis, but it is less likely in a patient with an established autoimmune disease like rheumatoid arthritis.

- **D. Systemic vasculitis:** Vasculitis can cause fever and organ dysfunction, but it typically does not present with the specific laboratory findings and bone marrow changes seen in MAS.

Additional Considerations:

- Early recognition and treatment of MAS are crucial for improving patient outcomes.

- Treatment typically involves high-dose corticosteroids, immunosuppressive agents, and supportive care.

- Mortality rates for MAS can be high, emphasizing the need for prompt diagnosis and management.

Understanding the clinical presentation and diagnostic criteria for MAS is essential for managing patients with complex inflammatory conditions.

431. Correct Answer:

A. Wernicke encephalopathy, thiamine replacement

Explanation:

The classic triad of confusion, ataxia, and ophthalmoplegia is highly suggestive of Wernicke encephalopathy, a condition caused by thiamine deficiency. This is a medical emergency that requires immediate treatment to prevent irreversible brain damage. Thiamine replacement is the cornerstone of management.

Why other options are incorrect:

• **B. Korsakoff syndrome:** While Korsakoff syndrome is also alcohol-related, it is characterized by memory loss and confabulation, not the classic triad of Wernicke encephalopathy.

• **C. Delirium tremens:** Delirium tremens presents with tremors, agitation, and hallucinations, not the specific neurological symptoms described in the question.

• **D. Alcoholic hepatitis:** While alcoholic hepatitis can cause confusion, it typically doesn't present with ataxia or ophthalmoplegia.

Additional Considerations:

• It's important to administer thiamine before glucose infusion in patients with suspected alcohol abuse to prevent precipitating Wernicke encephalopathy.

• Other supportive measures, such as correcting electrolyte imbalances and managing other alcohol-related complications, may be necessary.

Early recognition and treatment of Wernicke encephalopathy are crucial for preventing irreversible neurological damage.

432. B. Low tidal volumes, high PEEP

Explanation:

The cornerstone of ARDS management is **protective lung ventilation**. This involves using low tidal volumes to prevent ventilator-induced lung injury (VILI) and high positive end-expiratory pressure (PEEP) to recruit and stabilize alveoli, improve oxygenation, and reduce lung edema.

Why other options are incorrect:

• **A. High tidal volumes, low PEEP:** This strategy is harmful and can worsen lung injury.

• **C. High respiratory rate, low inspiratory flow:** While respiratory rate can be adjusted to maintain adequate ventilation, excessively high rates can lead to increased dead space and reduced tidal volume.

- **D. Low respiratory rate, high inspiratory flow:** High inspiratory flow can increase peak airway pressure and barotrauma, which is detrimental in ARDS.

Additional Considerations:

- Other ventilator strategies, such as prone positioning and neuromuscular blocking agents, may be considered in severe ARDS.
- Frequent assessment of lung mechanics and blood gases is essential to optimize ventilator settings.

By understanding the principles of protective lung ventilation, you can improve outcomes for patients with ARDS.

433. Correct Answer:

D. NSAIDs

Explanation:

NSAIDs (Non-Steroidal Anti-Inflammatory Drugs) can exacerbate heart failure symptoms by:

- **Reducing renal blood flow:** This can lead to fluid retention and worsening edema.
- **Inhibiting vasodilatory prostaglandins:** These prostaglandins help maintain renal blood flow. By blocking them, NSAIDs can exacerbate sodium and water retention.

Why other options are incorrect:

- **A. Furosemide:** A loop diuretic, furosemide is used to treat heart failure by reducing fluid overload.
- **B. Metoprolol:** A beta-blocker, metoprolol is used to improve heart function and reduce heart strain.
- **C. Lisinopril:** An ACE inhibitor, lisinopril helps to lower blood pressure and reduce fluid retention.

Therefore, in a patient with heart failure experiencing worsening symptoms, NSAIDs should be avoided.

434. **A. Acute pancreatitis, pain management and fluid resuscitation**

Explanation:

The patient's presentation of severe abdominal pain radiating to the back, nausea, vomiting, and elevated lipase is highly suggestive of **acute pancreatitis**.

Priority interventions for acute pancreatitis include:

- **Pain management:** Severe abdominal pain is a hallmark symptom and requires aggressive pain control with opioids.
- **Fluid resuscitation:** To prevent hypovolemic shock, which is a common complication of acute pancreatitis.

Other options are less likely based on the given symptoms:

- **Cholecystitis** typically presents with right upper quadrant pain and often has associated fever.
- **Peptic ulcer disease** can cause abdominal pain but usually not as severe or with radiation to the back.
- **Appendicitis** typically presents with right lower quadrant pain.

Therefore, based on the given information, acute pancreatitis is the most likely diagnosis, and pain management and fluid resuscitation are the priority interventions.

435. A. Norepinephrine

Explanation:

Norepinephrine is the first-line vasopressor for patients with septic shock who remain hypotensive despite adequate fluid resuscitation. It has a balanced alpha and beta-adrenergic effect, leading to increased systemic vascular resistance and improved cardiac output.

- **Dobutamine** is primarily an inotropic agent, used to improve cardiac contractility. While it may increase blood pressure, it is not the first choice for septic shock.
- **Phenylephrine** is a pure alpha-adrenergic agonist, which can increase blood pressure but may reduce cardiac output.
- **Epinephrine** has both alpha and beta-adrenergic effects, but it is generally reserved for refractory cases or when there is evidence of poor cardiac output.

Therefore, norepinephrine is the most appropriate initial choice for this patient.

436. A. Head CT scan

Explanation:

The patient's symptoms of right-sided weakness and facial droop are highly suggestive of a **stroke**. A **head CT scan** is the initial imaging study of choice to differentiate between ischemic and hemorrhagic stroke.

- **Ischemic stroke** is caused by a blockage in a blood vessel to the brain.

- **Hemorrhagic stroke** is caused by bleeding in the brain.

The treatment for these two types of stroke is vastly different, so it is crucial to determine the cause as quickly as possible.

While the other options may be considered later in the evaluation process, a head CT scan is the most important test to perform immediately.

437. A. Insulin and glucose

Explanation:

Insulin and glucose are the most effective agents for rapidly shifting potassium from the extracellular to the intracellular space. Insulin stimulates the sodium-potassium pump, drawing potassium into the cells. Glucose is administered to prevent hypoglycemia induced by insulin.

- **Calcium gluconate** stabilizes cardiac membranes but does not lower potassium levels.
- **Sodium polystyrene sulfonate (Kayexalate)** is used for long-term potassium removal but has a slow onset of action and is not suitable for acute hyperkalemia.
- **Hemodialysis** is a definitive treatment for hyperkalemia but is not the first-line therapy.

Therefore, in a patient with acute hyperkalemia, insulin and glucose are the preferred initial treatment to quickly lower potassium levels.

438. A. Unfractionated heparin

Unfractionated heparin is the initial treatment of choice for a confirmed pulmonary embolism (PE). It rapidly inhibits thrombin formation and prevents the extension of the clot.

- **Low molecular weight heparin** can also be used but is generally considered second-line therapy.
- **Warfarin** takes several days to achieve therapeutic levels and is not suitable for immediate treatment.
- **Thrombolytic therapy** is reserved for patients with massive PE who are hemodynamically unstable and at high risk of death.

Therefore, unfractionated heparin is the most appropriate initial treatment for a patient with confirmed PE.

439. A. Vertebral compression fracture, X-ray
Explanation:

Given the patient's age, history of osteoporosis, and sudden onset of severe back pain after lifting a heavy object, the most likely diagnosis is a **vertebral compression fracture**.

An **X-ray** is the initial imaging study of choice to confirm this diagnosis. It is quick, readily available, and often sufficient to visualize vertebral fractures.

While other conditions like spinal cord compression or herniated disc can cause back pain, they are less likely in this specific scenario.

440. A. Hypokalemia
Explanation:

Diuretics, especially loop diuretics, promote the excretion of potassium along with sodium and water. Therefore, patients receiving intravenous diuretics are at increased risk of **hypokalemia**. It is essential to monitor potassium levels closely in these patients and replace potassium as needed to prevent serious cardiac arrhythmias.

441. B. Infective endocarditis
Explanation:

The combination of fever, chills, a new heart murmur, and a history of intravenous drug use strongly suggests **infective endocarditis**.

- **Intravenous drug use** is a significant risk factor for this condition.
- The **new heart murmur** is often a result of vegetation formation on the heart valves.

While the other options are possible, they are less likely given the patient's history and presentation.

442. C. Computed tomography angiography (CTA) of the chest

A CT angiography of the chest is the most appropriate diagnostic test to confirm an aortic dissection. It provides a rapid and accurate visualization of the aorta, allowing for identification of the tear in the aortic wall and determining the extent of the dissection.

The other options are less likely to provide a definitive diagnosis:

- **Chest X-ray** may show mediastinal widening, but it's not specific for aortic dissection.
- **Electrocardiogram (ECG)** can rule out myocardial infarction, but it won't confirm or exclude aortic dissection.
- **Transesophageal echocardiogram (TEE)** is more invasive and requires sedation. While it can provide detailed images of the heart and aorta, CTA is generally preferred as the initial imaging study due to its speed and accuracy.

443. B. Esophageal varices

Explanation:

A patient with cirrhosis is at high risk for developing portal hypertension, which can lead to the formation of esophageal varices. These varices are prone to rupture and cause significant upper gastrointestinal bleeding, manifesting as hematemesis (vomiting blood) and melena (black, tarry stools).

While other options like Mallory-Weiss tear, gastric ulcer, and duodenal ulcer can cause upper GI bleeding, they are less likely in a patient with cirrhosis.

444. B. Short-acting beta-agonists

Short-acting beta-agonists (SABAs) are the first-line treatment for acute asthma exacerbations. They rapidly relax the airway muscles, relieving bronchospasm and improving airflow.

- Inhaled corticosteroids are for long-term control of asthma, not acute exacerbations.
- Long-acting beta-agonists are also for long-term control and prevention of exacerbations, not immediate relief.
- Leukotriene modifiers are used as add-on therapy for persistent asthma, not for acute attacks.

445. Correct Answer:

A. Appendicitis

Explanation:

While appendicitis is more commonly associated with younger individuals, it remains a significant differential diagnosis in older adults. The classic presentation of appendicitis includes:

- **Right lower quadrant pain:** Often starts as vague periumbilical pain that migrates to the RLQ.
- **Fever:** Indicative of inflammation.
- **Leukocytosis:** Elevated white blood cell count due to infection.

In this case, the patient's age and diabetes may complicate the clinical picture, as atypical presentations are more common in these populations. However, the given symptoms align closely with the classic presentation of appendicitis.

Why other options are incorrect:
- **B. Diverticulitis:** Typically presents with left lower quadrant pain, although it can occur anywhere in the colon.
- **C. Cholecystitis:** Usually associated with right upper quadrant pain, nausea, and vomiting.
- **D. Pancreatitis:** Characterized by severe epigastric pain radiating to the back, along with nausea, vomiting, and elevated lipase.

Additional Considerations:
- **Atypical presentations:** In older adults, appendicitis may present with less typical symptoms, such as anorexia, constipation, or vague abdominal discomfort.
- **Diagnostic challenges:** Due to atypical presentations and increased risk of comorbidities, diagnosing appendicitis in older adults can be challenging.
- **Prompt diagnosis and treatment:** Early diagnosis and surgical intervention are crucial to prevent complications such as perforation and sepsis.

Case Study: A 68-year-old female with type 2 diabetes presents with a 2-day history of vague abdominal discomfort that has worsened to right lower quadrant pain. She complains of decreased appetite, low-grade fever, and chills. Physical exam reveals right lower quadrant tenderness, guarding, and rebound tenderness. Laboratory results show leukocytosis. A CT scan confirms acute appendicitis.

Knowledge Candidate Should Know:
- Classic and atypical presentations of appendicitis
- Differential diagnosis of acute abdominal pain
- Diagnostic modalities for appendicitis (e.g., CT scan, ultrasound)
- Management of appendicitis, including surgical and medical treatment.

446. Correct Answer:

C. Spironolactone

Explanation:

Spironolactone is a potassium-sparing diuretic, meaning it promotes potassium retention in the body. This effect is particularly pronounced in patients with impaired renal function, such as those with chronic kidney disease. Therefore, administering spironolactone to a patient with hyperkalemia and chronic kidney disease would likely exacerbate the hyperkalemia.

Why other options are incorrect:

- **A. Furosemide:** This is a loop diuretic that promotes potassium loss, which would be beneficial in the setting of hyperkalemia.
- **B. Hydrochlorothiazide:** A thiazide diuretic, it also has a mild potassium-wasting effect.
- **D. Acetazolamide:** A carbonic anhydrase inhibitor, it has a minimal effect on potassium levels.

Additional Considerations:

- Hyperkalemia is a serious condition that can lead to cardiac arrhythmias and potentially death.
- Careful monitoring of potassium levels is essential in patients with chronic kidney disease, especially those on diuretics.
- Other medications, such as angiotensin-converting enzyme (ACE) inhibitors and angiotensin receptor blockers (ARBs), can also contribute to hyperkalemia, particularly in patients with impaired renal function.

Case Study: A 55-year-old male with type 2 diabetes and chronic kidney disease presents with fatigue, weakness, and muscle cramps. Laboratory results reveal hyperkalemia. His medication list includes lisinopril, metformin, and spironolactone for heart failure. The spironolactone is identified as the likely culprit for the hyperkalemia and is discontinued.

Knowledge Candidate Should Know:

- The mechanism of action of different diuretics and their impact on potassium levels.
- The risk factors for hyperkalemia, including chronic kidney disease.
- The management of hyperkalemia, including dietary modifications, medications, and dialysis.

447. Correct Answer:

B. Tissue plasminogen activator (tPA)

Explanation:

The patient's presentation is highly suggestive of an ischemic stroke, likely due to a cardioembolic event given her history of atrial fibrillation. Tissue plasminogen activator (tPA) is the gold standard treatment for acute ischemic stroke when administered within a specific time window (usually 4.5 hours) from symptom onset. It works by dissolving the blood clot blocking blood flow to the brain.

Why other options are incorrect:

- **A. Aspirin:** While aspirin is important for stroke prevention, it is not the initial treatment for acute stroke. It does not have the rapid clot-busting effect of tPA.
- **C. Warfarin:** Warfarin is an anticoagulant used for stroke prevention in atrial fibrillation but does not have a role in the acute treatment of stroke.
- **D. Heparin:** While heparin is an anticoagulant, it does not have the rapid onset of action needed for acute stroke treatment.

Additional Considerations:

- Time is critical in stroke treatment. Early recognition and rapid intervention are essential to maximize patient outcomes.
- Eligibility for tPA requires strict inclusion and exclusion criteria.
- Other treatment options for ischemic stroke include mechanical thrombectomy and endovascular therapy.

Case Study: A 72-year-old woman with atrial fibrillation is brought to the emergency department with sudden onset of right-sided weakness and difficulty speaking. A CT scan of the head is negative for hemorrhage. The patient is determined to be eligible for tPA and receives the medication within 3 hours of symptom onset. She shows significant neurological improvement within the next few hours.

Knowledge Candidate Should Know:

- The signs and symptoms of stroke
- The importance of time in stroke treatment
- The role of tPA in acute ischemic stroke
- The eligibility criteria for tPA
- Alternative treatment options for ischemic stroke

448. Correct Answer:

A. Laryngeal cancer

Explanation:

The combination of hoarseness, dysphagia, and weight loss in a smoker is highly suggestive of laryngeal cancer. The larynx is located in the upper respiratory tract, and its involvement often leads to voice changes (hoarseness). As the tumor grows, it can obstruct the airway, causing difficulty swallowing (dysphagia). Weight loss is a common symptom of advanced cancer.

Why other options are incorrect:

- **B. Esophageal cancer:** While dysphagia is a hallmark symptom, hoarseness is less common and weight loss is not as pronounced early in the disease.
- **C. Lung cancer:** While smoking is a significant risk factor for lung cancer, the classic presentation doesn't typically include hoarseness and dysphagia as early symptoms.
- **D. Thyroid cancer:** Hoarseness can occur due to involvement of the recurrent laryngeal nerve, but dysphagia and weight loss are not typical early symptoms.

Additional Considerations:

- Early detection and treatment of laryngeal cancer are crucial for improved outcomes.
- Other potential causes of hoarseness, such as vocal cord nodules or gastroesophageal reflux disease (GERD), should be considered and ruled out.
- A thorough head and neck examination, including laryngoscopy, is essential for diagnosis.

Case Study: A 62-year-old male with a 40-pack-year smoking history presents with a two-month history of progressive hoarseness. He also complains of difficulty swallowing solid foods and unintentional weight loss of 10 pounds. Laryngoscopy reveals a mass on the left vocal cord. Biopsy confirms squamous cell carcinoma of the larynx.

Knowledge Candidate Should Know:

- The classic symptoms of laryngeal cancer
- Risk factors for laryngeal cancer
- Diagnostic procedures for laryngeal cancer
- Treatment options for laryngeal cancer

449. Correct Answer:

D. All of the above

Explanation:

All of the listed laboratory tests are associated with SLE and are likely to be positive in a patient with an established diagnosis of the disease. Let's break down each test:

- **Antinuclear antibodies (ANA):** This is a general screening test for autoimmune diseases, including SLE. While not specific to SLE, a positive ANA is often the first indication of an autoimmune disorder.

- **Anti-dsDNA antibodies:** These antibodies are highly specific for SLE and their presence supports the diagnosis. They are also associated with disease flares.

- **Anti-Smith antibodies:** This is another highly specific antibody for SLE. Its presence confirms the diagnosis.

Why other options are incorrect:

Given that all three tests are associated with SLE, there is no single "most likely" positive test. They all contribute to the diagnosis and management of the disease.

Additional Considerations:

- While these antibodies are important for diagnosing SLE, they do not determine disease severity or predict flares.

- Other laboratory tests, such as complement levels (C3 and C4), antiphospholipid antibodies, and blood cell counts, may also be abnormal in patients with SLE.

- The diagnosis of SLE is based on a combination of clinical manifestations, laboratory findings, and other criteria.

Case Study: A 42-year-old woman with a history of fatigue, joint pain, and a malar rash is evaluated for suspected SLE. Laboratory results reveal a positive ANA, anti-dsDNA antibodies, and anti-Smith antibodies, supporting the diagnosis of SLE.

Knowledge Candidate Should Know:

- The diagnostic criteria for SLE
- The role of autoantibodies in the diagnosis of SLE
- The clinical manifestations of SLE
- The management of SLE

450. Correct Answer:

C. Testicular cancer

Explanation:

The most common presentation of testicular cancer is a painless testicular mass. While other conditions can cause scrotal masses, testicular cancer should always be considered until proven otherwise in this age group. It's important to emphasize that early detection and treatment of testicular cancer significantly improve outcomes.

Why other options are incorrect:

- **A. Testicular torsion:** This is a painful condition caused by the twisting of the spermatic cord, leading to decreased blood flow to the testis.
- **B. Epididymitis:** Usually presents with pain, swelling, and tenderness of the epididymis, which is a structure behind the testicle.
- **D. Hydrocele:** A painless collection of fluid around the testicle, typically translucent and without a solid mass.

Additional Considerations:

- All scrotal masses require prompt evaluation by a healthcare provider.
- Ultrasound of the scrotum is often used to differentiate between solid and cystic masses.
- If testicular cancer is suspected, referral to a urologist for further evaluation and management is essential.

Case Study: A 28-year-old male notices a painless lump in his left testicle. He has no history of trauma or urinary symptoms. Ultrasound confirms a solid testicular mass. The patient undergoes surgical removal of the testicle, and pathology confirms testicular cancer.

Knowledge Candidate Should Know:

- The importance of early detection of testicular cancer
- The classic presentation of testicular cancer
- The differential diagnosis of scrotal masses
- The diagnostic workup for testicular cancer
- The treatment options for testicular cancer

451. Correct Answer:
C. Computed tomography (CT) scan of the head
Explanation:

Before performing a lumbar puncture, it's crucial to rule out increased intracranial pressure (ICP). This is because performing an LP in the presence of increased ICP can lead to herniation of the brain stem, a life-threatening complication. A CT scan of the head can quickly and effectively evaluate for signs of increased ICP, such as brain swelling, hemorrhage, or mass lesions.

Why other options are incorrect:

- **A. Complete blood count (CBC):** While a CBC can provide information about the patient's overall health status, it does not help to rule out meningitis or assess intracranial pressure.

- **B. Lumbar puncture (LP):** As mentioned, an LP should not be performed before ruling out increased ICP.

- **D. Magnetic resonance imaging (MRI) of the brain:** While MRI can provide more detailed images of the brain than CT, it is not as readily available in emergency settings and takes longer to perform.

Additional Considerations:

- If the CT scan is normal, a lumbar puncture can be performed to confirm or rule out meningitis.

- Other tests, such as blood cultures and cerebrospinal fluid (CSF) analysis, are essential for the diagnosis and management of meningitis.

Case Study: A 22-year-old male presents with fever, severe headache, stiff neck, and photophobia. A CT scan of the head is performed and is negative for any abnormalities. A lumbar puncture is then performed, and the CSF analysis confirms bacterial meningitis. The patient is promptly started on appropriate antibiotic therapy.

Knowledge Candidate Should Know:
- The classic symptoms of meningitis
- The importance of ruling out increased ICP before LP
- The role of CT scan in the evaluation of meningitis
- The diagnostic criteria for meningitis
- The management of meningitis

452. Correct Answer:

D. Metoprolol

Explanation:

In a patient with acute decompensated heart failure and atrial fibrillation, the priority is to control the ventricular rate to improve cardiac output and reduce symptoms. Beta-blockers, such as metoprolol, are the first-line agents for rate control in this setting. They effectively reduce heart rate, improve left ventricular function, and decrease myocardial oxygen demand.

Why other options are incorrect:

- **A. Digoxin:** While digoxin can be used for rate control in atrial fibrillation, it has a narrower therapeutic index and is associated with increased risk of toxicity, especially in older adults with impaired renal function.
- **B. Amiodarone:** Amiodarone is primarily an antiarrhythmic agent used for rhythm control, not rate control. It has a long half-life and can accumulate, leading to toxicity.
- **C. Diltiazem:** Calcium channel blockers like diltiazem can be used for rate control, but they have a negative inotropic effect, which can worsen heart failure.

Additional Considerations:

- The choice of medication for rate control should be individualized based on the patient's hemodynamic status, comorbidities, and response to treatment.
- Other medications, such as diuretics and vasodilators, are essential in the management of ADHF.
- Close monitoring of heart rate, blood pressure, and renal function is crucial during treatment.

Case Study: A 70-year-old woman with a history of atrial fibrillation is admitted with shortness of breath, orthopnea, and peripheral edema. Her heart rate is 130 beats per minute and irregular. She is started on intravenous diuretics and metoprolol for rate control. Her symptoms improve significantly within 24 hours.

Knowledge Candidate Should Know:

- The pathophysiology of acute decompensated heart failure
- The importance of rate control in atrial fibrillation with ADHF
- The different classes of medications used for rate control and their indications
- The potential side effects and risks of these medications

453. Correct Answer:

B. Non-contrast computed tomography (CT) of the abdomen and pelvis

Explanation:

A non-contrast CT scan is the most accurate and rapid diagnostic test for confirming nephrolithiasis. It can visualize kidney stones with high sensitivity and specificity, even small ones. Additionally, it can rule out other potential causes of flank pain, such as appendicitis, pyelonephritis, or hydronephrosis.

Why other options are incorrect:

- **A. Abdominal ultrasound:** While ultrasound can detect kidney stones, it is less sensitive than CT, especially for small stones. It is also less effective in visualizing the ureters, where stones often become lodged.
- **C. Intravenous pyelogram (IVP):** This test involves injecting contrast dye into the bloodstream, which can be harmful to kidney function, especially in patients with suspected kidney stones. It has largely been replaced by CT scans.
- **D. Kidney, ureter, and bladder (KUB) X-ray:** This test has low sensitivity for detecting kidney stones, especially small ones. Many stones are radiolucent and cannot be seen on X-ray.

Additional Considerations:

- While CT is the preferred initial imaging study, other tests may be necessary depending on the clinical presentation and patient factors.
- Blood tests, such as complete blood count (CBC) and basic metabolic panel (BMP), can help assess for infection or kidney injury.
- Urine analysis can detect blood, crystals, and bacteria.

Case Study: A 35-year-old male presents with severe right flank pain radiating to the groin. He reports nausea and vomiting. A non-contrast CT scan reveals a 5mm stone in the right ureter. The patient is managed conservatively with pain medication and hydration, and the stone passes spontaneously.

Knowledge Candidate Should Know:

- The classic presentation of renal colic
- The differential diagnosis of flank pain
- The role of imaging studies in diagnosing kidney stones
- The management of nephrolithiasis

454. Correct Answer:

A. Vitamin B1 (thiamine)

Explanation:

The classic triad of confusion, ataxia, and nystagmus is highly suggestive of Wernicke's encephalopathy, a condition caused by thiamine deficiency. Chronic alcoholism is a common risk factor for this condition due to poor nutritional intake and malabsorption of nutrients, including thiamine.

Why other options are incorrect:

- **B. Vitamin B12 (cobalamin):** Deficiency of vitamin B12 can lead to neurological symptoms, but the presentation is typically different, involving peripheral neuropathy, megaloblastic anemia, and subacute combined degeneration of the spinal cord.
- **C. Vitamin C (ascorbic acid):** Deficiency of vitamin C (scurvy) primarily affects connective tissue and manifests as bleeding gums, easy bruising, and fatigue.
- **D. Vitamin D (calciferol):** Deficiency of vitamin D is associated with bone health issues, such as osteomalacia and osteoporosis. Neurological symptoms are not typically seen.

Additional Considerations:

- Wernicke's encephalopathy is a medical emergency, and prompt treatment with thiamine is crucial to prevent permanent neurological damage.
- Other neurological complications of alcoholism include Korsakoff's syndrome (amnesia), peripheral neuropathy, and cerebellar degeneration.
- It's essential to assess for other vitamin deficiencies in patients with chronic alcoholism.

Case Study: A 55-year-old man with a history of heavy alcohol use is brought to the emergency department with confusion, difficulty walking, and abnormal eye movements. He is diagnosed with Wernicke's encephalopathy and is treated with intravenous thiamine.

Knowledge Candidate Should Know:

- The nutritional deficiencies commonly associated with alcoholism
- The clinical manifestations of Wernicke's encephalopathy
- The importance of early recognition and treatment of Wernicke's encephalopathy
- The management of alcohol withdrawal syndrome

455. Correct Answer:

B. Magnetic resonance imaging (MRI) of the foot

Explanation:

MRI is the most sensitive imaging modality for detecting early-stage osteomyelitis in the foot. It can visualize bone marrow edema, which is an early sign of bone infection. MRI is particularly useful in patients with diabetes due to the potential for neuropathy, which can mask the typical signs and symptoms of osteomyelitis.

Why other options are incorrect:

- **A. X-ray of the foot:** While X-rays can show advanced changes in bone, such as bone destruction or periosteal reaction, they are often insensitive for early-stage osteomyelitis.

- **C. Bone scan:** Bone scans can detect areas of increased bone metabolism, which may suggest osteomyelitis. However, they lack the specificity of MRI and are less effective in visualizing soft tissue involvement.

- **D. Wound culture:** While important for identifying the causative organism, a wound culture does not provide information about the extent of bone involvement.

Additional Considerations:

- Other diagnostic tools, such as ultrasound and white blood cell count, may be used to assess for soft tissue infection and inflammation.

- Early diagnosis and treatment of osteomyelitis are crucial to prevent complications, such as amputation.

- Optimal management of diabetic foot infections involves a multidisciplinary approach, including podiatry, infectious disease, and vascular surgery.

Case Study: A 50-year-old diabetic patient presents with a non-healing foot ulcer and increasing foot pain. An MRI of the foot reveals bone marrow edema, consistent with early-stage osteomyelitis. The patient is started on intravenous antibiotics and undergoes surgical debridement.

Knowledge Candidate Should Know:

- The risk factors for diabetic foot infections
- The clinical presentation of osteomyelitis
- The diagnostic workup for osteomyelitis
- The treatment options for osteomyelitis
- The importance of prevention and foot care in diabetic patients

456. Correct Answer:

B. Administer tissue plasminogen activator (tPA)

Explanation:

The patient's presentation is highly suggestive of an ischemic stroke. Time is of the essence in treating ischemic stroke, as brain cells begin to die rapidly after blood flow is interrupted. Tissue plasminogen activator (tPA) is a thrombolytic agent that can dissolve the blood clot blocking blood flow to the brain, but it must be administered within a specific time window (usually 4.5 hours) from symptom onset.

Why other options are incorrect:

- **A. Administer aspirin:** Aspirin is important for stroke prevention but does not have a rapid clot-busting effect and is not the most time-sensitive intervention in this acute setting.
- **C. Initiate intravenous heparin:** Heparin is an anticoagulant used to prevent blood clot formation but does not dissolve existing clots and is not the first-line treatment for acute stroke.
- **D. Start antihypertensive therapy:** While blood pressure management is important in stroke care, it is not the most time-sensitive intervention in the acute phase.

Additional Considerations:

- Early recognition and rapid activation of the stroke code are crucial for optimizing patient outcomes.
- Eligibility for tPA requires strict inclusion and exclusion criteria.
- Other treatment options for ischemic stroke include mechanical thrombectomy and endovascular therapy.

Case Study: A 68-year-old man is brought to the emergency department with sudden onset of right-sided weakness and difficulty speaking. A CT scan of the head is negative for hemorrhage. The patient is determined to be eligible for tPA and receives the medication within 3 hours of symptom onset. He shows significant neurological improvement within the next few hours.

Knowledge Candidate Should Know:

- The signs and symptoms of stroke
- The importance of time in stroke treatment
- The role of tPA in acute ischemic stroke
- The eligibility criteria for tPA

- Alternative treatment options for ischemic stroke

457. Correct Answer:
B. pH 7.48, PaCO2 30 mmHg, HCO3- 22 mEq/L
Explanation:
Respiratory alkalosis is characterized by a decreased PaCO2 (partial pressure of carbon dioxide) and an increased pH. This occurs when hyperventilation leads to excessive carbon dioxide elimination.
- **pH 7.48:** This value is above the normal pH range of 7.35-7.45, indicating alkalosis.
- **PaCO2 30 mmHg:** This value is below the normal PaCO2 range of 35-45 mmHg, indicating hypocapnia (low carbon dioxide levels) and respiratory alkalosis.
- **HCO3- 22 mEq/L:** The bicarbonate level is slightly low but does not significantly contribute to the acid-base imbalance in this case.
Why other options are incorrect:
- **A. pH 7.30, PaCO2 50 mmHg, HCO3- 24 mEq/L:** This represents respiratory acidosis, as the pH is low and the PaCO2 is high.
- **C. pH 7.35, PaCO2 40 mmHg, HCO3- 28 mEq/L:** This is a normal ABG result.
- **D. pH 7.25, PaCO2 60 mmHg, HCO3- 26 mEq/L:** This represents respiratory acidosis, as the pH is low and the PaCO2 is high.
Additional Considerations:
- Acute asthma exacerbations often lead to hyperventilation and respiratory alkalosis due to increased respiratory effort.
- Compensatory mechanisms may eventually lead to metabolic acidosis to offset the respiratory alkalosis.
- . The ABG results should be interpreted in conjunction with the patient's clinical presentation and other laboratory findings.
Case Study: A 25-year-old woman with asthma presents to the emergency department with shortness of breath, wheezing, and tachypnea. An ABG is obtained, which reveals a pH of 7.52, PaCO2 of 28 mmHg, and HCO3- of 24 mEq/L, consistent with respiratory alkalosis. The patient is treated with inhaled beta-agonists, corticosteroids, and oxygen therapy.
Knowledge Candidate Should Know:
- The acid-base balance system and the role of the respiratory system

- The interpretation of ABG results
- The pathophysiology of asthma and its impact on acid-base balance
- The management of acute asthma exacerbations

458. Correct Answer:

A. Decreased FEV1/FVC ratio

Explanation:
- **FEV1** is the forced expiratory volume in one second, which measures how much air a person can forcefully exhale in one second.
- **FVC** is the forced vital capacity, which measures the total amount of air a person can forcefully exhale after taking a deep breath.
- The **FEV1/FVC ratio** is calculated by dividing FEV1 by FVC.

In COPD, there is a significant obstruction to airflow, making it difficult to exhale quickly. This results in a **decreased FEV1** while the FVC remains relatively normal or may even increase due to air trapping. Consequently, the **FEV1/FVC ratio is significantly reduced.**

Why other options are incorrect:
- **B. Increased FEV1/FVC ratio:** This would indicate a restrictive lung disease, not obstructive.
- **C. Normal FEV1/FVC ratio:** This would suggest normal lung function, which is not consistent with COPD.
- **D. Increased total lung capacity (TLC):** While TLC can be increased in COPD due to air trapping, it is not the most specific finding for COPD.

Additional Considerations:
- Other PFT findings in COPD may include decreased FEV1, decreased forced expiratory flow (FEF25-75), and increased residual volume.
- Pulmonary function tests are essential for diagnosing COPD, assessing disease severity, and monitoring response to treatment.

Case Study: A 60-year-old male with a history of smoking presents with chronic cough, shortness of breath, and wheezing. PFTs reveal an FEV1 of 50% predicted, an FVC of 80% predicted, and an FEV1/FVC ratio of 55%. These findings are consistent with a diagnosis of COPD.

459. Correct Answer:

B. Brain natriuretic peptide (BNP)

Explanation:

BNP is a hormone released by the heart in response to increased pressure or stress. It is a highly sensitive and specific marker for heart failure. In patients with worsening heart failure, BNP levels typically rise. Therefore, monitoring BNP levels can help assess the severity of heart failure, monitor response to treatment, and predict outcomes.

Why other options are incorrect:

• **A. Serum creatinine:** While important to monitor kidney function, especially in patients with heart failure, it is not the most critical test for assessing the acute worsening of heart failure.

• **C. Troponin:** Primarily used to diagnose myocardial infarction, troponin is not the most relevant test for monitoring heart failure exacerbation.

• **D. Complete blood count (CBC):** A CBC can provide information about the patient's overall health, but it is not specific for assessing heart failure.

Additional Considerations:

• Other laboratory tests, such as electrolytes, liver function tests, and thyroid function tests, may also be helpful in assessing the overall status of the patient with heart failure.

• BNP levels can be used to differentiate between heart failure and other causes of dyspnea.

• Regular monitoring of BNP levels can help optimize treatment and prevent hospitalizations.

Case Study: A 70-year-old woman with a history of heart failure presents with worsening shortness of breath and leg swelling. Her BNP level is elevated, confirming the diagnosis of decompensated heart failure. She is treated with diuretics, intravenous loop diuretics, and inotropic support.

460. D. Prednisone

Explanation:

The patient is presenting with a severe flare-up of ulcerative colitis, characterized by abdominal pain, bloody diarrhea, and fever. In such cases, **high-dose corticosteroids like prednisone** are the mainstay of treatment for inducing remission quickly. They work by suppressing the immune system and reducing inflammation.

Why other options are incorrect:

- **A. Mesalamine and B. Sulfasalazine:** While these are effective for mild to moderate ulcerative colitis, they are generally not sufficient for inducing remission in severe flare-ups.
- **C. Infliximab:** This is a biologic agent used for moderate to severe ulcerative colitis that has not responded to conventional therapy. It is not typically the first-line treatment for induction of remission in a severe flare.

Additional Considerations:

- Once the patient's condition stabilizes with corticosteroids, the goal is to taper the steroid dose gradually and introduce maintenance therapy with aminosalicylates or biologics to prevent relapse.
- Severe ulcerative colitis can lead to complications such as toxic megacolon, which is a medical emergency.